Bodystat

. . . . .

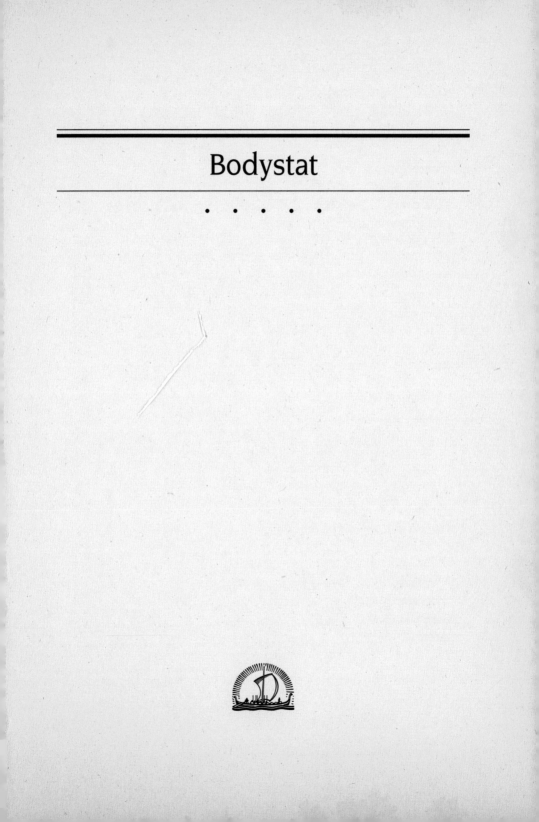

BODYSTAT

How to Reset
Your Fat Thermostat
Permanently

ERIC WITT, Ph.D.,
and CAROL WIRTH

VIKING

VIKING
Published by the Penguin Group
Penguin Books USA Inc., 375 Hudson Street,
New York, New York 10014, U.S.A.
Penguin Books Ltd, 27 Wrights Lane, London W8 5TZ, England
Penguin Books Australia Ltd, Ringwood, Victoria, Australia
Penguin Books Canada Ltd, 10 Alcorn Avenue, Toronto, Ontario, Canada M4V 3B2
Penguin Books (N.Z.) Ltd, 182–190 Wairau Road, Auckland 10, New Zealand

Penguin Books Ltd, Registered Offices:
Harmondsworth, Middlesex, England

First published in 1996 by Viking Penguin,
a division of Penguin Books USA Inc.

1 3 5 7 9 10 8 6 4 2

A NOTE TO THE READER

The ideas, procedures, and suggestions contained in this book are not intended as a substitute for consulting with your physician. All matters regarding your health require medical supervision.

Grateful acknowledgment is made for permission to reprint excerpts from *The 10% Solution for a Healthy Life* by Raymond Kurzweil. Copyright © 1992 by Raymond Kurzweil. Reprinted by permission of Crown Publishers, Inc.

LIBRARY OF CONGRESS CATALOGING IN PUBLICATION DATA
Witt, Eric, Ph.D.
Bodystat / Eric Witt, Ph.D., and Carol Wirth.
p.   cm.
Includes bibliographical references and index.
ISBN 0-670-85955-9
1. Weight loss.   I. Wirth, Carol.   II. Title.
RM222.2.W56   1996
613.2'5—dc20   95–38803

This book is printed on acid-free paper.

∞

Printed in the United States of America
Set in Simoncini Garamond
Designed by Victoria Hartman
Illustrations by Gale

We would like to dedicate this book to the memory
of Harold Witt, to Beth Witt, and to Pat and Mike Wirth—
our parents, who were wonderful role models.
We have long appreciated and depended upon your love,
support, and understanding, as well as your keen
minds and quick humor. Thank you.

Acknowledgments

• • • • •

There are many people without whose help this book would not have been possible. We would like to thank our friends and family for their loving support and patience. In particular, we would like to thank: Beth Witt, Shelly McKeirnan, and Sharon Correia for their wonderful recipes; Lori Butterworth, Ian and Jolie McTavish, Darlene Molesworth, Jessamyn and Mark Vinzent, Beth Witt, Emily Witt, Pia Larson, Maurizio Podda, M.D., Nicole Podda, M.D., Thomas Kelso, M.D., Ph.D., Pat and Mike Wirth, and Janet Provensal for the many hours they spent reading various versions of this book and giving us invaluable feedback on its content; Suzann Photography and Steve Underwood and Adrian Ordenana for their wonderful photographic work; Trina Oliver for making us look pretty; Bob and Joan Grazzini for being our witnesses; Juel Herbranson for his inspiring and humorous slides for our workshops; and Mindy Werner, Carolyn Carlson, Patti Kelly, and the gang at Viking Penguin for their tremendous job of coaching, editing, and hand-holding us through this incredible process.

Contents

· · · · ·

Introduction

· · · · ·

I f you're like most Americans, you weigh more than you want to. You may have struggled with your weight all your life. Or it may be something that crept up on you in adulthood. But whether it's recent or a lifelong constant, your weight problem is probably puzzling to you. You may be an expert on diets, having been on dozens—none of which have worked permanently. The usual ways of thinking about fat and why we store it in our bodies lead to unsuccessful strategies for its control. Diets don't work. Focusing only on the psychological aspects of eating doesn't work. Even the current rage, low-fat eating, may have left you *fatter*.

When you have a problem that you can't control, you start to think about it. All the time. Your body, your weight, and, especially, *food* become the source of an overwhelming portion of your conscious and unconscious thoughts and emotions.

You may judge entire days and weeks by the amount of food you eat. But you get caught in a double bind. If you eat so little that you're happy with the amount, you're miserable because you're hungry. And if you eat enough to satisfy your hunger, you're miserable because you feel fat and out of control. Yet there doesn't seem to be any other way of losing fat besides cutting calories. So, with no alternative, you try and fail over and over again. Even doctors and scientists, who unanimously agree that the major effect of dieting is not weight loss, but rather a profound sense of failure and despair, rarely have anything else to offer. Until now cutting calories has been the dominant model for weight control.

But a new light is gradually dawning. A little-known explanation for the reasons that we carry fat on our bodies (proposed decades ago) is now gaining widespread acceptance. Once you understand that explanation, you can easily see what strategies will work for becoming lean. Powerful new research is showing just how incredibly effective these strategies are.

We discovered these principles almost by accident many years ago. We've both struggled with weight and body image, and our own stories, which you'll read about in chapter 1 and throughout the book, exemplify many of the issues that men and women encounter regarding fat and body image. Although we're both lean now, and have been for years, it wasn't always this way.

We began teaching others the principles we discovered because one of us (Carol) was being teased at school. No, they weren't teasing her about being fat. At the time, she was lean, as lean as she is now. And no, it wasn't in grade school. It was in the high school where she teaches chemistry and biology, and the people who were teasing her (good-naturedly) were her fellow teachers. They were teasing her about the size of her lunches, which were enormous. On a typical day she brought a plastic shopping bag half-filled with leftovers from dinner, salads, bagels, apples, bananas, crackers, gummy candies . . . and she *ate it all* during the day. Even students started to notice, saying things like "Ms. Wirth, every time I see you you're eating! What gives?" People couldn't believe that she could eat so much and stay lean.

It was out of the interest of these friends that we developed and began teaching a workshop, titled Living Lean in a Fat World. The workshop follows very closely the outline of this book, and, in fact, this book grew out of the workshop. In the three years since we've started the class, the experiences of hundreds of people have convinced us that people learn these principles quickly and easily, and even after just one day, they can start practicing them in their own lives, often with dramatic results.

In fact, in the early days of teaching the workshop, people were reporting such rapid weight loss that we didn't believe them. We'll tell many of their stories here (unless otherwise noted, all names are real). One man reported losing five pounds a week, another lost thirty-five pounds in three months. Although such weight-loss rates are reported for people on liquid protein fasts, the people from our workshops accomplished it *while eating all they wanted.* We knew you could lose weight without going hungry—in fact, it's a key principle of our program. But so fast?

That led Eric into the scientific literature about weight control—or, rather, *back* into the scientific literature. He'd studied it in graduate school, when he got his Ph.D. in physiology. He'd seen that convincing studies done in the 1960s and 1970s showed that calorie cutting didn't work for weight loss, but that simple life-style modifications did. These classic studies helped us develop the principles by which we lived, and which we then taught to others. When Eric, now a research biochemist at the University of California at Berkeley, started examining the scientific studies that had been done in the 1980s and 1990s, he was astonished.

Hundreds of studies, many of them completed only in the past few years, support the ideas that you will read about in this book. Not only can people lose weight at the rates we'd heard at our workshops, in some studies people lost weight at the rate of *almost one pound a day,* while eating as much as they wanted! These weren't claims from "diet doctors," either. They were reports of carefully designed experiments, appearing in the most prestigious scientific journals.

This, for us, was the most exciting aspect of our program. The fact that we were able to stay lean in the midst of hectic lives might just be luck. The fact that we saw so many people become lean using the same principles might just be temporary. But these studies, involving thousands of people, were unanimous: these principles work! Simple life-style changes lead to permanent reduction in body fat. Even more exciting, these are exactly the same changes that will protect you from heart disease, breast cancer, and a host of degenerative diseases. While we were writing this book, several exciting new studies have emerged that further support the ideas you will read about here. We'll tell you about some of the most convincing in these pages.

This new way of looking at fat and how to lose it is what this book is all about. In it you will learn:

• *Why you get fat.* You're *not* fat because of a personality defect, or because of a lack of willpower. You're fat because everything in our modern world activates mechanisms in your body for storing fat. These mechanisms for storing—and losing—fat are controlled by brain centers that, collectively, we have called the "bodystat."

• *How to get lean.* To become lean, you must live differently. You must learn the strategies that will activate your bodystat's program for *leanness,* and integrate these strategies into your life.

Now, anyone can change his or her life radically for a few months and lose weight. In our program you will learn, instead, to change your life subtly, forever—and lose fat *permanently.* Specifically, you will learn to modify your eating habits to eat *more* (not less) of the types of food that lead to fat loss. And you will learn to modify your activity patterns.

And we make one unequivocal statement: *human beings are naturally lean.* You've heard about "fat genes." What you haven't heard is that those very same genes can make you *lean,* naturally and healthfully, if you follow simple life-style modifications.

At this point, you expect the gimmick. Medical breakthrough! Diet secrets uncovered in our laboratory! Use our cream and thin your thighs, watch our video and drop a size, fat melts off before your eyes!

Of course, there are no gimmicks. This is a book for people who have had enough of the gimmicks, who are ready for the truth about weight loss. Instead of gimmicks, this book relies on three sources: our own experience, the experiences of hundreds of people to whom we have taught these principles, and the experiences of thousands of people recorded in the scientific literature.

Our workshop participants have often asked us if there were any books they could read explaining our principles. While there are several that covered one or two aspects, there were none that completely explained these concepts of weight control. And there were none that offered the flexible program that we had found through experience was necessary to help people in all situations to fit these principles into their lives.

So we've written such a book. It's the book we wish we could have read when we were struggling with our own weights. We hope that you'll enjoy it, and that you'll apply these ideas to your life, to discover, as thousands of others have, that your natural state is to be lean.

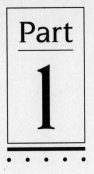

Part

1

What
Your Mother
Never Told You
About
Weight Control

1

Our Dinner with Lori

• • • • •

I f you'd told us five years ago that we would be giving workshops and writing a book about weight control, we would have been flabbergasted. Eric had just finished his Ph.D. in physiology, and was a research scientist at Berkeley, studying nutrition and health. Carol was a high-school biology-and-chemistry teacher. It was true that we'd uncovered some interesting scientific studies about weight loss, and we'd found that they helped us stay lean without dieting, hunger, or willpower. For Carol these ideas had helped end a lifelong obsession with food and struggle with weight. We both felt more energy and optimism as a result of changing our eating habits. But we really didn't think anyone else would be interested. In fact, we didn't think about it much at all. It was just the way we lived.

Then along came Lori.

Lori is our friend and Carol's teaching colleague. Like Carol, she had struggled all of her adult life with her weight. It's not that she's fat. It's just that, to stay as slim as she wished, she had to engage in a daily battle with food. She could never eat as much as she wanted or what she wanted. She was obsessed with food. When her weight crept up an extra ten or fifteen pounds, she'd go on a diet—and she'd tried them all.

"I've been on the pineapple diet and the Beverly Hills diet, I've used metabolic-breakthrough plans and endocrine-control plans," says Lori. "They all worked, for a while. Then it was as if I just couldn't help myself. No matter how hard I tried, the weight came back, every time. I alternated between starving but being the weight I wanted, or having my hunger satisfied but being ten or twenty pounds overweight—and hating myself for my lack of willpower. No matter what I did, I was unhappy, and I couldn't see any way out except the next diet."

But Lori noticed that Carol didn't seem to go through these cycles. Carol brought lunches to school that were so big they became a running joke. She ate all her lunch, every day, as well as several large snacks. She never seemed to be embarrassed about the amount she ate, and she never talked about her latest diet. Yet she stayed lean.

One day, Lori had had enough. "Look, Carol," she said, "it's driving me nuts. Either you're one of those awful people who don't gain weight no matter what they eat, or you're taking some pill that burns fat, or you're secretly cutting calories. Whatever it is, I want to know about it."

"Well, I'm certainly not one of those people who've never had a weight problem, or a problem with food," said Carol. "In fact, at one point in my life I was bulimic, and hating myself for the way I looked and the way I couldn't stop thinking about food. But I'm not that way anymore. And there aren't any secret pills or calorie-cutting routines. I have no idea how many calories I eat each day. Why don't you come over for dinner, and Eric and I can tell you what we've learned over the years about weight control."

"You're on," said Lori. "I've seen your lunches. I can't wait to see your dinners."

What Is Wrong with This Picture?

A few nights later, Lori arrived for dinner. While we were having drinks and hors d'oeuvres (bread sticks and carrots dipped in a cream-cheese–garlic fondue), Carol pulled out a photo album.

"I just want to show you a picture of me taken about six or seven years ago, so you'll know that I really did have a weight problem," she said, turning the pages. "Here it is. I was nineteen or twenty when this picture was taken."

Lori looked closely at the photo. "Wow. I can't believe it. Now I really want to know what diet you're on."

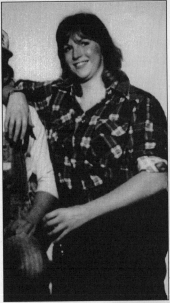

COURTESY OF AUTHOR

Carol: before and after

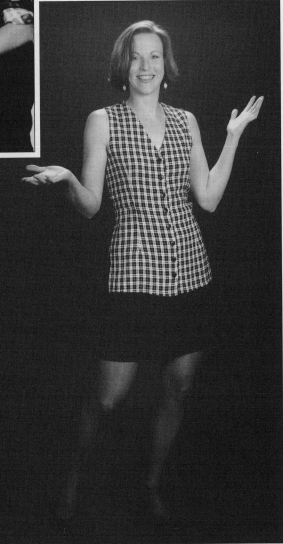

"Actually, I was probably on a diet when that picture was taken," said Carol. "And I may have been smiling, but I wasn't happy. Those were the days when I was obsessed with food. I'd go on diet after diet, then blow it by bingeing. I'd go through phases where I would work out for hours a day, but I was still fat. I pretty much felt that I was a failure, that I had no control over my eating, and that I was destined to be fat. Obviously you can see that I've changed. One key was to realize that diets were never going to work, *ever*. Also, since that picture was taken I was in a car accident and broke my back, and my exercise has been quite limited."

"Now I'm really confused," said Lori. "You no longer diet, and you can't exercise as much as you did before, yet you're obviously much thinner than you were."

"Let's talk about it over dinner," suggested Carol.

We settled down to dinner: lasagna, French bread, salad, and mixed vegetables.

"Okay," said Lori, "now tell me about your ideas for weight control."

"Well," said Carol, "why don't you tell us first how *you* lose weight."

Lori told us ideas that we've since heard dozens of times. You have to cut calories to lose fat. When you lose all the weight you want to, you can go back to normal eating. You just have to be careful not to pig out. That's where Lori had trouble—she didn't feel she had the willpower to resist her urges to eat. She thought it might be all psychological. She reported that sometimes she ate when depressed, or when really happy, or sometimes when she was just bored.

• • •

Lori, like millions of others, was seduced by the calorie-cutting method for weight loss. It's a seductive idea, because cutting calories to lose weight makes perfect sense—in theory.

You look in the mirror and see that you are fatter than you want to be. You know that fat is the way your body stores energy. If you eat fewer calories (less energy) every day, your body has to make up the difference by burning its own fat. A pound of fat produces about 3,500 calories of energy when it burns. That means that, if you cut out 1,000 calories each day, you should burn off a pound of fat in three or four days. That's about two pounds a week, or eight to ten pounds a month.

It should be easy for your body to process its own fat, which is sitting right there on your thighs or hanging down as love handles. It should be just as easy as getting the calories from, say, a double cheeseburger, so you shouldn't get too hungry—you look in the mirror and see you've got a *lot* of double cheeseburgers on you. And even after you lose the first five or ten pounds, you look in the mirror and see plenty of fat left, so, if you continue to cut out the same number of calories, you should continue to lose weight and you still shouldn't get very hungry.

Finally, when you've lost as much fat as you want, you should be able to go back to your previous way of eating. As long as you use a little restraint and don't pig out, as long as you just eat until your hunger is satisfied (rather than until you're bursting at the seams), you should be able to maintain your new, lower weight. All it will take is a little willpower. If you just pay attention when you eat, you should be able to avoid overeating, and not gain back the weight you lost.

It sounds so reasonable. It is still the model for weight loss used by many doctors, dieticians, and nutritionists. *It is completely contradicted by the experience of every dieter who has ever squinted at a calorie chart.*

Let's take a look at the dieting experience step by step and discover how this seemingly commonsense theory is contradicted by the realities of a diet.

First, at the start of a diet you may see *weight* loss on the scale but disappointingly little *fat* loss from your body. Fat is not the only source of calories your body uses when you go on a diet. It also burns a substantial amount of muscle. Why? Because your brain and spinal cord *must* have glucose, and only glucose, as a fuel source. The flow of glucose can't be interrupted, even for a few minutes, without coma or death resulting. You don't store much glucose, only about a day's worth, and when it's gone, your body must convert some other fuel into glucose. Muscle protein can be converted to glucose, *but fat can't,* so you start burning your muscles to feed your brain. Because of this biochemical quirk, the more calories you cut out of your daily diet, the more muscle you lose, to keep your brain fueled. And muscle loss is not pretty. It leads to the concentration-camp look of pencil-thin arms and spindly legs.

Second, even though you may be very strict about maintaining your low-calorie diet, you inevitably reach a point at which weight loss slows or even stops. It can happen after you lose as little as five pounds. This doesn't fit into normal dieting theory at all. The conventional diet picture is that your body requires a fixed number of calories per day, so, if you eat fewer than that number, you must burn fat (and, as we just saw, some protein). But, in fact, when your body senses that it is losing some of its fat, it activates a number of mechanisms that cause it to use *fewer* calories each day (more on this in a moment). Every dieter knows that the first few pounds are relatively easy to lose, but no matter how strictly you are staying on your diet, the more weight you lose the harder it gets to take off additional weight—even if you can look in the mirror and see gobs of fat left. As you lower your caloric intake, your body lowers caloric expenditure, sometimes to the point where you stop losing weight altogether, though you are still very carefully restricting calories.

Third, you don't just get a *little* hungry on a diet. You get ravenously hungry, all the time. And the more you lose, the hungrier you get. Even though, according to the conventional model, your body should be able to easily burn its own fat to make up the calories that you've cut from your diet, and your mirror tells you that there is plenty of fat to burn, you get hungry. If you slip up and really gorge yourself one day, and eat (on that one day) far more calories than your body needs, after your feast you still feel that constant, gnawing hunger—while you look down at your painfully swollen belly. That's not explained by the conventional diet model. How can you be hungry after you just ate double the number of calories that you need for one particular day?

Fourth, after you go off the diet you regain the weight you lost, despite eating sensibly. This, again, goes completely against conventional dieting ideas. After all, if you have lost, say, twenty pounds of fat, you should be able to return to normal eating and remain at that new weight. By "normal eating" we mean that you now consume as many calories as you use each day. By all rights, you should not be hungry, because you're not dieting anymore.

But you are hungry. And that hunger is constant. It will make you eat just a few more calories than you use in a day, or it may trigger binges during which you eat a lot more calories than you use in a day. Either way, the weight comes back. If you exert great willpower, continually monitor your eating, and always stay a little hungry, it may come back slowly. If, like most people, you just don't have the energy to be constantly vigilant, it comes back astonishingly quickly. But sooner or later, 95–98 percent of former dieters find that they have regained the weight they lost.

And finally, and most discouragingly, even though you go on diet after diet, as the years go by you see yourself getting fatter. A pound this year, a couple of pounds next year, and soon you are twenty pounds heavier than you were a decade ago, despite trying perhaps twenty or thirty diets during those years.

· · ·

"Everything you say rings true," said Lori. "Now that I think about it, I realize that diets and calorie-counting never have worked for me in the long run. But what else can I do besides go on another diet? I still think it's just a matter of willpower. How else am I going to keep from ballooning up?"

"Let me ask you some questions," said Carol. "Didn't you tell me that you went to college on your own, and worked your way through UCLA?"

"Well, yes," said Lori.

"And then went to graduate school and completed a master's degree?"

"Well, yes."

"Aren't you a single mother, raising a young son while holding down a full-time job?"

"Well, yes."

"Do you really think you don't have much willpower?" asked Carol.

"When you put it that way," said Lori, "I guess I'd have to say that I do have willpower for some things. But I don't get it. If it's not a matter of counting calories, how do you do it?"

Eric was eyeing the lasagna. A third helping? Why not?

"You know, women aren't the only ones who worry about their weight," he said. "I was fat enough as a kid that I used to look at my legs and wonder if I could have surgery to remove the excess flab. My mother and older sister went on diets and I went right along with them. In high school and college I was active in competitive sports and managed to stay fairly lean, but after college I came down with a rare form of arthritis, and I couldn't exercise very much. I was starting to fight the battle of the bulge again, and I started going on diets again. And just like everyone else, I gained the weight right back.

"Then, when I was in graduate school, working on my doctorate, I started to read some scientific studies about weight control. They had to do with a concept called 'set point,' something I'd heard about in my physiology classes. I'd never heard it applied to weight before, but as soon as I read those studies I realized that this idea was right. Lately I've been seeing a lot more studies coming out in the medical and scientific journals to support the idea. Since the day I read about the concept of set point, I have never gone on another diet, but I've kept my weight exactly the same as when I graduated from college."*

The Bodystat

All of the seeming paradoxes of dieting are explained if you consider the idea that your body has a certain amount of fat that it wants to keep, and it's not happy unless you're carrying around that amount of fat. This is the *set-point concept.*

The idea of set point is very common in engineering and physiology, and we use it all the time in our everyday lives. In fact, the easiest way to understand it is to think of your thermostat on the wall at home. Whether it is a simple thermostat or a fancy one, the basic concept is the same.

Your thermostat has two parts. The first is a knob, or a lever, or maybe a set of buttons, that you can manipulate. This is how you set the temperature that you want your house to be. This temperature that you set is the set point. The second part is some way of keeping track of the actual temperature. In your thermostat, this is the thermometer.

The thermometer and the set-point mechanism "talk" to each other. When the temperature is at the set point, the house is quiet. The furnace

---

*For a fascinating and highly readable account of the history of set point, see William Bennett, M.D., and Joel Gurin, *The Dieter's Dilemma* (New York: Basic Books, 1982). For a further description of this book, see Bibliography.

is off; the air conditioner is off. The house has to "expend" no "effort" to remain at the proper temperature.

Sometimes the actual temperature will be lower than the set point. For example, during the winter you may turn your thermostat down at night to 50 degrees. When you wake up in the morning the temperature in your house may be 50 degrees, and you turn up the set point on your thermostat to around 70 degrees. So the actual temperature is now 20 degrees lower than the set point. The thermostat sends out a signal that turns on the furnace, and that signal continues until the house temperature is the same as the set point, 70 degrees.

And sometimes the opposite happens, and the actual temperature is higher than the set point—when you come home from work on a hot day having left the thermostat off, and find the temperature in your house is about 90 degrees, you turn the set point on the thermostat down to 70 degrees. If you have a fancy modern house, the thermostat will activate the air conditioner. The air conditioner stays on until the house has cooled off to the set point (70 degrees); then the signal to the air conditioner stops.

So, whenever the temperature is different from the set point, some mechanism is activated to bring it back to set point, automatically. When set point and temperature are equal, everything is quiet.

Our bodies contain many analogous systems. You have a "thermostat," located in the lower parts of the brain, that monitors body temperature. The set point for body temperature is 98.6 degrees. If your actual body temperature goes below the 98.6 degree set point—when you go out on a winter day without a jacket on and you shiver—that's your "furnace," producing heat to get your body temperature back up to set point. If your body temperature goes above the 98.6 degree set point—when you run around on a hot day and sweat—that's your "air conditioner," cooling you off until your body temperature has come back down to set point.

Neither shivering nor sweating is under your conscious control; these processes start when your body temperature moves away from set point, whether you want them to or not. Next time it's a hot day, try to stop sweating by exerting your willpower.

You also have a mechanism that monitors the body's fat stores. We call this the "bodystat."

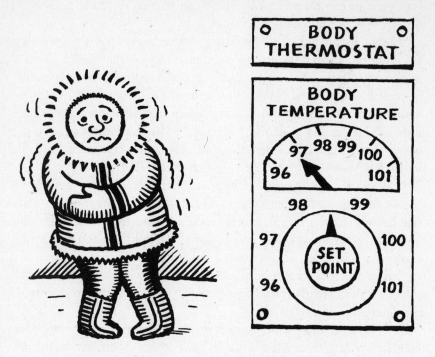

If your temperature gets too low (below the 98.6-degree set point),
you shiver—that's your "furnace."

Just like the thermostat, the bodystat is located in lower brain centers, beneath conscious control, and has a set point—in this case a certain number of pounds of fat that your body should be carrying—and a "fat-o-meter," a way to keep track of the actual number of pounds of fat.

"Wait a minute," said Lori. "I can see why I have a body thermostat. If my body temperature goes too high or too low, I'd die. But why a bodystat? Why does my body want me to carry around twenty or thirty extra pounds of ugly lard?"

"You have to remember," replied Eric, "that you're wearing ten-thousand-year-old genes. That is, genetically you're still almost identical to our ancestors living ten thousand years ago. Evolution acts so slowly that a thousand years is just the wink of an eye. Our ancestors evolved at a time when famines were a constant threat. During a famine, those who

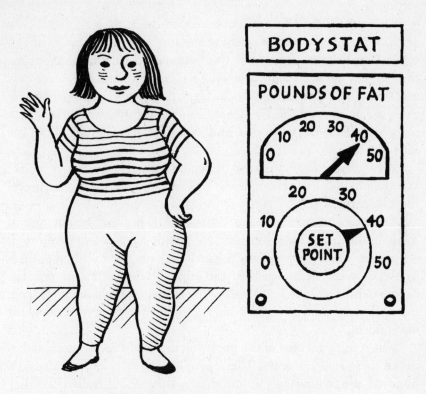

*When you're at your set point, your bodystat is not
sending out any signals to gain or lose fat.*

hadn't kept some fat on during times of plenty perished. On the other hand, *too much* fat interfered with hunting and gathering when food was available—tribes of people who carried around too much fat tended to perish, too, because they weren't very efficient at getting food. The people who survived and passed their genes on to us were those whose bodies could regulate the amount of fat they carried, never letting fat stores get so low that they couldn't survive short periods without food, but never letting them get so high that they couldn't move around to get food during normal times. Thus, the bodystat."

"But I see all sorts of people around, some skinny, some fat," said

Lori. "It seems like there must be a lot of leeway in the bodystat setting."

"That's true," said Eric. "People vary in the settings of their bodystats. Some people are naturally at the low end of the range of settings. We all know people like this, who are just naturally thin even though they eat everything that's not nailed down and are completely inactive. These people can be so lazy that they have someone else push the buttons on the TV remote control, yet they remain maddeningly lean. They're exceptions, and won't care very much about the set-point idea."

Lori smiled. "That's the kind of person I thought Carol was, until I saw the picture. I just thought she was naturally slim. And I figured I must be naturally fat."

"There *are* people who are naturally fat, but you're not one of them," said Eric. "Those unfortunate people have exceptionally high set points. These are people who carry perhaps two hundred pounds or more of fat. Although they can probably lose some of that fat, maybe quite a bit of it, by following the guidelines we'll tell you about, they will never be comfortably slim. But, again, this sort of person is exceptional.

"Ninety-nine percent of the people in the world fall somewhere between these two extremes. These people may carry around five to a hundred and five pounds more fat than they would really like. They have a ten-thousand-year-old set point responding to the modern world."

"Okay," said Lori. "So you're telling me that *my* set point is about twenty pounds higher than I want it to be. So why can't I just stay twenty pounds below it? It's not going to kill me—there's no threat of famine in *my* life."

"Oh, yes, there is," said Carol. "Every time you diet, your body sees it as a famine. And it responds as if you were facing a life-and-death situation. To your body, losing that reserve of fat has to be fought by every trick it can muster. . . ."

Why Cutting Calories Never Works

The concept of set point explains why conventional dieting is doomed to failure.

In a conventional diet, you cut down the number of calories that you eat. And you lose fat. Unfortunately, you have done nothing to change your set point. As a result, your body's fat stores go below, sometimes *far* below, your set point.

It's like having your house thermostat set to 70 degrees on a winter day, then deciding you want the house to be 50 degrees. But instead of lowering the thermostat, you open all your doors and windows. Sure enough, the actual temperature of your house drops to 50 degrees and stays there. The thermostat, still set to 70 degrees, will send constant signals to keep the furnace on. But as long as the doors and windows are open, the house can't get back up to 70 degrees, and the thermostat will keep the furnace on indefinitely.

Similarly, when your body's fat stores have dropped below your fat set point, the bodystat sends out continuous signals for fat conservation—three signals that you cannot control or override.

The first signal goes to all the cells in your body, telling them to lower their basal metabolic rate. This is the rate at which you use energy (calories), just to do the basic biochemical chores that keep you alive, like breathing. There's a little play in this basal metabolic rate, so when the body senses that it's losing fat it will drop the basal metabolic rate to dead low. You will use fewer calories just in the act of staying alive. This is one reason why dieting is so difficult after you lose the first ten pounds or so—you stop using as many calories as you did before. (Another reason that initial weight loss on a low-calorie diet is so easy is that most of that initial weight isn't fat—it's water and carbohydrate, which can be lost extremely rapidly. But after that weight is gone, the loss has to come from fat plus muscle. And fat loss is slow.)

The second signal is sent to behavior centers. Your bodystat tells you to slow down, because slowing down uses fewer calories. As the diet goes on day after day, you find yourself walking instead of running, standing instead of walking, sitting instead of standing, lying down instead of sitting, and falling asleep instead of staying awake. This further conserves the remaining fat stores. The signal also gets stronger the further below set point your body's fat stores go. You can fight the signal, but you can't stop it.

The third signal is to activate your hunger drive. All the time. Day and night. Even after eating a large meal, when your distended stomach may be telling you you're full, you don't feel satisfied. And the further below your set point you get, the stronger the activation.

Hunger is one of three basic, primal drives, along with the drive to breathe and the drive to drink. You might think the sex drive is basic. Sex is nice, but you can live without it. You can't live without air, water, or food. So lack of any one of these triggers an urgent, constant need that is not satisfied until the lack is remedied.

You have a reserve of oxygen—in your lungs and in your blood— enough for a few minutes without air. But when you use up even a few seconds of that reserve, you feel an overpowering need to breathe. Your body is taking no chances with your precious oxygen supply. You have a reserve of body water in the tissues of your body, enough for a few days without water. But if you fail to replenish it for even a day, you will experience an overpowering thirst. Your body can't risk becoming even a little dehydrated. You have a reserve of calories in your fat, enough for a few weeks. But after you lose just a few pounds of that fat, you start to experience overpowering hunger. Your body just can't take the chance of letting its calorie stores get too low.

Now you can see why the idea of willpower for the dieter is so misleading. Got a minute? You can demonstrate how much stronger these primal drives are than your willpower. Try holding your breath. Set a goal: you will hold your breath for ten minutes. Hold it as long as you can—exert all your willpower! Can you do it? Of course not. The same thing is happening when your body's fat stores go below set point, only it happens over a period of days and weeks rather than seconds. You activate a powerful drive; the more fat you lose, the more insistent the drive becomes. It doesn't matter how much willpower you have: that hunger is going to overpower you and you are going to eat, and continue eating, until you are back at your set point.

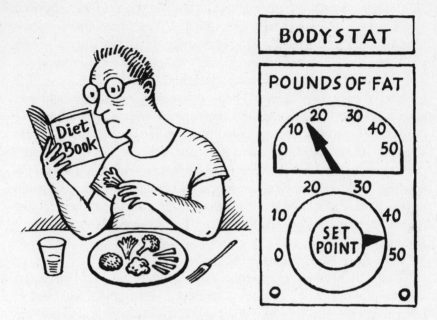

When you're below your fat set point (as is the case at the end of a diet),
the bodystat sends signals to regain fat by lowering the
metabolic rate, decreasing physical activity, and increasing hunger.

All three of the signals—for lower metabolic rate, for more sluggish behavior, for hunger—will continue to go out even after you have stopped dieting, because they're not activated by your day-to-day calorie intake, but by comparisons that your body continuously makes between your fat set point and the actual amount of fat on your body. Many, many people you see who are apparently thin are actually far below their set point and experiencing constant hunger and a battle of will. *Inside many a thin person is a fat person screaming to get out.*

When you look at dieting from the point of view of set point, its paradoxes are explained—the slowing of weight loss, the constant hunger, the weight gain at the end of the diet.

• • •

"It certainly sounds convincing," said Lori, "and it does explain what I've always experienced on a diet. But if I understand this set-point idea, I should have a hard time *gaining* weight, too. My body wouldn't want me to go *above* set point, either. And I put on ten pounds at the drop of a Twinkie. How do you explain that?"

"You're right," said Eric. "The fact that you can't lose weight and keep it off is only half of it, and everyone believes that half, because everyone's been on a diet and failed. But that ten pounds that you gain so easily can also be explained by set point. When was your last diet?"

"Oh, about three months ago. It was the citrus-fruit diet. I ate grapefruit for breakfast, grapefruit for lunch, and oranges for dinner. I could have unlimited snacks of lemonade made with artificial sweetener. I lost fifteen pounds in six weeks. Of course, I'm gaining it back, just like I always do."

"How much have you gained back?" asked Eric.

"Well, I've been pretty careful, watching what I eat, and I've gained only five pounds back. . . . Oh, I get it now. Even though I feel like I'm fatter than I want to be, right now I'm still about ten pounds *below* my set point. Come to think of it, I'm always either on a diet or just coming off one. I must *always* be below my set point. No wonder I'm always thinking about food."

"Are you happy with how much you weigh now?" asked Eric.

"No," said Lori. "Like I said, I gained five pounds back already."

"Yet you're still ten pounds below your set point," said Eric. "This is a really important point. *You can be fatter than you want to be and still be below your set point.* That's what happens when you're going on diets all the time. There's only one time on a diet when you are as thin as you want to be, and that's at the very end. Before the end, you're fatter than you want to be—otherwise you wouldn't be on the diet. And after the diet, as you gain the weight back, you're fatter than you want to be. But the whole time, until you've gained back *all* the weight, you're below your set point.

"And it's not just you, Lori. This is the situation with about two-thirds of the people in America," said Carol. "Did you know that at any given time 40 percent of American women and 25 percent of American men are trying to lose weight, almost always by going on a diet? That means that all those people are below their set points. Plus an equal number have probably just come off a diet, and are still below *their* set points. So 80 percent of American women and 50 percent of American men are below their set points. You can see why people get confused and think that gaining weight is easy. Most people are in a constant state of semistarvation, even if they feel they're fatter than they should be. From their perspective, the idea that it would be hard to gain weight is absurd."

"The trick," said Eric, "is to find some people who aren't chronic dieters and see how hard it is for *them* to gain weight—because they will probably start at their set point, rather than ten or twenty pounds below. Set-point theory predicts that these people will have just as hard a time gaining weight as dieters have losing weight.

"Actually, I've had this experience myself.

"When I was a junior at Berkeley, I started rowing on the crew. Now, with the kind of workouts the rowing team did, sometimes two or three hours of hard rowing each day, my problem suddenly became keeping weight *on,* not off. I was getting so thin that at the end of my first year my coach took me aside. 'Witt,' he said, 'you look a little skinny. I want you to gain twenty pounds over the summer.' "

" 'This should be easy,' I thought. 'I won't be working out much during the summer. All I have to do is eat a lot and get fat.' But it wasn't easy. In fact, it was quite a chore to gain that twenty pounds. I ate a midnight snack of two or three hot dogs every night, washed down by a big milk shake. I upped my already considerable beer consumption. But gaining that weight was a slow, painful process. In its way, it was as bad as any diet I'd been on—the constant worry about food (was I eating enough?), the daily weighings (oh my God, I actually *lost* a pound yesterday!), the jubilation when I finally reached my goal (I broke the two-hundred-pound barrier!).

"But after that summer I relaxed my vigilance, stopped eating so much, and lost most of those hard-earned pounds. I haven't been within ten pounds of two hundred pounds in the twenty years since that summer. Although I didn't know anything about set point at the time, when I later read some of the scientific studies of overfeeding that support the idea of set point, I could really feel for the subjects in the studies. *Real* overeating isn't anywhere near as much fun as you'd think it would be. . . ."

You Can't Be Too Fat in Cameroon

In a classic 1964 study, prisoners were asked to gain weight to a level 20 to 25 percent above their normal weight. So a 150-pound man would be trying to go to about 185 pounds. Since these men were not chronic dieters, they started out at their natural set points. A special kitchen was set up, and the men ate the equivalent of five meals a day. The volunteers were able, with enormous effort, to gain the weight. But it wasn't easy. One of the volunteers simply couldn't gain the amount of weight required for the experiment (just as some dieters simply can't lose large amounts of weight). All who did gain the required weight had to eat *far more calories* than would be theoretically necessary to add the amount of fat they were trying to gain. It was as if their metabolisms were speeding up to use the unneeded calories (just as a dieter's metabolism slows down). And as they gained fat, it became difficult to put on more.

Not only that: when they reached their target weight, they had a terribly difficult time keeping the weight on. They had to consume 2,000 *extra* calories per day, beyond their normal meals, just to maintain their overweight! When they were allowed to go back to normal eating, they dropped naturally, with no dieting, back to their original weight in a matter of months.

An even more convincing study comes from Cameroon, where societal values about body fat are the opposite of our values. Among the Massas, an ethnic group from northern Cameroon, *fatness* is a highly valued, socially encouraged trait. To achieve a desirable, fat body, young men participate in a traditional fattening session called Guru Walla, during which they force-feed themselves for four to six months, gaining an average of forty-three pounds. After the fattening session, they return to their normal eating patterns. When a group of these young men was carefully studied by a team of scientists, it turned out that, although fatness is prized, and although they have expended quite a bit of effort in achieving their rotundity, the men couldn't remain fat. The blubber melted away, quickly at first, then more slowly. They lost an average of twenty pounds in the first three months after the fattening session. By three years after their "reverse diet," the men weighed *exactly* the same as they did before they started.

The stories of Eric, the prisoners, and the men from Cameroon all show that it is just as hard to gain weight as it is to lose it. Once you're above set point, your bodystat activates mechanisms to slow your fat gain, and to take the fat off once you stop force-feeding yourself.

Lest you think that this applies only to men (since all of the examples were men), or it applies only to people who are naturally lean, you should know about a landmark study reported in 1995, one of the most carefully designed studies of set point ever conducted.

The researchers deliberately chose both men and women, and both obese and lean people, as subjects. The average weight of the obese people was almost three hundred pounds. The researchers first had the subjects gain weight, to 10 percent above their normal weight, then had them lose weight, to 10–20 percent below their normal weight. When the subjects were above their normal weight, their bodies started burning more energy, over 500 calories a day more, in an attempt to burn up the extra fat. This was true for both the obese and the lean subjects, and for men and women. When they were below their normal weight, their bodies burned less energy, over 300 calories per day less, in an attempt to bring fat stores back up to normal. Again, obese and lean, men and women, all experienced the same result.

So it doesn't matter whether you're a man or a woman, fat or thin. When fat stores differ from set point, your body tries to correct the situation. The fascinating thing about the 1995 study is that it almost seems as if the body resists being above set point even more than it resists being below—people were burning 500 calories a day more when above set point, but only 300 calories a day less when below.

To use the analogy of breathing again, if you were to hyperventilate for several minutes (we do *not* suggest that you try this), your body would sense that your breathing was out of balance. You would feel a very strong urge to *stop* breathing for a while; in fact, you might pass out—a safeguard mechanism to let your body return to normal without your conscious interference. It's just the opposite of what happens when you hold your breath. Any abnormalities in your breathing pattern, whether holding your breath or hyperventilating, activate corrective behaviors.

In the same way, overfeeding activates mechanisms that are the opposite of those activated by underfeeding (dieting). Your metabolic rate goes up (you burn extra calories even if you're just sitting still), you tend to want to be more active, and you experience fewer hunger signals—and, unlike the signals you experience during a diet, these tend to make you feel more energetic.

$$\bullet \quad \bullet \quad \bullet$$

"I've got to admit I'm a little depressed by all this," said Lori. "It's not that I don't believe this set-point idea. These studies are pretty convincing. But it looks like I either have to be hungry all my life, or settle for being fat. It just doesn't seem fair that, because there might have been a famine ten thousand years ago, I have to be fat now."

"Ah, but that's the nice thing about set point," said Carol. "Human beings are designed to carry a little bit of fat, that's for sure. But ancient cave paintings show that our ancestors were quite lean. And primitive hunter–gatherer tribes in the world today show no signs of obesity. The fact that there are so many fat people in America doesn't mean that we have set points that are permanently stuck on 'blimp.' What it means is that the set point can go up or down. *YOU CAN RESET YOUR SET POINT.* When I realized this, I knew that I finally had control over my body weight. The first thing I realized is why I had always had a tendency to be fat. . . ."

How to Get Fat Without Really Trying

There are two ways to raise your set point: have an inactive life-style or eat a high-fat diet.

Inactivity resets the set point upward. Dozens, probably hundreds, of studies have consistently shown that the less active you are, the fatter you are. It's true for humans, it's true for dogs, it's true for laboratory rats. The invention of the TV remote control probably put another half-pound of fat on everyone in America, because no one even walks to the TV anymore.

A hundred years ago, if you wanted to visit a friend who lived a mile away, you walked. If your friend was ten miles away, you rode a horse or hitched up the wagon. All of these are very active things to do. And people were active like that all day, every day. Our great-great-grandparents were much leaner than we are, and they didn't belong to fitness clubs. Their whole lives were one big fitness club; there was no choice. Now we have a choice, and we choose to be inactive. And we weigh, on average, over twenty pounds more than our great-grandparents did. We love the convenience of all our gadgets, yet demand to be thin. That's unrealistic.

Why would inactivity tend to make your body hold on to fat? About the only time our remote ancestors were inactive was during a famine. When food was plentiful, people *had* to be active, to gather the berries or to hunt the animals. When food was scarce, people became inactive—if the winter was long and hard, there was no food to be had and all you could do was wait it out. So your body interprets activity as a sign of plenty (no need to keep a lot of extra fat on, it will just interfere with food-gathering) and inactivity as a sign of famine (turn every available calorie into fat, we don't know how much food we'll be getting). It made perfect sense ten thousand years ago, and our genes are very slow to get the message that in the late twentieth century there are twenty-four-hour convenience stores on every corner.

Lack of activity also explains why people seem to get fatter as they get older. They become more inactive. Watch children at play sometime; they're *always* running. Watch teenagers; they don't run as much, but they are still constantly moving, fidgeting, wiggling. Watch young adults; they're starting to slow down. Stuck now in jobs, eight to ten hours a day, they tend to indulge in any leisure activity, including dancing or playing sports, less often. Just too tired from work. And when they have children, there seems to be no time for anything besides the kids. By the time the kids are out of the house, people have lost all concept of an active life-style. So there is a constant decrease in activity levels. It's imperceptible on a day-to-day or even a year-to-year basis. But not to your set point. Your set point is keeping perfect track. And your body fat reflects what your set point sees, as it increases a pound here, two pounds there.

High-fat eating also raises set point. Gradually, over the decades, our diet has gotten higher and higher in fat, and we've gotten fatter and fatter—Americans weigh more now than at the turn of the century, and we now eat 40 percent of our calories from fat, whereas in 1910 it was 30 percent. Of course, we're also less active, so it's difficult to separate the two effects.

But recent research is making it very clear that eating fat, with no other changes in life-style, makes you fat. Fat people have been found to eat no more calories than thin people, but they do eat more fat in their diets. They're not overeating—they're overfatting.

And when people change their fat intakes, their weight changes accordingly. For example, in one study women ate foods that contained 20 percent fat for two weeks, foods that contained 30 percent fat for two weeks, and foods that contained 40 percent fat for two weeks, for a total of six weeks. The order of the various eating regimes was random. The women who entered the study normally ate foods that contained 30 percent fat (which is lower than the national average of 40 percent). *They were told to eat as much as they wanted, as often as they wanted.* They were also told not to alter their activity levels. As you would expect, while eating 30 percent fat, the women neither gained nor lost weight. During the two weeks of eating 40 percent fat, however, the women gained an average of one pound. During the two weeks of eating 20 percent fat, they lost a pound. Remember, this is just two weeks. Imagine how much they would have gained (or lost) if the diets had been permanent.

Again, to our bodies this makes perfect sense. In the natural world, not many foods are high-fat; in fact, it's estimated that our ancestors, eating a natural diet, ate about 10–15 percent of their calories from fat. Even the meat they ate, from wild game animals, was only 10–20 percent fat. Encountering a particularly high-fat food, such as a crop of nuts, was a rare event. Foods high in fat can't be stored for long, because they go rancid easily, and our hunter–gatherer ancestors couldn't carry the weight of stored food with them anyway, at least not in its normal form. The best, most efficient way to store and carry those calories was as fat on the body. When your body encounters foods that average 40 percent fat, its ten-thousand-year-old brain is thinking "Hey, we must have found a bunch of nuts. We better turn up the bodystat set point to store as much of this as quickly as possible."

Unfortunately, your bodystat is getting that message at every meal, every day, year after year.

Taken together, these two powerful set-point modifiers answer the question "Why are Americans so fat?" The number-one reason we are so fat is that we are the most inactive society that has ever existed on the face of the earth, and we are constantly devising ways to become more inactive (leaf blowers rather than rakes, power lawnmowers instead of hand mowers). The number-two reason we are so fat is that we in North America eat one of the highest-fat diets that any group of human beings has ever consumed. It's a wonder we aren't fatter than we are; everything we do seems to raise our set points.

What Goes Up Can Come Down

Now let's look at the good news, how to reset the set point downward. There are three ways.

The first is through drugs. Nicotine, diet pills, and amphetamines all lower set point. They are not merely "appetite suppressants." They lower set point, and weight drops to a new, low level, where it stabilizes. Nicotine, of course, is in cigarettes; for women who smoke, the number-one reason they give is weight control. Diet pills are available at your friendly supermarket. Amphetamines are available from your friendly doctor. All three of these "diet aids" are potentially deadly; all will not merely lower your set point but shorten your lifespan. And all stop working the minute you stop taking them. We include them here for the sake of completeness, but please don't use them (we'll have more to say about "diet aids" in chapter 10).

Exercise is a second way to lower set point. Exercise, of course, is just the opposite of inactivity. If you raise your set point by not moving a muscle, you must be able to lower it by moving your muscles. And the more muscles you move, the more often, the lower the set point goes.

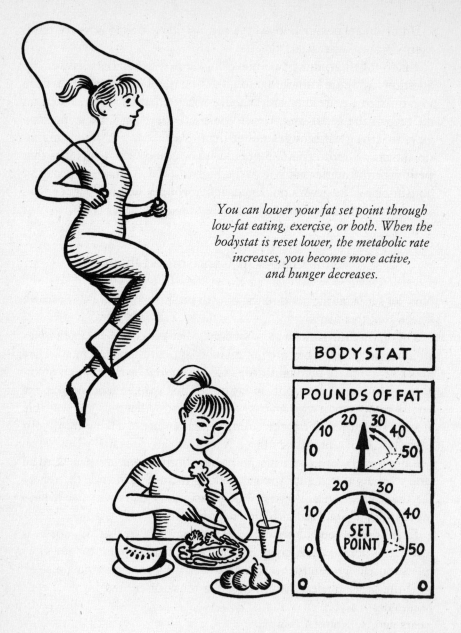

You can lower your fat set point through low-fat eating, exercise, or both. When the bodystat is reset lower, the metabolic rate increases, you become more active, and hunger decreases.

BODYSTAT

POUNDS OF FAT

10 20 30 40

0   50

20   30

10   40

SET
POINT

0   50

It has always been obvious that physical activity decreases fat stores, because most cultures, from the ancient Greeks to modern Americans, have had groups of people that are more active than the norm: athletes. Everyone knows that athletes tend to be leaner than the general public. The leanest are the ones engaged in the most energetic sports—runners and cross-country skiers, for example. But even football players tend to be lean. They may be huge, but they generally don't carry around much fat. And when athletes retire from competition and their activity level drops to normal, they get just as fat as everyone else. So it's quite easy to accept that exercise does something to make you leaner, and lack of exercise does something to make you fatter.

And it's not just the "extra" calories you burn while you're exercising, which is the conventional explanation for why exercise causes fat loss. Let's say you start walking two extra miles a day, which requires about 200 extra calories of energy. You will lose weight. Conventional wisdom has it that you are using 200 extra calories, which come from your fat stores, each day, so in about three weeks you lose a pound of fat, in a year about seventeen pounds. So far, so good—if you did start walking two extra miles a day you might, indeed, lose about seventeen pounds in a year, and stabilize at a new, lower weight. The question is, if you keep walking two miles a day after that first year, why don't you keep losing weight? By conventional reasoning, you should lose 170 pounds in ten years. For most people, that means that, if they start walking two miles a day, in ten years they will cease to exist! The bodystat concept explains the actual result of losing for a while, then stabilizing at a new weight—you've increased your activity level and your set point dropped accordingly. When you reach your new set point you stay there; your bodystat adjusts caloric expenditure and intake to keep you there as long as you maintain that activity level.

The third way to lower set point is through low-fat eating. If high-fat eating raises set point, then low-fat eating will lower it.

This *hasn't* been so obvious, because there haven't been, until a few years ago, substantial numbers of people eating low-fat. *Everyone* ate high-fat. People who ate low-fat weren't admired, as athletes are. They were thought to be crazy. So not very many people ate low-fat. But ever since Nathan Pritikin began popularizing the idea of eating low-fat for health reasons, groups of people have appeared who eat low-fat foods on a regular basis. And these groups consistently lost weight, and kept it off.

For example, Dr. Dean Ornish, who recently wrote the best-seller *Eat More, Weigh Less*, has been investigating low-fat eating for over a decade. In his first study, done in the 1970s, he asked heart patients to eat low-fat, about 10 percent calories from fat, and to practice stress-reduction techniques. He wanted to see what effect these two measures would have on their heart disease; though he wasn't interested in weight loss, he did keep track of their weight. *The participants lost an average of over ten pounds in the first month of the study.*

They were not asked to restrict their eating; in fact, most ate more than they had before the program. Also, in this first study Ornish did not ask them to exercise (which we know would help them lose weight). So their weight loss had to be due to the low-fat eating or the stress reduction, and numerous other studies indicate that it was the low-fat eating that was important.

In chapter 5 we'll talk about many more examples of weight loss through exercise and low-fat eating.

For some people, low-fat eating may be all it takes—some people's set points are particularly sensitive to the fat content of the foods they eat. For others, exercise might be enough—some people's set points are particularly sensitive to activity levels. For most people, some combination of the two is the most workable, and most effective, method for becoming and staying lean.

"So you see," said Carol, "it's a matter of lowering your set point. If you can do that, you'll be like those Cameroonians after their fattening session. You'll be *above* your set point. The weight comes off effortlessly, just as it did for them. In fact, they *wanted* to stay fat and couldn't. And the best thing is that you aren't hungry, ever, and your energy levels are high. That's my 'secret,' and that's Eric's 'secret.' We've changed our life-style to one where we keep our set points low, not high. The fat takes care of itself."

Dinner was over and it was time for dessert. Carol brought on the Bavarian Black Forest Chocolate Cake.

"Wait a minute," said Lori. "You two have been talking about how exercise and low-fat eating are the keys to lowering set point. But we just had cheese fondue and lasagna for dinner, and now we're about to have fudge cake for dessert. And I know you guys don't belong to a health club, and you've both told me that your exercise is limited. Come to think of it, I don't see any evidence that you two eat low-fat, or work out much."

"Yes, that's the second part of staying lean," said Eric. "We realized that these strategies for lowering set point wouldn't work for us unless we made them part of a normal life. We didn't want to eat such weird foods that we could never have friends over for dinner, or sacrifice our family life or careers to four hours a day of working out. Neither one of us is capable of working out that much any more, anyway. We had to find ways to make low-fat eating and exercise fit *us*. And you have to find ways to make them fit *you*."

"For example," said Carol, "this dinner, even with the chocolate cake for dessert, is less than 10 percent fat.* And both of us still exercise regularly, but a lot of it is stuff we fit into the nooks and crannies of our days, things you wouldn't even think of as exercise."

"That makes me feel a little better," said Lori. "When you started talking about low-fat eating, I pictured rice and beans, or some exotic dishes. And exercise? I can't see myself puffing away on an exercise bike for an hour a day. What excruciating boredom. I'm totally convinced by the set-point idea, but I can see there's still a lot to learn.

"One thing bothers me, though. I asked my doctor about losing weight, and she said to cut calories, just like all the diet books say. Why hasn't she heard about this idea of set point?"

"The chances are less than one in four that your doctor was even required to take a course in nutrition in medical school," said Eric. "So it's unlikely that your doctor knows much about the connections between life-style and obesity—or between life-style and disease, for that matter. Among nutrition experts, the idea of set point is well accepted. And exercise physiologists have known for decades about exercise's ability to make people lean. The ideas of low-fat eating are starting to gain acceptance, too. Not many people have put all these ideas together, though. We think in the next decade or so these ideas will become the

---

*You will find recipes for the lasagna, chocolate cake, and cream-cheese fondue in the recipes appendix.

dominant way of thinking about weight control. And perhaps then we'll finally start doing the things that really work, and stop wasting time on calorie cutting."

"I don't want to wait a decade," said Lori. "I want to start learning exactly how to incorporate these ideas in my life, starting tonight."

"Well," said Carol, handing Lori a piece of cake, "you can start by having some dessert. . . ."

Five Years After Dinner

After that dinner, over five years ago, we spent perhaps a day discussing a program for Lori in more detail with her. And that was all it took. Lori has never gone on another diet. She adopted the principles that we'll discuss in the rest of this book, and dropped two dress sizes. She no longer goes hungry or worries about how much she eats. Yet she stays lean.

Even better, she told us, "Six months after I started changing my life-style the way you showed me, I suddenly realized that I was no longer obsessed with food. I didn't feel guilty about eating, I didn't worry about overeating, I just ate. Diets were always a disruption of my 'normal' eating, and they always failed me. Now, for the first time in years, I feel in control of my eating and my weight. I'm finally over the obsession, after so many years of pain."

Other friends asked about these ideas, and eventually we began giving workshops. We took people, step by step, through customizing a program that would work for each individual. The rest of this book is based closely on our workshops and workbook, which have been refined through working with hundreds of people and listening to their feedback.

We've also witnessed the explosive growth of interest in low-fat eating as a means of weight loss. When we had dinner with Lori, low-fat eating was still considered somewhat bizarre, the practice of a few health nuts. But then some popular books appeared, and the low-fat bandwagon gathered steam. It seemed to accelerate from zero to sixty in seconds flat.

Can Eating Low-Fat Make You Fatter?

In the modern world, any new idea generates skepticism, then hype, then frenzy, and finally backlash. In late-twentieth-century America, the stages are sometimes only weeks apart. That seems to have happened with the idea of low-fat eating for weight loss.

After the first several hundred reports of weight loss through low-fat eating, the media were looking for something new. Along came a few reports of people *gaining* weight while on low-fat diets. The old-school diet experts shook their fingers. "See, we told you so. You must always count calories in order to lose weight. It just stands to reason." And, quicker than you can say "media feeding frenzy," we were into the low-fat backlash. *The New York Times* even ran an article that stated, "While foods like pasta may be perfectly healthy and even free of fat, people still gain weight if they consume them in large quantities." As "proof" of such claims, the media offered testimony from people who had started to eat low-fat diets and actually gained weight. One woman interviewed for a newspaper article said, "I went went from a size 8 to a size 12 on 35 fat grams a day."

We believe these people's stories. On the other hand, we also believe the enormous body of scientific evidence that shows that switching from eating high-fat to eating low-fat will cause weight loss, even if you eat as much as you want. In fact, we have yet to see a single scientific study, out of dozens that we have reviewed in preparing this book, that shows that, in the long run, low-fat eating of any type causes weight gain. How can we reconcile these people's stories with the scientific evidence?

Let's consider Lori again. Because Lori was the first person we heard about who gained weight while eating low-fat. And we weren't surprised.

Within a matter of days after our dinner, Lori stopped limiting the amount she ate, and instead concentrated on limiting the amount of *fat* she ate. She started working out several times a week. She couldn't wait for the fat to melt away.

But it didn't happen at first. Initially, Lori *gained* several pounds.

She called Carol. "You said I could forget about counting calories, so I did. Now I'm ballooning! Cow city! What's going on here?"

"Be patient," said Carol. "You've got to realize that, before you started this life-style change, your weight was ten to fifteen pounds *below* your set point, because of chronic dieting. The first thing that will happen when you start eating as much as you want, even if it's low-fat food, and even if you're exercising too, is that your body will be saying, 'Finally, she's eating. Let's put the fat on to get back up to set point, where we should have been all along.' So you gain a few pounds right away, even though you're eating low-fat foods. But meanwhile, the low-fat eating and exercise are lowering your set point. It just takes time. For a few months or so, you'll be fatter than you want, but slowly, inevitably, your set point will continue to drop. One day, it will drop below your present weight, and you'll start to lose, even though you continue to eat as much as you want. And it will continue to drop. Trust me. You will never have to be hungry again, and you will become lean."

That was what happened. After those first couple of months, Lori began losing, and never regained the weight.

The woman in the newspaper article who went from a size 8 to a size 12 said that, before low-fat eating, "I was always watching my calories." But after going on a low-fat diet, "I just went wild. I was having so much fun eating all the food I wanted. . . ." This woman probably began the low-fat diet weighing twenty, thirty, or even forty pounds less than set point. She had maintained her weight there for years, always feeling a little hungry, always counting calories, always being miserable. Her low-fat diet lowered her set point, but it's a gradual process, taking months to a year or more. So, for at least several months, her weight continued to be below set point, but now she could eat as much as she wanted. The result? She gained weight initially. When chronic dieters are finally allowed to eat normally, to respond to their hunger signals, they can gain weight remarkably quickly, putting on several pounds a week. So this woman was getting fatter *even as her set point was coming down.* She just didn't continue on the low-fat program long enough.

Without understanding the concept of set point, you are very unlikely to stay with a low-fat eating program beyond those first few months if you gain a few pounds initially.

And, to make matters worse, many people think they're eating low-fat when they aren't. This is due to confusing labeling laws that allow manufacturers to lie about the fat contents of their food (more on this when we talk about label-reading in chapter 8). You can switch to foods labeled "low-fat" and "97% fat-free" and wind up eating *more* fat than you were before. When we question people in our workshops who say they're already eating low-fat, it usually turns out that they're eating high-fat products while under the belief that the products are virtually fat-free. We wonder if the woman quoted in the newspaper was doing the same thing while eating "35 grams of fat a day." (By the way, even 35 grams of fat a day is not truly low-fat. Truly low-fat is about 20 grams a day, as we'll explain.)

There are three reasons scientific studies of low-fat eating don't find the same weight gain that Lori and the woman in the newspaper article exhibited.

One is that in scientific studies researchers take the average of what happens to all subjects. If there are five hundred subjects in a study of low-fat eating, and 495 lose weight while five gain weight, the average for everyone will overwhelmingly show weight loss. But guess which of those subjects in the study is going to get an interview on a talk show? Losing weight by eating low-fat isn't news anymore; gaining weight is.

The second reason is that the best studies of low-fat eating are long-term, lasting several months. Any initial weight gain is reversed and becomes weight loss as the study progresses.

The third reason is that most of the shorter studies are deliberately designed to exclude people who have recently been on a diet and are thus below their set points. When you are only going to be looking at people for a few weeks, you can't afford to have your results confused by someone who is on a "diet rebound." Researchers typically ask volunteers questions like "Have you been on a diet in the last year?" People who answer "yes" are rejected, under the assumption that they are still below set point.

So, if you find yourself getting a little fatter at first on a low-fat, all-you-want-to-eat diet, follow these guidelines:

- *Make sure you are REALLY eating low-fat.* The number-one reason people don't lose weight while eating low-fat is that they're not really eating low-fat. In this book we are concerned with making sure you know where the fat really is in your diet. Make sure you take our diagnostic quizzes.

- *Don't give up.* You will become leaner as your body responds and lowers your set point. That will take months, even a year in a few cases. But if you stop the low-fat eating, you stop the signal to your set point to decrease. Give yourself a chance.
- *Use exercise.* Don't forget, there are two ways to lower set point. Exercise can help you combat any initial weight gain as your hunger is finally being satisfied, keeping the weight gain to a minimum and hastening the day when you start to lose.

But we're getting ahead of ourselves. You need to find out a bit more about how a program based on set point differs from others, and what effects on your life in addition to weight loss such a program will have.

2

Heresies

• • • • • •

As we started giving workshops on the idea of focusing on the set point and letting the fat take care of itself, we found that we were describing a number of ideas that would be considered heresies in a conventional calorie-cutting program. Yet they are crucial to your success in becoming leaner.

These are:

Throw Away Your Scale

Conventional diets encourage you to weigh yourself and to keep track of your progress by your weight. The sleazier ones take advantage of tricks to make your body lose water so that you lose weight rapidly, and the weight loss appears on your scale. So scales and weights are very important in conventional diets. But there are two reasons why you should get rid of your scale.

First, a scale makes you focus on *weight,* when you should be focusing on *fat.* If you change your life-style to lower your set point, you will lose fat permanently. But if part of that life-style change is to exercise more, you may well replace the fat with muscle. Muscle is more compact than fat and makes you look better (it shapes and tones), but it does have weight. So, even though you are losing *fat,* and your body shape is changing, and clothes are fitting that didn't fit before, and people are complimenting you on your appearance, you may not lose any *weight* for months. In fact, you can completely change your shape with little change in your weight. This is especially true for men. If you make weight your primary focus, you may feel discouraged for a long time.

The second problem with scales is that they encourage impatience. The scale is sitting there in the bathroom every time you take a shower. There you are with no clothes on to add extra weight. The temptation to weight yourself is overwhelming. So you do. Every day. Maybe twice a day. But true fat loss takes place over a period of weeks and months, not days. Even if every ounce of fat lost were reflected as an ounce of weight loss, the greatest fat loss you could reasonably expect would be about two to four pounds a month (and for many people it's less than that). Your weight fluctuates two to four pounds *a day,* because of varying water retention, the quantity of your last meal that is still with you, etc. This means that your fat loss will be masked by your normal daily fluctuations until you've lost about four pounds, which will take at *least* a month and often two or more months. Think about something you did two months ago. Seems like a long time ago, doesn't it? Imagine weighing yourself every day in that two months and only today seeing something that looks as if it *might* be weight loss. Most of us would never make it.

And remember, if you've been dieting all your life you will probably start out by *gaining* a few pounds, as Lori did. It will disappear as your set point comes down, but if weight is your entire focus you'll get discouraged.

Throw away your scale and remove the temptation to focus on this meaningless issue. Weight is completely unimportant. In a later chapter we'll give you more valid ways of measuring your progress. If you can't stand the thought of throwing away your $500 Super Digital Mass Evaluator, at least give it to a friend. That way you'll only be tempted to use it when you're at your friend's home (so maybe it shouldn't be a close friend).

Don't Count Calories

Forget calories. Studies show that even the most vigilant calorie-counters, people who keep track of every last morsel that they eat, usually can't estimate the number of calories that they have eaten on a given day to within 30 percent. That's an error of 600 calories! Your body is perfectly able to control your caloric intake so that your fat level will match your set point—in fact, it will insist on it, no matter what you do. If you stuff yourself one day, your appetite automatically decreases over the next couple of days to compensate. So change your set point and forget about calories—like the fat on your body, the number of calories you consume each day will take care of itself with no effort on your part. Stop being obsessed with the quantity you eat. If you want to be obsessed, be obsessed with the *quality* of what you eat. Your set point will drop, and the weight will disappear automatically.

Don't Psychoanalyze the Reasons Why You Eat

We're so accustomed to thinking of fatness as a failure of will, rather than as an inevitable biological consequence of our life-style, that we come up with all sorts of bizarre reasons why we "eat more than we should." Many diets focus on remaining aware of why you are eating, making sure you eat only when you're hungry, stopping when you're "satisfied" rather than "full," etc. The idea is that, if only we would just eat for the "right" reason (true hunger) and not for the "wrong" reasons (because we're stressed, or depressed, or happy, or bored, or whatever), then we would stop "overeating" and stop being "overweight."

There is little or no evidence that this kind of behavior modification helps people become permanently thinner, but the mythology persists that there are "right" and "wrong" reasons for eating. We consider fat people lazy, and lacking motivation or self-control. And yet there are countless examples of people who are highly successful but can't control their weight. CEOs of major corporations get fat. Nobel Prize winners get fat. Presidents of the United States end up chubby. These people are hardly lazy or lacking in motivation and self-control. How could they be so strong in the rest of their lives and so weak when it came to food?

Darlene, one of our early clients, was a member of a fasting group for two years before she started our program. She lost over a hundred pounds through the periodic fasting, yet, when she began eating a prudent, normal diet, the weight started coming back. Try fasting for just one day and you will see what kind of willpower Darlene must have. Why would her willpower suddenly desert her when she returned to normal eating? And what psychological process could explain the fact that, now that she is eating a low-fat diet and exercising, she is slowly losing the weight permanently, without hunger?

In truth, we should be looking at physiology, not psychology. Many people wonder what awful psychological secrets are causing their constant desire to pig out. But when you carry around less fat than your bodystat is set for (and most people, thanks to constant dieting, are below set point), you are constantly hungry, and pretty much any signal that makes you temporarily drop your vigilance will make you eat. So you might gorge yourself for any reason—an upsetting phone call, a big promotion, a fight with your spouse, a good grade. If you focus on these events, and try to build a psychological theory as to why you eat, you will come up with some bizarre ideas—and psychologists have indeed come up with some laughable explanations for "overeating." On the other hand, if you realize that many people, *even fat people,* are far below their set points and constantly exerting their willpower to restrain their eating in the face of unceasing hunger signals, it's easy to see that anything that temporarily distracts you, good or bad, could trigger an eating binge.

Your body will override your brain every time. It will make you eat just the right amount to remain at your set point. If your set point is high, you'll be fat, no matter how much or how little your mother loved you. It really doesn't matter what you are thinking or feeling at the time you eat, so don't worry about it. Just worry about lowering your set point.

Bingeing and bulimia

In chapter 1 we suggested that you try holding your breath to see how powerful basic drives are. Bingeing is the dieting equivalent of taking a deep breath after you've been holding your breath for a minute or so.

You take a deep breath because your body senses that you don't have enough oxygen. People binge after cutting calories because their bodies sense that they don't have enough fat stored. It is perfectly natural—in scientific studies of people who are deliberately underfed for extended periods, then allowed to eat as much as they want, bingeing is the norm, not the exception. It will continue until the person reaches set point.

Bingeing with purging (vomiting or using laxatives to get rid of the meal just eaten), the pattern in bulimia, is just one step beyond this. The difference is that, whereas most dieters binge, feel guilty about it, and get a little fatter (a little closer to set point), the bulimic binges, giving in to hunger and craving (which is completely normal), but then immediately releases all those calories by vomiting or other means, so that there is no fat gain. The bulimic is just as far away from set point after the binge as before the binge. So, for the bulimic, hunger signals continue unabated, leading to another binge, another purge, in a vicious cycle.

One of us (Carol) can talk about bulimia from personal experience. Like many young girls, Carol was highly conscious of her weight. She is tall for a woman, five feet ten, and always felt big and unfeminine. She tends to carry any excess weight on her hips and thighs. As a young woman she looked around at her shorter, smaller peers, and the beautiful willowy models on magazine covers, and knew that she had to be thin or she would be ugly and completely unappealing to men. She began to diet during her senior year in high school. Looking back, she can see that she was not fat, but the fear of being unattractive warped her perspective. She tried many diets. She'd stay on the diet for a few weeks and lose weight, but ultimately couldn't maintain the loss. She always wanted to eat more than those diets recommended and would eventually lose control and binge.

Then she found another and, she thought, better way: she'd eat everything she wanted and just throw it all back up. It made perfect sense to her—she could enjoy eating without gaining weight. But she became constantly obsessed with food, and started having stomach and intestinal problems. She hated throwing up. It really was kind of disgusting, and she felt so guilty. She tried to hide it from her family. Luckily, however, they found out and helped her stop.

Once she stopped, she got even fatter. She felt lousy most of the time, was tremendously obsessed with food, and had feelings of self-hate and disgust. She had at least rid herself of the potentially fatal habit of bulimia. But she was still miserable, as she fought against her natural set point. Though bulimia wasn't the solution, neither were conventional diets.

Obsession with food

Obsession with food is extremely common among those who try to control their weight through conventional dieting. Obsessional thinking is another of your body's methods of getting you to eat, like constant hunger. These are not, in the vast majority of people, signs of abnormal psychology, but of abnormal *physiology,* of a body desperately trying to regain the fat that it is set to store.

At the end of World War II, experiments were conducted to study starvation, and how best to renourish large populations that had been on very low calorie diets for years due to food shortages. Volunteers were subjected to very low calorie diets in order to get them to extremely low body weights. During the starvation part of the experiment, these volunteers reported experiencing insatiable hunger, as well as fatigue and lethargy. Interestingly, when the volunteers were allowed to eat normally, their hunger persisted. They reported being hungry even after stuffing themselves with a big meal; the hunger and the obsession with food did not go away until they reached their normal weight. Just as with those volunteers, when you diet, your body acts as if it's starving, and makes food *the* focus of your life.

After abandoning bulimia, Carol blundered around for many years trying to control her weight, at times exercising as much as three hours a day to stay thin. She tried all sorts of diets—the pineapple diet, the grapefruit diet—she tried diet pills, she tried eating only when she was hungry, she tried thinking only "correct" diet thoughts. Sometimes she was thin enough, but most of the time she wasn't. Even when she perceived herself as being thin she was miserable, because she was obsessed with food and lived in constant fear of gaining weight. And with good reason, since it always happened—she always regained whatever weight she'd lost.

It was not until she began to eat low-fat consistently, and established regular exercise habits, that her weight stabilized at a level she was satisfied with.

Something else happened, though, that took her completely by surprise. One day, at work, she realized that she no longer thought about food all the time. She also realized she couldn't remember the last time she'd binged. The bingeing and obsessional thinking had just gone away. She hadn't tried to think or feel differently, it just happened. That's when she became convinced that the obsession and bingeing are primarily physiologically based. Take away the physiological cause (contantly trying to stay below set point) and all the "bad reasons" for eating simply disappear.

An experiment

Try this: Drop the fat content of your diet to 20 percent (or, better yet, 10 percent) and exercise for half an hour to an hour daily. Do this for the next six months, and promise yourself that you won't worry about why you eat in that period. If you want to worry about something, worry about *what* you eat. At the end of this time, you will probably find that your clothes are looser, you look better, you feel better, and your obsession with food is gone. After all, if you can eat any time, any amount you wish, and still get thinner, what's there to be obsessed about? Don't try to lose fat by going below your set point; *then* you will be obsessed. Instead, lower your set point.

If we could get everyone in the country off of diets and on to weight-lowering eating and exercise programs, the collective brainpower that would be freed from obsession with food would probably be enough to find a cure for cancer in a matter of months.

If you're still not convinced, read on. . . .

Never Go Hungry

This is the one that people seem to have the most trouble with, and yet it is very important to understand.

We have it deeply ingrained from all those diet programs that hunger is good, that it will lead to our being lean, even though that idea flies in the face of every dieter's experience of regaining all the weight he or she lost through enduring weeks of hunger.

When you look at it from the set-point view, going hungry can be seen for what it really is—evil. By allowing yourself to get hungry, you set yourself up to sabotage the two habits that will allow you to truly lose weight, low-fat eating and exercise.

Low-fat food is like jet fuel—it burns clean and makes you feel sky-high, but it burns fast, and you need to anticipate that. If you switch to eating low-fat, but still maintain the "no snacks, careful not to eat too much at any meal" mentality, you will find yourself hungry within an hour of your last meal. When you get hungry, you want to eat any-thing. Since most food choices available to you out in the big bad world are still high-fat, you stand a good chance of pigging out on a high-fat option. Not the end of the world, but if it happens constantly you are defeating yourself. It won't happen much if you don't let your-self get hungry.

Snacking is not only not forbidden on a low-fat diet, it must become a habit. Instead of making you fat, it helps get you lean and keep you that way—as long as the snacks are low-fat. If you ate breakfast an hour ago but you're hungry, eat a bagel, or a banana, or whatever (low-fat) snack it takes to stop the hunger signal. We have lots of sugges-tions for low-fat snacks in chapter 9.

Going hungry also tends to defeat your exercise efforts. As you get hungrier, you focus more and more on the simple act of getting food, and less and less on anything else. Your unconscious mind views procuring food as a far higher priority than working out on a Nautilus machine. It easily overrides your conscious desires. If you normally ex-ercise after work, you may instead find yourself drawn into the nearest fast-food restaurant, where you stuff yourself with burgers, fries, and milk shakes. And after that, with a lump of grease in your gut, the idea of exercise is distasteful. If, instead, you had a big low-fat snack in the middle of the afternoon, not only would you not be hungry, but you would be fueled and ready to go for your exercise.

So do not go hungry. Don't skip meals if you can avoid it.

If you're like most of our workshop participants, you will resist this idea. You'll want to speed things up by skipping a few meals. Please don't. When you are losing weight permanently through permanent life-style changes, you must take the long-term, not the short-term, view. Which leads us to our last heresy.

Be Patient

If you cut down the amount of fat you eat (from a typical American diet of 40 percent fat to a more natural 10 percent fat), and you exercise regularly, we guarantee that you will lose fat. But for many people, the fat loss may be imperceptible at first, *maybe even for several months.* Be patient! At the end of a year, the fat loss will be very noticeable, perhaps (depending on your physiology and how far you want to go) profound.

But you *must* be patient. If you keep your scale (shame on you) and you notice that you have lost fifteen pounds in the first two weeks, by conventional diet standards that is wonderful. By the standards of this program it is *horrible.* Very, very few people lose fat at this rate, and those who do are generally very obese to begin with. If you didn't weigh three hundred pounds or so at the start of your new habits, it is extremely unlikely that you can lose weight that quickly. You are doing something wrong, probably going hungry (shame on you again) to "speed things up." A more typical rate of loss is two to five pounds of fat in two weeks, so the other eight to ten pounds of that miraculous fifteen-pound loss must be water, or carbohydrate stores, or muscle protein. People don't function well when they are dehydrated, or when they are not carrying around the proper amount of carbohydrate stores, or when their muscles are wasting away. Get back on the program. Stop going hungry. Rapid weight loss, even rapid fat loss, is a *bad* sign for almost all people. You may be able to do it for a while, but your set point never sleeps. It will make you hungrier and hungrier, make you crave fattier foods, until you give in, give up, and get fat again.

Let's examine more closely the rewards of patience and the folly of impatience.

We'll look at two women, Patient Penelope and Impatient Irmagard. They both want to lose about twelve pounds of fat. Patient Penelope follows the guidelines we will talk about. She decides that she'll eat about 20 percent calories from fat (a little higher than optimum for weight loss, but Patient Penelope prudently predicts positive pound-loss promotion) and she'll exercise about two hours more per week. She starts the program, within weeks is comfortable with it, and just lets it be a part of her life. Impatient Irmagard irrationally insists that the latest fad diet, in which you eat nothing but ten bonbons a day, is the one that will take the fat off and keep it off.

Let's follow them for a year and a half, looking at the number of pounds of fat each woman carries, and how that changes. Let's say that, at first, both women carry a little over forty pounds of fat, not unusual among American women.

After a month, Impatient Irmagard has lost ten pounds of fat by more or less starving herself. (We're exaggerating the amount that Irmagard could lose in a month. But she's in for a rude surprise, so let's let her lose this much.) Definitely thinner, able to fit into clothes she couldn't fit into before, she happily returns to normal eating, confident that her newfound thinness will last.

After a month, Patient Penelope has lost a pound of fat. She's also gained a pound of muscle because of her increased exercise. She threw away her scale, so she can't see that her weight has remained the same, but she really doesn't notice any difference yet.

Six months after the two women have begun their fat-loss programs, however, the tables have turned. Irmagard, off her diet, has regained all the fat she lost. Penelope has now lost six pounds of fat. She has also gained four pounds of muscle, so even at this point, if she were relying on her scale to show progress, she probably wouldn't see much. But she's starting to be able to fit into clothes that were too tight before, and people are asking her if she's lost weight.

Hope springs eternal, so Irmagard now goes on the new Physician's Rapid Weight Loss Diet that she saw advertised in a newspaper at the supermarket checkout stand. You take these magic diet pills (only $9.99 per dozen—order now!) and the fat melts away.

A month later, Irmagard has again managed to lose ten pounds. She's thin again! Those diet pills really work. Unfortunately, they make her irritable, upset her stomach, and give her constipation and insomnia. Oh well, now that she's lost the weight she can stop taking the pills.

Penelope continues with her life-style of low-fat eating and exercise. It's just the way she lives.

Another five months pass, bringing us to one year from the start of the women's fat-loss programs. Irmagard has been on two gimmick diets. Of course, as soon as she went off the diet pills, her fat returned. In fact, because she's been neglecting exercise in favor of her gimmick diets, her set point has gone up a bit, and she's fatter than ever. On the other hand, Penelope has lost twelve pounds of fat. She's had to buy new clothes, because none of her old things fit her. *Everyone* now comments on how much better she looks.

Irmagard decides that the liquid-protein fast is the only way she will truly lose weight. She presents herself at a clinic and pays several hundred dollars to go on the program, which is so dangerous that it must be done under a doctor's supervision. But it must really work. After all, a doctor wouldn't lie to you, at the expense of your health, just to make money—would he?

And Patient Penelope? Well, you know the story.

After a month of protein fasting, Irmagard has lost those ten pounds again. But the nice doctor at the clinic tells her that she has to stop because of irregularities in her heartbeat. Good thing she didn't just drop dead, as have many people who have tried this approach. We'll bet you can guess what happens to her fat stores in the next six months. Balloon city.

After a year and a half, Irmagard is fatter than ever. Her health has probably suffered from the diet pills and the protein fast. Let's hope she's a little wiser now and will give up on the diet routine. Also, note that, during the entire year and a half, her body fat was constantly below set point—she was either losing fat or regaining it, but she was never at her set point except on the days between diets. Obsessed with food, constantly hungry, she weighed herself three times a day, tended to binge, felt guilty about her bingeing, and sometimes wondered if she was deliberately building a wall of fat to be unattractive. In light of set-point theory, all of this is to be expected of a perfectly normal person whose body-fat content has been artificially lowered below set point.

Penelope has stabilized at a new set point twelve pounds below her old one. That's twelve pounds of fat, which is a lot. She was never in danger of going off her "diet," because she was never on one. She was never hungry—Penelope was always *above* set point during her weight loss. She stopped worrying about how much she was eating or how often. She feels better than ever, and her health has improved. Her friends want to know how she lost all that weight and are very curious about her new way of eating (they can't believe she can eat so much and still lose weight; there has to be a gimmick). If Penelope wants to lose more fat from her body, she can switch from eating 20 percent fat to eating 10 percent. Or she can exercise more. Or both. It depends on what fits into her life.

You may be thinking that Penelope didn't lose all that much, that twelve pounds of fat really isn't such a great loss. If so, you're still thinking about *weight* loss, not *fat* loss. On a typical quick weight-loss diet, you may lose twelve pounds quite rapidly. But remember, only about two or three of those pounds are fat. The rest is water, carbohydrate stores, and protein, which isn't what is hanging from your thighs.

How much is twelve pounds of *fat* loss?

Go look at a pound of butter or margarine, one of the standard cartons with four cubes in it. Butter is 100 percent fat. So is margarine. When you lose a pound of fat, you've lost a volume of fat equal to one of those cartons. One pound may not be noticeable, but twelve is a lot—very noticeable, even on a fairly tall person. In our workshops, Carol holds twelve cartons of butter next to her body to demonstrate the added bulk of such a quantity of fat; people are astonished to see the difference. When you're at the store sometime, take twelve cartons of butter or margarine out of the dairy case and heft that weight. It's substantial. Try padding your body with it, if you like (but don't get arrested for shoplifting!). You can lose at least that much bulk, and for most people twice that much or more, in a year. All it takes is patience and the proper program.

3

Side Effects

• • • • • •

Most people are interested strictly in the weight-loss aspects of our program. But you should keep in mind that, any time you change your eating and exercise patterns, you will affect your health. Conventional, calorie-cutting diets have side effects. So does a program of low-fat eating and exercise. You should be aware of them.

Side Effects of Calorie-Cutting

Very low calorie diets can cause fatigue, hair loss, dizziness, gallstones, and acute gallbladder disease

These side effects were listed by the National Institutes of Health, the largest biomedical-research organization in America. If you're dieting to become more attractive, you may be a bit alarmed at the image of yourself staggering down the street moaning from the pain in your gallbladder, clutching your bald head. Severe dieting gives you bad breath, too. (No, we're not kidding. Metabolic changes during severe calorie restriction cause the formation of bad-smelling ketone bodies, which you exhale, much to the dismay of anyone near you.)

Dieting increases the risk of heart disease

A few years ago, researchers discovered an alarming connection: people who underwent large fluctuations in weight had increased risk of heart disease.

In the town of Framingham, near Boston, scientists have been keeping track of the most minute details of the lives of five thousand people since 1948, to find out what aspects of a person's life are most likely to be associated with various diseases, especially heart disease. One factor that the Framingham researchers have followed is people's weights. The researchers found the people who had experienced the most fluctuations in their weight, and compared their rates of death from heart disease with those whose weights didn't fluctuate. These researchers were pretty sure they had eliminated anyone whose weight fluctuated for other reasons, such as illness.

The results were shocking. People whose weights fluctuated the most (almost certainly chronic dieters, whose weight fluctuates as they lose, then regain, then lose . . . sound familiar?) had a risk of heart disease that was 30 to 100 percent greater than for those whose weight was steady! Those whose weight yoyoed also had a risk of cancer 5 to 33 percent greater than that of nondieters, though the increase was not statistically significant.

Precisely why dieting might cause such an increase in the risk of these major killers is not known, and the exact connection is still the subject of intense research and debate in the scientific community. But it makes sense. Every time you drastically cut calories, you also drastically cut your intake of natural substances in foods that are protective against cancer and heart disease—and you can't make up for this by taking a vitamin pill. Many of the most powerful of these substances are just starting to be identified (we'll talk about one of the most powerful later in the chapter). For now, they come only in food, not pills. It's not natural for your body to be subjected to famine several times a year, and it's not surprising that it breaks down if you do this year after year. Maybe you should stop.

Common diet programs,
supervised by doctors, kill people

The liquid-protein fasts (Doctor supervised! They must be safe!) have helped more than fifty people enter a state in which they need never again fret about being overweight. These people died while on liquid-protein fasts. The nice diet-clinic doctors assure us that they keep better track now, that the liquid-protein diets are much safer these days. That's like the builders of the *Titanic II* assuring you that this time they really have that iceberg problem licked. The difference is that on the *Titanic II* you know that—if it doesn't sink—you will reach your destination. On a liquid-protein diet, even if you don't die, you won't keep the weight off.

Anyone want to buy a ticket?

Dieting while pregnant (or even before)
may harm the developing baby

These days, doctors tell pregnant women in no uncertain terms *not* to diet. The fetus will be harmed by the life-or-death stress of a famine, which is what a diet is. So almost no woman would go on a diet after she knew she was pregnant.

But the time of most rapid brain-cell division is the first few weeks after conception. The developing embryo is particularly vulnerable to the mother's nutritional state at this point, because the placenta has not yet formed. Ironically, this is the time when most women are unaware that they are pregnant. You may be on a diet at the time when your baby can least afford to suffer any lack of nutrients. In fact, some experts think that the nutritional state even before you conceive is crucial, because it takes some time to recover from the malnutrition of a severe calorie-restricting diet.

We don't mean to imply that if you skip breakfast occasionally you will have a mentally handicapped child. The deficits are generally more subtle. The main point is that dieting puts your body in a state of malnutrition, a state from which it cannot recover quickly. So play it safe. If you are a woman of childbearing age, don't diet. Ever. That way, you know that any baby you conceive, even an "accident," has the best chance for normal development. If you want to lose weight, you can do so in a way that will actually improve your nutritional state and your health. That's what this book is all about.

This section may have scared you. We hope it did. You've probably been on a few diets; in fact, if you are at all typical, you've been on a dozen or more. You can't do anything about those past diets, and if you're not dead yet, you probably didn't ruin your health (by the way, how's that hair loss?). But *please, please, don't go on any more diets.* Whenever you are tempted to do so, read chapter 1 and this section again.

Side Effects of Low-Fat Eating and Exercise

You may be thinking that losing weight is a dangerous proposition no matter how you do it. Perhaps you should avoid any program that promises weight loss, even a program like low-fat eating and exercise. Do low-fat eating and exercise have side effects?

They do, and in all fairness we should warn you of them before we go any further. Low-fat eating and exercise work together to produce some dramatic changes, not only in your weight, but in your health and well-being. But, unlike the side effects of low-calorie diets, the side effects from low-fat diet and exercise are all positive: greater sense of energy and well-being; decreased medication needs for adult-onset diabetes; reduced blood pressure; decreased risk of heart disease; and decreased risk of cancer.

We've arranged these more or less in the order in which you will notice them.

Greater energy and sense of well-being

Within days of starting a low-fat eating program, people notice that they no longer are so sleepy after meals, and they just generally seem to feel better. Exercise also has positive effects on mood. These aren't just psychological, either. Low-fat eating and exercise cause different biochemical changes that lead to mood elevation.

When we first considered doing workshops to teach people how to eat low-fat and exercise, we asked our friends what they thought.

"What will people get out of it?" our friends asked.

"Well," we replied, "besides losing weight, they can slash their risk of heart disease, cancer, diabetes. . . ."

"Yuk!" replied our friends. "Let's talk about something more pleasant."

That made us think. Why did we eat low-fat and exercise? What *really* made it worthwhile, on a day-to-day basis? The answer wasn't our near-immunity to heart attacks and cancer—those diseases generally strike in late middle age at the earliest, still more than a decade away for us. That would be a nice dividend for the future, but it certainly didn't provide motivation to turn down a dish of ice cream *now*.

We began to realize that we live this way because we get two sources of quick gratification. The first is becoming and staying lean, and that is what this book is mainly about. The second is a feeling of greater energy and well-being, more optimism, a feeling of "something in reserve" to get us through stressful times. Some people report that they need less sleep when living this way. We've found that, although we still need the same amount of sleep on a nightly basis, we can tolerate an occasional very late night with much greater ease.

It's these internal effects, just as much as the external effects of greater attractiveness, that motivate us. That they are due to diet and exercise is dramatically demonstrated on our "feast days," the occasions such as Thanksgiving and Christmas when we eat high-fat (more on this concept in chapter 6). And suddenly we're feeling sluggish, bloated, a bit dyspeptic. The energy is gone in an instant. And the next day, when we return to our usual fare, the energy returns. It's as simple—and as fast—as that.

This feeling of energy doesn't happen just because you're doing something good for yourself and you feel good about it. There are three profound biochemical changes that occur. Low-fat eating causes two of these changes; exercise causes the third.

First, as mentioned, when you start eating food that is lower in fat than your usual fare, you may notice that you no longer have an intense desire to nap after lunch and other meals. The effect is more pronounced as you cut more fat out of your diet, because it is directly due to the *lack* of fat in your diet. If you eat a high-fat meal, the fat goes right into your bloodstream, and blocks oxygen delivery to the tissues. One of us (Eric) has taken hundreds of blood samples from subjects in the lab, and he can tell if the subject has just eaten a high-fat meal—a white scum forms on the top of the blood after it has been processed to make the blood cells settle. That's fat (fat floats, so it rises to the surface). Since the fat causes blood cells to clump together, they have a harder time getting through the small blood vessels that feed the tissues with oxygen and nutrients. As a result, you feel sluggish and dull after a high-fat meal. On the other hand, if the meal is low in fat, the blood cells circulate freely to all parts of the body and you remain alert and awake. When Eric takes a blood sample from someone who has just eaten a low-fat meal, there is little or no white scum.

But eating meals that are low in fat may do more than just prevent an after-lunch coma. It may also actually improve your mood, through a second mechanism.

Scientists have known for decades that food influences mood. The effect is based on the amino acids in foods. Amino acids, the building blocks of protein, have many functions in the body. One is familiar to everyone—to repair and maintain muscle tissue and other protein components of the body. But certain amino acids also act in the brain, as the building materials for some types of neurotransmitters, the chemical messengers by which nerve cells in the brain and elsewhere communicate. One amino-acid-derived neurotransmitter that is almost certainly related to mood is serotonin; it seems to cause calmness, optimism, a general feeling of well-being. Many common antidepressants work by increasing brain serotonin levels.

By a complicated biochemical chain, eating meals high in carbohydrates can increase the body's serotonin levels, and elevate mood. Now, we don't mean to imply that you can cure major clinical depression by dietary manipulation. But there is no doubt that food influences mood, and the way to influence it in a positive direction is to increase carbohydrate consumption. But we suggest a more personal experiment. Simply study the principles of low-fat eating in this book, then try eating low-fat. You'll be convinced.

The third mood-influencer is exercise. Exercise stimulates the release of endorphins, powerful natural painkillers and tranquilizers. One clever way to show that mood elevation from an activity is caused by endorphins is to have people take a drug that blocks the natural endorphin-receptors in the brain. The blocking agent acts like a key that breaks off in a lock—it won't unlock the door to pleasant feelings, nor will it let the real key, the endorphins, unlock the door. When people exercise after taking such a blocking agent, they no longer report the pleasant mood elevation that they usually get from exercise. Since we're normally not taking endorphin-blocking-agents, we get the mood-elevating effects. And your exercise doesn't have to be a marathon, either. A simple half-hour walk can have noticeable mood-elevating effects.

Remember—these are not some weird biochemical manipulations that you're putting your body through. Low-fat eating and exercise are natural activities, for which we've been genetically programmed over millions of years of evolution. It's natural to feel good, energetic, and optimistic. It's unnatural to feel sluggish, depressed, and tired.

Decreased medication needs for diabetes or high blood pressure

Within weeks of starting a low-fat diet or an exercise program, people with diabetes or high blood pressure may find their medication needs dropping dramatically.

Millions of Americans suffer from diabetes, and millions more suffer from high blood pressure. Diabetes, with its complications, is the seventh-highest cause of death in the United States. You may not suffer from either of these conditions. But if you do, you need to know that living according to the principles in this book may have a dramatic effect on your condition, and you need to be prepared.

A low-fat diet and exercise are thought by many doctors to be two of the most effective ways of decreasing, even eliminating, the medication needs of many people with high blood pressure. An exercise program can also be highly effective in helping some diabetics (Type II diabetics, also known as "adult-onset diabetics," or "non-insulin-dependent diabetics," who constitute the majority of diabetics) to decrease medication needs. Studies have also shown a dramatic effect from low-fat eating on Type II diabetes, but some doctors feel that the mix of fat, carbohydrate, and protein must be carefully monitored.

As you begin to eat low-fat and exercise, you will move back toward normal—that is, if you have diabetes you may require less and less medication to control your blood sugar, and if your blood pressure is high it may become lower (it may even become completely normal). If you continue to take your medications at the same dose you were on before the program, it could be quite harmful, even fatal. These are for unhealthy people; if healthy people take them, the drugs can be devastating.

This leads to an extremely important warning:

> If you are taking medication for high blood pressure or diabetes, or if you take any other medication regularly, *make sure your doctor knows you are going on this program and monitors your condition carefully.* You may get too healthy to take the dangerous drugs your doctor prescribes.

This is especially important if you decide to decrease the amount of fat in your diet to 10 percent, the level you reach in our Phase 2 (see chapter 8). Your blood pressure and blood sugar may start changing toward normal within *days,* so be sure your doctor knows right from the start. Diabetics, especially, should consult with their doctors about the fat and carbohydrate levels in their diets, which may require some fine tuning based on individual blood chemistry.

• • •

The changes in energy and mood occur within days, and the changes in diabetes and blood pressure can happen in months. *But it may take decades to notice the major health effects of low-fat eating and exercise.*

As you continue to eat low-fat and exercise your way into a vigorous and vital middle and old age, you will notice that you aren't dying or disabled by heart disease (the number-one killer in the United States) or cancer (the number-two killer in the United States). Such a program is the surest way to avoid these killers. You probably already know that. What you may not know is just how dramatic a difference a relatively small change in your life-style can make.

Heart disease, diet, and exercise

By now everyone has heard that low-fat eating and exercise prevent heart disease. Other books which primarily deal with the health effects of such a life-style go into great detail on the connection. Four that we highly recommend are *The Pritikin Promise* by Nathan Pritikin, *The McDougall Plan* by John A. McDougall, M.D., and Mary A. McDougall, *The 10% Solution for a Healthy Life* by Raymond Kurzweil, and *Dr. Dean Ornish's Program for Reversing Heart Disease* by Dean Ornish, M.D.

What most people *don't* know is how dramatic the connection between diet and heart disease really is. We think one illustration, from epidemiological data, will make clear the link between the two. Epidemiology is a branch of medical science in which large populations are studied to see if certain life-style habits correlate with higher risk of certain diseases. If there is a correlation, it doesn't *prove* that the life-style factor is the cause of the disease. But it certainly makes you suspicious, and you do other experiments to test for a causal link. Epidemiological evidence provides a real eye-opener for those who are skeptical of the link between dietary fat and heart disease.

HEART DISEASE AND FAT CONSUMPTION

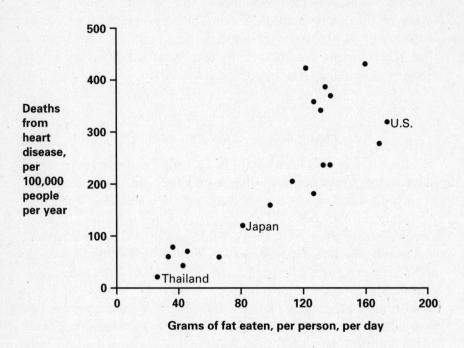

Figure adapted from Raymond Kurzweil, *The 10% Solution for a Healthy Life*.
Data from the World Health Organization.

Fig. 1 *Rates of death from heart disease versus fat consumption in twenty countries. Each point represents a different country; to avoid clutter, only the points for the United States, Japan, and Thailand are labeled.*

The graph shows fat consumption on the horizontal axis—the farther to the right you go, the higher the amount of fat in the diet for a particular country. On the vertical axis is the rate of death from heart disease, mainly from heart attacks. The higher you go, the more people die each year (per 100,000) from heart disease.

You can see that there is a very strong correlation between fat consumption and death from heart disease. As we go away from countries that eat little fat and toward countries that eat a lot of fat, we see higher and higher rates of death from heart disease. The correlation isn't perfect; some countries have higher rates of heart disease than others where almost exactly the same amount of fat is consumed, especially among the countries where people eat a lot of fat. That's because other factors also cause heart disease (smoking, lack of exercise, stress, etc.). Still, it's quite striking that in *all* the countries in which people eat low-fat the rates of death from heart disease are low, and in *all* the countries in which people eat high-fat the rates of death from heart disease are high.

For example, here in the United States we consume a lot of fat in our diets. And a lot of us die each year from heart attacks—almost half a million people a year. Compare the United States with Thailand. People in Thailand eat very little fat, probably around 10 percent calories from fat. Death from heart disease in Thailand is rare.

The astute student will object, "Sure, the rate of death from heart disease is lower in Thailand, but they don't have a very good medical system compared with the United States. Most people die before they get old enough to die of heart disease." To counter that argument, you look at a country like Japan, which has a medical system comparable to ours and where people live about as long as we do in the United States (in fact, they live longer in Japan). Japan is right along the trend. They consume less fat than we do, and they have less heart disease. The Japanese consume more fat than people in Thailand, and they have more heart disease. Where is *your* diet on this graph?

Many other studies, on animals and on humans, conclusively show that excess fat in the diet *causes* heart disease. (Specifically, the type of fat that causes heart disease is saturated fat. But if you lower the overall fat content of your diet, especially to 10 percent calories from fat, you will almost certainly lower the saturated-fat content, so we don't worry about the distinction.) The most important thing you can do to decrease your chances of dropping dead from the number-one killer of Americans is lower the fat content of your diet.

Exercise will also help, and it doesn't have to be marathon training. In one study, a group of men was asked to eat a diet that was slightly lower in fat than the American average—they dropped from about 40 percent calories from fat to about 30 percent (you can go much, much lower than these men did, and we'll show you how). This group decreased their risk of heart disease by about 20 percent. Another group cut the same amount of fat from their diet and, in addition, walked or ran about nine miles a week (that averages out to about fifteen minutes a day—not very much by any standards). This group's risk of heart disease dropped 37 percent.

Cancer and diet

Cancer is probably the most feared disease in America, because there seems to be no rhyme or reason as to whom it will strike, and it seems to strike more than it should. Cancer is the second-highest killer in this country, just behind heart disease. But most people are now aware of the connections between life-style and heart disease, whereas cancer still seems to invite confusion. Is getting cancer just a chance event, like getting in an accident? Or is it due to all the toxic chemicals in our modern environment, all the pesticides we eat? Or is it genetic?

Adding to the confusion is that there are many different forms of cancer and many different parts of the body that are susceptible. Let's limit our discussion to the top four types of cancer in the United States, which kill more people each year than all the other forms of cancer combined. They are lung cancer, breast cancer, prostate cancer, and colon cancer. We'll look especially closely at breast cancer, because it is the number-one cancer killer among young women, and because it's an example of how much confusion exists about the causes of cancer.

Lung cancer is the number-one cancer killer of both men and women (when all ages are considered together). The major cause here is quite obvious. Ninety percent of the cases of lung cancer are caused by smoking, and lung cancer is a particularly lethal form of the disease. It should be equally obvious how you avoid this one.

The other three types of cancer—breast, prostate, and colon cancer—are strongly correlated to fat content of the diet. *In countries where people eat little fat, these cancers are uncommon. In countries where people eat a lot of fat, these cancers are common.*

Does excess fat in the diet contribute to breast cancer?
Let's take a close look at breast cancer, since most women are understandably concerned about it. The latest statistics show that one in eight American women will get breast cancer. Media reports make it seem that we are in the midst of an unexplained epidemic, that every woman is at risk, and that you might as well adopt a fatalistic attitude. We think if you look at the evidence you'll see that the causes of breast cancer are quite clear, and that there is a lot you can do.

Let's examine the reasons why *eating high-fat* can be considered a major risk factor for breast cancer.

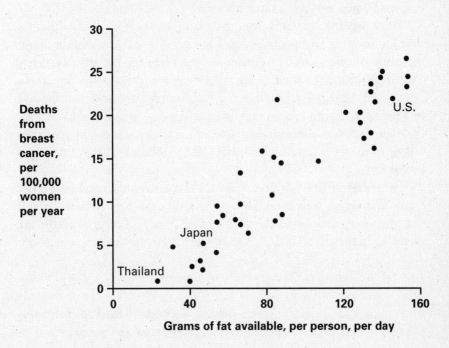

BREAST CANCER AND FAT CONSUMPTION

Figure adapted from Raymond Kurzweil, *The 10% Solution for a Healthy Life.*

Fig. 2 *Rates of death from breast cancer versus fat consumption in thirty-nine countries. Each point represents a different country; to avoid clutter, only the points for the United States, Japan, and Thailand are labeled.*

*The amount of fat eaten in different countries is strongly
correlated with their rates of death from breast cancer.*
Figure 2 is exactly the same type of graph as for heart disease, except
now we're looking at deaths from breast cancer (per 100,000 women).
You can see the incredibly strong relationship between fat consumption and breast-cancer deaths. We can compare the United States and
Thailand again, and see that death from breast cancer is virtually unknown in Thailand. The lower breast-cancer rates in Japan show that
this difference is not just due to a better medical system in the United
States, allowing women to live long enough to get breast cancer.

As the Japanese adopt more Western food habits, their fat consumption is going up—from 16 percent of total calories in 1965 to 26
percent in 1988. The Japanese rate of death from breast cancer has increased 50 percent in the same period.

We said before that this kind of graph makes you very suspicious
that fat *causes* a particular disease. But you have to be careful about
jumping to conclusions. For example, you often see fire trucks at fires.
The bigger the fire, the more fire trucks you are likely to see. There is a
very strong association between the number of fire trucks and the size
of a fire. That doesn't mean that fire trucks *cause* fires. In the same way,
the fact that you almost always see more breast cancer in countries
where more fat is consumed doesn't necessarily mean that fat causes
breast cancer.

We could test whether fire trucks really caused fires by sending a fire
truck to a house that is not on fire. Does the house catch on fire? If
not, then fire trucks probably don't cause fires. This sort of test is the
next link in the chain of evidence for the fat–breast-cancer connection:

*Animals fed a high-fat diet get more mammary (breast)
cancer than animals fed a low-fat diet.*
The equivalent of the fire-truck–fire test above is to feed animals varying levels of fat. Almost a hundred experiments have been done with
mice and rats that show that increasing the amount of fat in the diet increases the chances of mammary-gland (breast) tumors in these animals. This makes the case for the fat-cancer connection much stronger;
unlike our fire-truck example, where there's fat there's cancer.

Still, it would be nice to know *why* fat might increase the cancer rates in countries where people eat a lot of it. If we can explain why eating a lot of fat may cause breast cancer, the case becomes almost airtight.

There are at least three ways that high fat consumption can contribute to breast cancer.

1. *Fat consumption increases estrogen exposure.* Certain forms of the female hormone estrogen are known to cause breast cancer, and excess fat in the diet increases a woman's lifetime exposure to estrogen in several ways.

Women who eat a lot of fat in their diets start menstruating at a younger age and stop at a later age. Estrogen is a hormone of the menstrual cycle, and is present only at low levels before the onset of menstruation and after menopause. So eating a high-fat diet means you are exposed for a larger portion of your life to estrogen—which increases the risk of breast cancer. It's like the increase in the risk of lung cancer from smoking. If you smoke for twenty years during your life, your risk of lung cancer is higher than if you smoke for only ten years.

Eating a high-fat diet increases estrogen levels in the body, and eating a low-fat diet lowers those levels, so not only are high-fat eaters exposed to estrogen for a *greater portion* of their lives, they are exposed to *higher levels* during that portion. Continuing the lung-cancer analogy, people who smoke two packs a day for twenty years have a higher risk of lung cancer than people who smoke one pack a day for twenty years.

Eating a high-fat diet also leads to obesity, which increases estrogen levels even further.

Thus, in countries where the fat consumption is high, women tend to have greater estrogen exposure over the course of a lifetime than in countries where fat consumption is low. Fat consumption may not be the *direct* cause of breast cancer, but it causes increased exposure to estrogen over the course of a lifetime, which *does* cause breast cancer.

2. *Fat may cause the formation of molecules that encourage cancer to grow.* A breast tumor starts from a single cell that, for reasons that aren't completely clear, changes into a potentially cancerous cell. This process, called "initiation," turns the cell into a "tumor seed." It takes

years, even decades for it to develop into a life-threatening tumor. How quickly it develops, or whether it develops at all, depends on the hospitality of its environment. A high-fat diet may lead to the formation of molecules called "promoters," which provide "tumor seeds" with a very hospitable environment. This has been shown by studies in which researchers have given animals chemicals that cause breast cancer (planting the "tumor seed," in our metaphor), then put them on low-fat or high-fat diets. Animals kept on a high-fat diet (35–40 percent fat) have *three times* the rate of breast-tumor formation as animals kept on a low-fat diet (10–20 percent calories from fat).

3. *High-fat foods displace low-fat foods that may protect against cancer.* If you get most of your calories each day from high-fat foods such as meat and dairy products, you tend to eat fewer of the low-fat foods, such as fruits and vegetables. On the other hand, if you decrease the amount of fat in your diet, you must replace it with something else. In Phase 1 of the program (chapter 7), we're going to recommend that you replace at least a little of that fat with fruits and vegetables. We'll talk in detail about how this will improve your overall health (not to mention promoting weight loss), but we'd like to zero in on one specific aspect right now.

Not only are fruits and vegetables low in fat, they are high in chemicals called "phytochemicals." Scientists have much to learn about phytochemicals, but some of them appear to be extremely powerful anticancer agents. For example, broccoli and other cruciferous vegetables (cauliflower, brussels sprouts, cabbage) contain a substance called sulforaphane. When mice were injected with a chemical that causes breast cancer, 68 percent developed mammary tumors. But if they were also given sulforaphane, *it lowered the cancer rate by almost two-thirds!* So, if you replace just a little bit of the fat in your diet with just a few vegetables and fruits, you may get a great deal of protection against cancer. This particular study looked at sulforaphane, but there are literally hundreds of such chemicals in all sorts of fruits and vegetables.

• • •

You can see that women in countries where fat consumption is high are hit by a triple whammy: (1) They are exposed to more estrogen for a greater portion of their lives. (2) Their high-fat diet promotes cancer once it's started. (3) Because they eat lots of fat, they tend to consume fewer low-fat items, like fruits and vegetables, that may have a potent cancer-preventive effect.

If fat were on trial, it would be convicted of murder.

The case for the defense

You may say, "But wait a minute. Didn't I see some headline in the paper a while ago about how researchers didn't find any connection between the amount of fat women in America eat and their chances of getting breast cancer? It must be something else. We must just have bad genes here in America."

There were such headlines in 1992. Typical was this one, in the *Los Angeles Times*: "Study finds no link of fat in diet to [breast] malignancy risk." The research study that generated the confusion had looked at a group of American women and found that those who consumed the lowest-fat diets had no lower incidence of breast cancer than those consuming the highest-fat diets.

The study, however, had a fatal flaw: *Truly* low fat diets are so rare in America that the group with the lowest level of fat consumption in this study ate an average of 27 percent fat. Though this is certainly lower than the American average, it's a far cry from the 10 percent fat eaten by people in countries with low breast-cancer rates. So the researchers couldn't follow anyone who *really* ate low-fat. They looked at the very upper end of the fat-consumption range (where everyone gets sick) and concluded that they had found no evidence that fat intake is a major cause of breast cancer.

This is like studying the factors that contribute to death from drowning among nonswimmers and seeing that just as many people drown in pools that are ten feet deep as in pools that are fifteen feet deep. You *can't* jump to the conclusion that the depth of water must not be important in determining how likely people are to drown. If you look at how many people drown in puddles, you might conclude that depth of water is a crucial factor.

But you have to have some puddles to study first. We hope that this book, along with others out now, will help you reduce your fat consumption from a swimming pool to a puddle. That way, when researchers want to study *low*-fat eating they can go to you, and study your health for years, and years, and years. . . .

To be fair to the scientists who did the study on which those 1992 headlines were based, they were aware of the possibility that they had not studied low enough levels of fat consumption to see an effect, and explicitly cautioned, "Our data do not exclude the possibility that fat intake earlier in life *or at substantially lower levels* could influence risk of breast cancer" (emphasis added). But that sort of careful analysis doesn't make for good headlines or sound bites, and was virtually ignored by the media.

What can women do to prevent breast cancer?
You can see that the occurrence of breast cancer is not simply a matter of chance. Except in a small minority of cases, it's not genetic (and even if you are at risk genetically, you can greatly improve your odds). You have a great deal of control over whether you are susceptible or not. How do the arguments we've given translate into specific suggestions? What, exactly, can you do?

1. Eat low-fat.
This one is obvious from what we've said. If you eat a truly low-fat diet, down around 10 percent calories from fat, you will lower your estrogen levels, lose weight (which decreases risk), and provide an inhospitable environment for cancer to grow. Because careful, long-term studies of women who reduce their fat consumption to 10 percent of fat have not yet been done, we can't say exactly what the reduction of risk will be. But take a look at figure 2 again and you will see that the decrease in risk is potentially very large.

2. Increase your intake of fruits and vegetables.
If you increase your consumption of fruits and vegetables, you will provide yourself with cancer protection, possibly substantial protection. Especially important are the cruciferous vegetables.

3. Exercise.
Exercise not only will help you lose weight, it will lower your risk of breast cancer. Studies show that women who exercise an average of

four hours per week have *less than half* the risk of breast cancer of women who do not exercise. Researchers believe that the decrease in risk is due to the decrease in estrogen exposure from menstruation in the exercisers—women who exercise regularly tend to begin menstruation later in life and to have fewer periods compared with women who are sedentary. Both of these factors reduce lifetime estrogen exposure.

4. *Reduce your alcohol consumption.*
There is some evidence that alcohol consumption, perhaps as little as one drink a day, may increase the risk for breast cancer. The evidence is not as strong as for other factors, but why risk it?

5. *Educate your daughters.*
Studies of the survivors of the atomic bombings of Hiroshima and Nagasaki showed an increased risk of breast cancer, as you would expect after exposure to a huge dose of radiation. Women who were between the ages of ten and fifteen at the time of the bombings were the most susceptible to the carcinogenic effects of the radiation. This indicates that there may be a certain critical period during puberty, when breast tissue is developing, during which breast cancer is most likely to start, though the actual disease doesn't appear until decades later.

It's scary to think that your daughters may be exposed to the causes of this deadly disease even before they graduate from high school. But it's also a message of hope.

Again, we urge you to look at figure 2. There are countries in the world where breast cancer is essentially unknown, and in all of these countries women grow up on low-fat diets. Add to that the powerful protective effects of exercise, and you can see that *lifelong habits of low-fat eating and vigorous exercise may virtually immunize your young daughters against breast cancer.* We might, over the course of a single generation, drop the lifetime risk of this disease from one in eight women to one in fifty, or fewer.

The best way to instill these habits is to adopt such a life-style yourself. Lead by example. We'll talk more about strategies for integrating low-fat eating and exercise with your family in chapter 10.

Prostate cancer and colon cancer

Almost all of the arguments that implicate fat as a cause of breast cancer in women also apply to prostate cancer, the second-highest cancer killer in men. In the case of prostate cancer, the culprit hormone is the "male" hormone, testosterone.

Fat in the diet is also strongly correlated with colon cancer, although here the connection is quite direct—carcinogenic products from fat sit right in the colon and cause the cancer directly. The graphs for fat consumption and risk of prostate cancer or of colon cancer look almost exactly the same as that for breast cancer. So, for these cancers as well, decreasing the amount of fat that you eat is probably the single most powerful method of protection. The other preventive steps outlined for breast cancer will also be protective against *these* cancers.

Side Effects

You can see that low-fat eating and exercise are going to have many other effects on you besides making you leaner. You'll find yourself going strong at the end of the day instead of dragging. You may have to clean out your medicine cabinet. You'll decrease your risk of major diseases and help yourself to live into a vigorous and active old age. You may find, as time goes on, that these effects are just as important as the weight-loss aspects. In fact, decades from now, as you celebrate your ninetieth birthday by going out dancing, you may reflect on the weight-loss aspect of low-fat eating and exercise as a minor side effect.

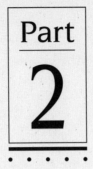

Part

2

Before You Begin

4

Design Your Own Program

· · · · ·

Long before we thought about teaching anyone else about low-fat eating and exercise, we had to teach ourselves. And we made every mistake possible. We forced ourselves to eat truly awful-tasting meals just because they were low-fat, because we didn't know how to modify our own favorite high-fat recipes. We boiled beans for hours because that's what the books we were reading said to do—even though we often only had minutes (or less) to prepare our meals. We missed exercise opportunities throughout the day because we were used to thinking of exercise only as "a workout," and there would often not be time in the day to get that workout in.

We were trying to change our lives to fit some "ideal" program, to fit somebody else's idea of how to do it. It wasn't until we started to do the "easy" things and forgot about the hard stuff that we really began to make progress. We started using canned beans instead of boiling our own. We found, through trial and error, a dozen or so meals that we really liked and that were very low in fat and nutritionally sound. We stopped making simple mistakes that were doubling the fat content of our daily menus. We started relying a lot on plain old walking to get some of our exercise.

Ten years after our first dietary experiments, we finally had an enjoyable, practical, flexible program—for us.

Lori's Story, Continued

Then Lori wanted to know how we did it, and she became our first student. After the dinner during which we told her about set point and the futility of dieting, Carol showed her how to cook low-fat. Even though Lori said that she couldn't see herself using one, we recommended that she get a stationary bicycle for exercise, because it was so practical and easy. Lori quickly learned the principles and started using them in her life. In the space of a few months, she completely integrated low-fat eating and exercise into her life—and she continues with these principles today, over five years later. Lori was the first success on our "program."

Except Lori didn't do anything exactly the way we'd told her.

Lori hated cooking, and ate at fast-food restaurants a lot. So she learned the low-fat items on the menus of half a dozen fast-food restaurants, and those became the core of her meals. Lori hated cooking for herself and her son because she didn't know how to cook for just two people. She was afraid that she would overeat. These days, Lori has learned to eat low-fat, and she's tried her hand at cooking low-fat. She reports that she loves it. And she no longer cares if she eats all the leftovers. What about the stationary-bicycle idea? She told us, "If I had gotten a stationary bike, I would have used it once and it would have ended up rusting in the closet. I really do *hate* exercising by myself." Instead, Lori does step aerobics at a local health club, where she exercises along with others and enjoys herself. She took the principles of what we taught her, and made them fit *her* life.

Different Strokes for Different Folks

Later, when we started giving workshops on our approach to becoming lean, we found that each individual had his or her own unique concerns and conditions, often as different from ours as Lori's were. We found that we had to present people with a flexible range of options, so that they could build their own, personalized programs.

Some just wanted to make small changes, and were satisfied with modest results. Tom, one of our early workshop participants, just wanted to find out if he could improve his eating habits. He was pretty much satisfied with his weight and with his eating patterns, but he wondered if there were any small changes he could make that would improve his health. Several months after the workshop, he told us:

"I really just wanted to start eating better, and I really didn't make any big changes. I now usually put jam on my morning bagels instead of butter, because I found out how much fat was in that butter. Even when I do use butter, I use a lot less. When I'm looking at a bag of potato chips, my new label-awareness makes it clear just how much fat they have. I eat a piece of fruit in my car on the way to work, and I feel I'm starting my morning off in a healthy way. At lunch sometimes I'll have a salad and bagel rather than lasagna. Really, it's just a matter of awareness.

"But the small changes I made gave me what I feel are large benefits. I feel better now, and it's easier to keep my weight stable. I really notice how bad I feel after I eat a high-fat meal. This is encouraging me to keep heading in a healthy direction."

Others wanted big changes and wanted them fast. They were willing to make large adjustments in the ways they ate and exercised to get fast results.

Mike exemplified this attitude. He attended a workshop in July, immediately made drastic cuts in his fat consumption, and began eating 10 percent calories from fat. He also started exercising. Three months later, in October, he had lost thirty-five pounds. There were dramatic effects on his health, too. He wrote to us, "I just got my blood-test results back. All blood chemistries are normal. A year ago [before the workshop], my total cholesterol level was 222, a bit above the 200 mark thought to be the dividing line [for risk of heart disease]. For my last tests, the cholesterol level was 188. The LDL/HDL ratio was also favorable. Much thanks, I think it really does work." A year later, at the age of sixty-six, Mike started a weight-training program. He's more enthusiastic than ever about the program.

How to Make This Program Work for You

Lori, Tom, Mike, and hundreds of workshop participants in the years since have taught us that principles are important, but these must be translated into the specifics of each individual's life.

So we've organized the rest of the book as a manual that will allow you to adapt low-fat eating and exercise completely to *your* life. You should determine whether you want to eat low-fat, or exercise, or both. Then you can decide how far you want to go with each. To do that, you need to know . . .

What to expect

In the next chapter, you'll find out just how much weight you can expect to lose by eating low-fat, by exercising, or by doing both. We've based this chapter on the best scientific studies currently available of low-fat eating and/or exercise. This will give you a basis for deciding how you want to approach your personal lean crusade.

More important, you can get an idea of how much weight loss people typically experience from different levels of each approach. It makes sense that, if you cut the fat you eat from 40 percent of calories to 10 percent, you will lose more weight than if you cut fat from 40 to 30 percent. But do you know how much more? How much will you lose if you add twenty minutes a day of exercise? How about an hour a day? After reading the next chapter, you'll have a good idea of the answers to these questions and will be able to tailor the program exactly to what you want.

Integrating low-fat eating into your life

Most people choose to use at least some degree of low-fat eating as part of their lifetime strategy for permanent weight control. But how to start? What's important and what isn't? What are the pitfalls. What are the shortcuts?

In our early days of low-fat eating, we often felt that the choice was between macrobiotics or McDonald's, carrot sticks or Cheez Whiz. A huge chasm yawned between eating the way we did (40 percent calories from fat) and eating the way we were "supposed to" (10 percent calories from fat). There often seemed to be no way to bridge the gap.

Part three of this book is your bridge. It's for those who want to make small changes as well as those who want to make big ones. You can change slowly or quickly (and we'll describe exactly how you can do it either way).

Chapter 6 will introduce you to the principles of low-fat eating. Whether you are just going to cut down a little, or want to slash the fat that you eat to the bare minimum, there are some concepts that will help you make the transition smoothly.

Next, you'll want to get into the nuts and bolts of changing your eating habits. To make things easier, in terms both of our teaching and of your conversion to a low-fat diet, we've divided the guidelines for eating into two phases.

In Phase 1, described in chapter 7, you take simple steps, virtual no-brainers, which will allow you to drop from the typical American diet, containing 40 percent fat, to one containing about 20 percent. You can cut your fat consumption in half—overnight, if you want—without counting calories or fat grams. It often surprises people how easy this is. You may want to stay at that level; many people do and are quite happy with the weight loss that results. Or you may want to cut even more fat out of your diet.

Phase 2, described in chapter 8, builds on Phase 1, teaching you the additional skills you need to get down to the optimum level of fat in the diet, 10 percent. You'll learn to restructure your habits to avoid *all* high-fat foods and to eat low-fat foods in their place. You'll learn to judge the *true* fat contents of food, cutting through deceptive food-labeling instantly. Then you'll use your new skills to eat truly low-fat meals at home, in restaurants, and as a guest.

We've found that many people at our workshops are so enthusiastic about the weight loss possible from eating low-fat that they decide to go all the way down to 10 percent fat. That's great! Chapter 9 gives you practical tips on making the changeover. It will help you plot a strategy to make such a change work for you. If you decide not to make such a large change right away, you can skip this chapter. You can always return to it later if you feel you want to take the total low-fat plunge.

People always have questions, concerns, and comments about changing their eating habits, and in chapter 10 we present the twenty most common questions we've been asked over the years. You'll find out about fitting low-fat eating in with your family, about nutritional requirements, and much more.

We've included diagnostic quizzes at several points to help you pinpoint exactly where there might be hidden fat in your eating habits.

An exercise in slimming

Most people fit into one of two categories: those who've never tried exercise because they think they'll hate it, and those who've tried it and are sure they hate it.

That's why part four, "Exercise Your Right to a Fat-Free Body," starts off with chapter 11, on myths about exercise. If you think of exercise as something painful, or boring, or complicated by worries about target heart rates, this chapter is a must-read. In fact, if you've decided not to try exercise in your weight-loss scheme, this chapter just might change your mind.

Exercise, like low-fat eating, can be divided into two types.

Chapter 12 will show you how to get exercise that doesn't even seem like exercise. We call this sort of exercise "opportunistic exercise." If you're put off by the idea of going to a gym, or sweating, or if you simply don't have the time each day for a regular exercise program, this chapter will be good news. You can get in a surprising amount of exercise without ever doing a workout or even breaking a sweat. Even if you already exercise regularly, this chapter will show you how to fit more exercise painlessly into the nooks and crannies of your day.

You needn't do any more than take advantage of opportunistic exercise to remain lean and fit. But a funny thing happens to some people. As they become more active in their daily lives, they being to crave even more activity. The walker becomes a jogger. Someone who started climbing a few flights of stairs a day finds himself buying a stepper, and loving it. Chapter 13 is for these people. It discusses structured exercise, what most people call a "workout." There's good news here, too. Workouts need not be painful or exhausting. In this chapter, you'll learn how to choose the optimum form of exercise for *you*. You'll learn the key reasons that most structured-exercise programs fail, and how to avoid them. If you're thinking of buying an exercise machine, you'll find one of the most complete guides to them ever offered.

Measuring up

We'll finish the book with some thoughts on measuring progress. You know that you should throw away your scale. But how will you know you're losing fat if you can't get on that little box every morning and read the number on the dial? We offer some alternatives, from the most high-tech to the humblest and simplest.

• • •

This book is a manual, a resource that we hope you'll use for a lifetime of leanness and health. We've organized it so that you can choose exactly where you'll start. Now turn to chapter 5 and you will see the sometimes astonishing changes that lie down the road.

5

What to Expect

· · · · · ·

Part one of this book was designed to answer the questions "How can I lose weight permanently? What really works?" If we've done our job, you are completely convinced that to lose weight permanently you have two weapons: You can eat less fat. You can exercise. Now the big questions become: "How much can I lose with each option?" "How much with both together?" and "How quickly?"

At this point it's customary to give either vague, general predictions ("You'll lose a lot, and you'll feel great. Trust us!") or stories of unbelievable weight loss ("Joe Schmo lost ten pounds in three hours! By the end of the first day, he had to buy a whole new wardrobe!").

We decided to break with tradition and give you, instead, answers based on the results of the *best scientific studies of low-fat eating and exercise.* We're not basing our answers on what Steve down at the gym told us, or how much weight Harriet lost on the latest fad diet.

Even so, you will indeed hear about some amazing rates of weight loss, especially with low-fat eating. And these are numbers you can trust. A good study contains enough people so that you get a realistic idea of what the *average* person can expect—some will lose more, some less, but if there are enough people it all averages out. Literally hundreds of experiments have focused on exercise and weight loss; the idea of low-fat eating is newer, but there are now dozens of good experiments and more emerging every month. We've examined these studies carefully. We were looking for answers to the following questions:

- Do men and women differ in their ability to lose fat?
- How effective is low-fat eating alone for weight loss?
- How effective is exercise alone for weight loss?
- How effective are low-fat eating and exercise together?
- Are there any factors that cause one person to lose more or less than another?

Before we get to the answers, a small note: we told you in chapter 2 to throw away your scale, to measure your progress by how much *fat* you lose. However, because it can be complicated and time-consuming to get really accurate body-fat measurements but very quick to weigh people, in many of the experiments we will discuss the researchers measured weight only. We'll give you the results of studies in terms of the amount of fat lost whenever the researchers did it that way; otherwise we have to talk about weight. But we still want you to throw away your scale.

Do Men and Women Differ in Their Ability to Lose Fat?

Conventional wisdom has it that women lose weight more slowly than men, and our everyday experience seems to confirm this. In fact, before we started the research for this chapter, we thought that the conventional wisdom was correct, that there was some basic difference between the ways the bodies of men and women hang on to fat. And that may actually be true *if you are looking at how they lose weight through conventional dieting* (that is, through calorie restriction). But as we looked at studies of weight loss through low-fat eating and exercise, we uncovered a big surprise.

Once you take into account differences in body size, *men and women lose weight at exactly the same rate* if on the same low-fat-eating or exercise program.

Researchers who examined and compared the results of hundreds of studies of exercise and weight loss concluded that exercise has almost identical effects on the amount of fat that men and women lose. The key factors were how much people exercised and how much fat they had to lose in the first place, not gender. And in our examination of dozens of studies of low-fat eating for weight loss, we could find no difference between men and women—when differences in body size were taken into account and it was possible to compare, both genders lost weight at about the same rate.

However, there are two factors that slow weight loss—and women end up affected by both of them in most studies.

First, smaller people lose weight more slowly than larger people, whether they lose the weight through a low-fat diet or through exercise. Since women in general are smaller than men, they will lose weight more slowly for this reason alone. For example, a woman who weighs 140 pounds might lose two pounds in a week, while her 210-pound husband loses three pounds, though both are on exactly the same low-fat-eating-and-exercise program. Relative to their body sizes, both are losing at the same rate: one pound of fat lost per seventy pounds of body weight. Please note that it doesn't usually work out this precisely—due to individual quirks of physiology, some people just naturally shed more weight than others (we'll discuss this later). We've heard of wives losing twice as quickly as their husbands, and we've heard of husbands losing four times as quickly as their wives. But, *in general,* both will lose at the same rate relative to body weight.

Second, in exercising, the more you exercise the more you lose (makes perfect sense). We noticed that exercise studies involving women usually prescribe less exercise than those involving men, averaging about 20–30 percent less exercise for the women. Sexism by the researchers? It's entirely possible—scientists are human. Whatever the reason, the result is that there is less likely to be a large weight-loss effect in studies on women, leading to the erroneous conclusion that it's the women, not the studies themselves, which are different. But when you correct for the smaller amount of exercise that the women did, you find that women lose *exactly* the same amount of fat per minute of exercise as do men.

So, when it comes to low-fat eating and exercise for weight loss, men and women are on equal footing. Now, how much can they lose?

How Effective Is Low-Fat Eating Alone for Weight Loss?

The idea of eating low-fat to lose weight is relatively new. But in the past several years, many careful scientific studies of low-fat eating and weight loss have appeared—enough for us to examine whether low-fat eating *really* works. We set strict criteria for a study to be included in our evaluation:

1. It had to be *a true scientific study,* not a self-serving report from a fat-farm.
2. People had to eat low-fat *without restricting calories.* Some studies tried to sneak in calorie restriction—even scientists are seduced by the promises of conventional diets. We rejected these.
3. People had to *keep their exercise levels constant* during the study (otherwise we wouldn't know which weight loss was due to exercise and which was due to low-fat eating).
4. The researchers had to *evaluate people's diets carefully* to find out how much fat the study subjects were *really* eating (not how much they wished they were eating).

We found about twenty studies that fit these strict criteria, enough to reach some firm conclusions. People in these experiments ate diets that ranged all the way from 7 percent fat to 35 percent (compared with a standard American diet of 40 percent fat), and were studied for periods ranging from two weeks to over a year. They included both men and women.

The results are exciting. *In every single study, people lost weight,* sometimes at an utterly incredible pace (as you'll see in the upcoming examples). When people were asked to rate how good the food tasted, low-fat food was consistently said to be better-tasting. When people were asked to evaluate the quality of their lives, the groups eating low-fat rated their lives as more satisfying after they started the low-fat program.

Let's take a look at just a few examples. You'll see how much weight was lost by people who dropped their fat consumption to 20 percent (which you'll learn to do in Phase 1 of low-fat eating), or to 10 percent fat (which you'll learn to do in Phase 2). You'll also see that even very small changes in your fat consumption can have noticeable effects. And keep in mind that these weight-loss effects come from changes in eating habits alone—adding exercise to your routine can help you to lose even more, and more quickly, than in these studies.

Eating 20 percent fat (our Phase 1)

Eating 20 percent fat represents a decrease of about half in the fat content of the average American's foods. It's relatively easy to do. Can something so easy really have any effect?

One of the longest (six months) and best-conducted studies of such modestly low-fat eating comes from the University of Minnesota. Moderately overweight women were divided into two groups. One group went on a conventional calorie-cutting diet, eliminating about 500 calories per day from their diet. The second group simply switched from their normal diet, which was about 35 percent fat, to a diet that was 20 percent fat. The conventional calorie-cutters had to do the usual scrimping on food and carefully watched what they ate so that they didn't "eat too much." The low-fat eaters ate as much as they wanted of their lower-fat food choices. During the study, both groups stuck to their habitual exercise patterns, neither increasing nor decreasing their activity.

The results? The moderately low fat eaters lost ten pounds during the six months of the study. The calorie-cutters also lost weight, but not as much as the low-fat eaters—only eight and a half pounds.

Not only did the low-fat eaters lose more weight than the conventional dieters, but they rated their 20-percent-fat diet *better-tasting* than their initial 35-percent-fat diet, said their food was *more satisfying* on the 20-percent-fat diet, and they rated the *quality of their life as better* on the low-fat diet. Meanwhile, the calorie-cutters said their food tasted worse, it was less satisfying, and their lives were worse during their calorie-restriction diet. It looks as if the conventional dieters were the big losers in this study in every way but the most important way—weight.

And remember, these low-fat eaters only cut down to 20 percent fat—it's possible to go a lot lower than that—and did not increase their exercise levels at all. Yet they lost ten pounds.

Eating 10 percent fat (our Phase 2)

Most studies of the effects of low-fat eating alone on weight have asked people to eat 20–25 percent fat. But a few researchers have looked at even lower levels, asking people to eat around 10 percent fat. That means cutting about three-quarters of the fat out of your diet, if you are an average American. It takes a little awareness, but it's not as difficult as most people think. The results are uniformly stunning.

The Ornish study

As we mentioned earlier, Dr. Dean Ornish is one of the pioneers of true low-fat eating, and has conducted some of the strongest research showing that a low-fat diet, combined with stress reduction and moderate exercise, actually *reverses* heart disease. His work is so convincing that a major insurance company pays for patients with heart disease to go on his program rather than undergo bypass surgery.

We already told you about his earliest study, where men eating 10 percent fat lost an average of *ten pounds in one month*. In this particular study, he did not ask the subjects to exercise; because of their heart disease, most could not exercise. He certainly didn't ask them to restrict calories; in fact, they ate more while in the study than before they started.

The breast-cancer study

Researchers at UCLA who were interested in discovering why a low-fat diet is protective against breast cancer put a group of twelve women on a diet in which 10 percent of calories were from fat, for one month. This was a study of changes in the chemistry of the breast ductal fluid that might be protective against breast cancer. It was not designed to be a study of weight loss, and the women who were subjects were not overweight. Yet *every single one* of the twelve lost weight during that one month on a 10-percent-fat diet. The smallest weight loss was one pound, the largest nine pounds.

This is an interesting study for several reasons. Because it was not a study of weight loss, the women probably were not trying, even unconsciously, to limit their caloric intake. They were just eating normally, yet they lost weight. As we said, they were not even "overweight" to begin with, yet every single one lost significant amounts of weight. After a single month on the 10-percent-fat diet, the women's cholesterol levels dropped by an average of 12 percent, and there were definite changes in the composition of their breast ductal fluid. The researchers concluded, "The fact that diet can modulate factors in breast ductal fluid raises the possibility that other factors in breast ductal fluid may also change with diet and therefore affect breast ductal cell proliferation and the risk of breast cancer."

This experiment shows that, especially for women, lowering the fat content of your diet is a lose-win-win situation: you lose weight, and win against heart disease and breast cancer.

The heart-disease study

At Tufts University, researchers investigated the effects of a 15-percent-fat diet on blood chemistry related to heart disease in both men and women. This is a little higher than the 10 percent that you can achieve, so you can probably do better than these people.

The design of this study dramatically illustrates the effect of eating low-fat on set point. The low-fat part of the study was divided into two phases. In the first, the subjects ate 15 percent fat but were asked to eat enough to keep their weights constant. Researchers did this because they wanted to look at the effects of low-fat diet alone, without weight loss, on the factors affecting heart disease. According to set-point theory, the subjects' set points should have dropped when they started eating the low-fat diet, so staying at their original weights (now higher than their set-point weights) should have required them to consume more food than they really wanted. Indeed, *the subjects reported that eating enough to keep from losing weight was uncomfortable, that they were eating more than they wanted.*

In the second phase of low-fat eating, the researchers "released the brakes." The subjects were still eating 15 percent fat, but now the researchers told them to eat to satisfy their hunger, rather than to maintain their weights. According to set-point theory, they would get the signal to eat much less, allowing them to drop to their new, lower set points. And that is exactly what happened. When they were allowed to eat to satisfy their hunger but not forced to stuff themselves, the subjects spontaneously ate less, and lost an average of twelve pounds in ten weeks. The study ended after ten weeks, so we don't know exactly how much they would have lost had they continued.

Imagine that—if you dropped to a fat content in your diet of 15 percent, you would have to stuff yourself uncomfortably full just to *maintain* your weight. If you ate normally, you would lose weight, automatically, spontaneously, easily, and quickly.

Now, the subjects in this study were slightly overweight, but not really obese. And although the fat content of their diet dropped pretty low, you can go lower still. One study shows the astonishing effects, on people who have a lot of weight to lose, of eating *really* low-fat.

The Hawaii study

The most incredible example of the kind of rapid weight loss you can expect from eating *very* low-fat comes from Hawaii. The subjects were native Hawaiians, both men and women, who were quite overweight—the average weight was 270 pounds! These people were selected for the study in part because they had diet-related health problems. They were put on a native Hawaiian diet, a very healthful combination of fish, chicken, taro (a native Hawaiian potatolike plant), sweet potatoes, yams, breadfruit, greens, fruit, and more.

The average fat content of the foods they were eating was 7 percent, which is a clue to the fat level our bodies evolved to deal with—this was the traditional native diet before Europeans came to Hawaii in 1778 (the present-day diet is about five to seven times *higher* in fat). The people in the study were encouraged to eat until their hunger was satisfied.

The experiment lasted only three weeks, but the participants lost an average of over seventeen pounds each. *That's over five pounds a week!* Their cholesterol levels dropped 14 percent and their blood pressures dropped an average of ten points. This shows the truly astonishing potential of a very low fat diet, especially for people who are quite overweight.

And that's the beauty of set point. Those who have the most to lose tend to lose most rapidly.

*Just cutting down 2 or 3 percent
can have a noticeable effect*

In any good scientific study there is a control group. In the case of low-fat-eating studies, this is a group that does not eat low-fat, but continues to eat their normal diet. In a few studies, even the control group ate a little less fat during the experiment, probably just because they became more aware of their diets as a result of participating in a scientific study. That's nice for us: we can see what happens to weight following even small changes in the fat content of the diet.

In one study, the control group lowered their fat intake just 2 percent (from 39 to 37 percent). You could reduce the fat you eat at least this much simply by switching to a nonfat salad dressing. This group lost an average of one pound in six months. In another study, the control group lowered their fat intake just 4 percent (from 39 to 35 percent). You could do this by switching from whole milk to 1-percent milk. They lost three pounds in three months. These aren't huge weight losses, but, again, the control groups achieved them without even trying.

How Effective Is Exercise Alone
for Weight Loss?

Studies of exercise and weight loss are a little tougher to analyze than those of low-fat eating and weight loss. There's only one way to eat low-fat—you cut fat out of your diet. And you can't go much lower than about 10 percent fat. On the other hand, there are innumerable types of exercise to choose from, and it seems as if researchers have used them all—walking, biking, swimming, running, tennis, weight lifting, dancing, cycling . . . ad infinitum. And there are almost limitless types of programs: forty-five minutes three days a week, an hour a day, half an hour two days a week, high heart rate, low heart rate. . . . All told, in the past forty years there have been *over five hundred scientific studies* of the effects of exercise on body weight in humans.

Fortunately, two brave researchers have waded through the morass.

Douglas Ballor and Richard Keesey looked at every single one of those five hundred studies, trying to find the ones that would give valid information about how much weight people *really* lose when they exercise. They rejected any studies that were too small, or that involved participants who were also dieting, or that lumped men and women together without giving the weight loss for each group (one of the things they wanted to see was whether there was any difference in the weight loss men and women can expect from exercise).

After ending up with forty-one studies of men and twelve studies of women, they performed a "meta-analysis," a sophisticated statistical analysis of all the studies, to find out whether exercise causes fat loss (and if so, how much), whether one form of exercise is better than another, and whether men and women are different in their weight-loss responses to exercise.

They found that exercise consistently caused fat loss, and at surprisingly high rates. As we mentioned earlier, in this landmark analysis they found that men and women lose about the same amount of fat from a given amount of exercise. That's no small matter: many researchers claim, even today, that women can't lose weight from exercise, or will have a very hard time.

They also found that the type of exercise doesn't matter much (more on this in part four). Brisk walking worked about as well as jogging, which was as effective as cycling, which gave about the same results as weight lifting. The main factor is simply using your muscles on a consistent basis. It turned out to be as simple as that.

Let's look at examples of studies of three levels of exercise, and the effects that they have.

Twenty minutes a day

A study from Stanford University shows that small, consistent amounts of exercise will produce a small but noticeable weight loss. Men and women were asked to exercise regularly, starting with three days a week and increasing to five. They ended up exercising—on average, over the course of the year—a little less than twenty minutes a day. Compared with a control group who didn't exercise, the exercisers lost about five pounds of fat over the course of the year. We'll talk in chapter 12 about how you can insert at least this much exercise in your day (and probably two or three times as much) without spending any extra time or doing any sort of regular workout.

An hour a day

In another study, moderately overweight women were asked to exercise for ninety minutes a day four or five days a week, which averages out to not quite an hour a day. After a little over a year, they had lost an average of nineteen pounds. The exercise was a combination of bicycling, swimming, walking, badminton, and aerobic dancing. Is there something in that mix that appeals to you? Get to it and start losing!

All day every day

Exercise is different from low-fat eating in one important way: there is really no limit to how far you can go. No matter how stringent you are in your diet, you can't get down below 10 percent, or maybe 5 percent, calories from fat. Nor would you want to: if you eat a diet much below about 5 percent calories from fat, you will run into health problems (see chapter 10). But, aside from the need for sleep, there is probably no limit to the amount of exercise you can do. What happens when people exercise at the extreme limits?

Let's take a look at the case of Mike Stroud and Sir Ranulph Fiennes. They decided to go cross-country skiing—across Antarctica. They made the trip completely under their own power, pulling sledges that contained all their gear. These sledges weighed 485 pounds each at the start of the trip.

Stroud, a doctor and nutritionist, was especially interested in the effects of this sort of extreme exercise on body fat. He knew that, no matter what they ate, they would inevitably lose weight: "In my job at the Army Personnel Research Establishment, I conduct research on the effects of different diets on physical performance and body composition. . . . We would lose weight while eating an enormous amount. It would be a strange situation, but one that would yield information that was pertinent to the normal. There is no way in which similar information can be gathered in the laboratory."

During their journey, the men ate 5,200 calories per day. They purposely ate an extremely high fat diet in order to be able to cut down on the weight of supplies they would need to carry to provide such an enormous calorie intake. "As anyone on a diet will know, fat contains more than twice as many calories as the same weight of protein or carbohydrate. Our day's ration was to consist of a hot cereal start, midday soups and a freeze dried evening meal, all fortified with butter and chocolate bars to make the contents almost 57% fat."

The extent and rate of the men's weight loss was astonishing. Pulling their heavy sledges all day, every day, caused the fat to melt off their bodies so fast that it must have been visible on a day-to-day basis. After thirty-seven days, they had each lost about twenty pounds. Stroud writes, "At that rate of loss . . . we would disappear completely before our hundred days [the time they estimated it would take to cross Antarctica] were up." After sixty-eight days, Stroud had lost forty pounds and Fiennes fifty. Bear in mind that they were doing everything possible to keep the weight on, but at such a level of exertion, they simply couldn't do it. This was the last time they weighed themselves on the journey.

Contrary to Stroud's prediction, the men did not disappear. They made it home, where Stroud found some interesting changes in their metabolisms. "While eating what by normal standards would be deemed excessive, we had lost weight by exercising continually. Our resting metabolism had gone sky high, but quite why this change occurred is beyond me. As an adaptation, it was enormously wasteful, burning more energy than was necessary." In other words, even at rest the men burned more calories than normal.

Although their experience was extreme, the men's journey illustrates what many people discover about exercise: it allows you to eat enormous amounts of food and still lose weight. These men lost weight so fast that it was actually their major concern about the journey—they literally didn't know if there would be enough of them left to continue. This despite eating almost three times the calories and twice the fat that a normal person eats!

We don't necessarily encourage you to jump on the next boat to Antarctica with your skis and your butter. But this story dramatically shows the kind of fat-burning potential that exercise alone has, even with an extremely high fat diet. Imagine what happens when you combine exercise and a *low-fat* diet.

How Effective Are Low-Fat Eating and Exercise Together?

The idea of combining low-fat eating and exercise is so new that almost no research has been done using both. One good, controlled scientific study in which they were used together, without any attempt to control calories, shows the potential.

•   •   •

Women lowered the fat in their diet to about 23 percent and walked briskly for an average of about forty minutes per day. The study only lasted four months, but the women lost an average of fifteen pounds in that time! That's almost four pounds a month, or about a pound a week—and we don't know how much *more* weight the women would have lost if the study had continued. This was pure fat they lost, not water, not muscle. You might want to try holding a pound of butter (as we suggested in chapter 2) and picture that amount of fat leaving your body every week, week after week.

The combination of low-fat diet and exercise used in this study is actually a fairly modest change. It's the equivalent of following our Phase 1 guidelines for eating (chapter 7), and taking advantage of opportunistic exercise (chapter 12). This may be as far as you want to go, and that's fine. You'll see that the results can be very rewarding.

It's quite possible, in fact enjoyable, to eat one-half the fat that these women were eating (i.e., about 10 percent fat), or to add more exercise to your day, or both. As of this writing, no reliable studies have been done of such programs, but if you do go to these levels, your fat loss will be even faster. You will probably *double* the rate at which these women lost (thus about two pounds per week, or eight pounds per month) and you will stabilize at a lower weight (at least thirty pounds below your present weight). This assumes that you are moderately overweight (twenty to forty pounds) to begin with, as the women in this study were, and as most of our workshop participants are.

Another way to look at it is this. In our experience, and that of others who teach people low-fat eating and exercise, those who drop to eating 10 percent fat each day, and exercise for about an hour a day, almost always lose fat and stabilize at a weight very close to their ideal weight. They become lean.

Are There Any Factors That Cause One Person to Lose More or Less Than Another?

You may read the preceding sections and calculate an exact weight loss that you expect. You make the necessary changes in your diet and/or exercise habits, and find that you are losing far more rapidly than predicted. Or less rapidly. What's going on?

Sometimes, it's an advantage to be fat

As we said earlier, the more overweight you are, the faster you lose. It's true for exercise—in fact, one of the most powerful predictors of how much weight a person will lose on an exercise program is how much he or she weighs before beginning. The fatter you are to start, the more fat you will lose. It may also be true for low-fat eating, although there is not enough research to give a definitive answer. But the Hawaiian study, where the starting weight averaged more than 250 pounds and people were losing at a rate of over five pounds a week, certainly indicates the same trend.

This is good news for people with a lot of weight to shed. It's also a caution for those who have perhaps ten or fifteen pounds to lose. Don't expect to lower the fat in your diet to, say, 7 percent (as the Hawaiians did), then lose fifteen pounds of fat in less than three weeks. You will certainly lose the weight if you decrease the fat in your diet to that degree, but a more realistic time expectation is six months to a year.

This makes perfect sense when you realize that all people are naturally lean. The ones who are furthest from that natural state (that is, the fattest) are the ones who are most sensitive to our modern high-fat, low-exercise life-style. They will also be the ones who are most sensitive to a change back to a natural low-fat, high-exercise life-style. They will lose weight most rapidly and dramatically.

You are unique

In weight loss, as in everything else, we are all different. Some people are extremely sensitive to the fat content in their diet. They balloon up during the holidays, for example, when we all tend to eat a higher-fat diet, but lose weight rapidly and painlessly when January 1 has passed. Others aren't so fortunate.

The same is also true for exercise. As an example, one long-term exercise study involved four women, each doing the same amount of exercise (a little less than an hour a day). They all lost fat weight over the course of this fifteen-month study, but each lost a different amount. One lost twenty-seven pounds, one lost twenty-two pounds, one lost fourteen pounds, and one lost only twelve. Exercise consistently causes weight loss, and the more you do the more you lose. But if you insist that you must lose a certain amount or you'll quit, you're taking a gamble. You're gambling that your physiology matches or beats the average.

If you've been dieting, be prepared to gain at first

You must be very honest with yourself about this. If you consistently watch how much you eat, and are a little proud of the days when you are hungry all day (and ashamed of the times when you eat enough to satisfy your hunger), you are probably below your set point, maybe as much as twenty pounds below. When you change your eating habits to allow yourself to satisfy your hunger, there will be a rebound up toward your set point.

Expect it, and give your new habits of low-fat eating and exercise at least six months to reverse the rebound. You will find at that point that you are losing fat, and you're finally doing it the right way, the healthy way, and the permanent way.

You Are Built to Be a Lean Machine

No matter what, remember that the *natural state of men and women is lean.* Scientific studies of the few primitive cultures remaining on earth, such as in Papua New Guinea, bear this out. In such cultures, obesity is almost unknown. It's also quite rare to see overweight people in places such as rural China, where people still eat their traditional diet, containing less than 20 percent fat, and are, simply through the necessities of everyday life, very active. They eat 30 percent *more* calories than the average American, so they certainly aren't going hungry, yet they are far leaner than Americans. When eating a diet of 10–20 percent calories from fat, and moving around during most of the day, no one stays fat.

You can certainly eat as hunter-gatherers eat (their diets are about 10 percent fat) without a great deal of effort. You may not be stalking an antelope for your daily exercise, but you can get a surprising amount of exercise during your day, even if you never do a formal workout. And if you change both your diet and your exercise habits, you will come to the natural state for a human being, which is lean and healthy. How far you want to go toward this state is up to you—but it really is your choice. It's not a matter of genetics. We are genetically programmed to be *lean.*

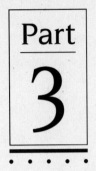

Part

3

Eat, Drink, and Be Lean

6

Principles of Low-Fat Eating

• • • • • •

Whether you've decided just to cut a little fat out of your foods, or to take the plunge all the way to 10 percent fat, there are some principles that inform everything we will say in the next few chapters. Keeping these in mind will help you to integrate low-fat eating into your life so that it *increases* your satisfaction with food. The principles are:

- Don't approach it as a diet.
- Concentrate on eliminating high-fat foods, not on counting fat grams.
- Don't allow it to take more time than your present way of eating.
- Make it fit *you* and *your* tastes.
- Schedule occasional "feast days."
- Don't make this a holy crusade.
- Start with the easy stuff.

Don't Approach It as a Diet

Most people have it permanently engraved in their brains that losing weight involves a temporary change in the way they eat (a diet), followed by a return to their "normal" way of eating. Weight goes down on the diet, and comes back up on the return to "normalcy." This approach clearly doesn't work. If you want to lose weight and keep it off, you need to make your *normal* way of eating one that lowers your set point; that is, you need to eat low-fat. As long as you eat low-fat, your set point stays low.

If you start eating low-fat, you will initially lose weight, then level out at some lower level (often quite a bit lower). The weight loss can take as long as a year or more, but eventually it stops. You have reached your new, lower set point. There is a very great temptation at this point to think, "Ahh! I've lost a lot of fat. Now I can go back to the way I used to eat and just be a little more careful about how much I eat. I know I was just overeating before." This is the old dieting mentality, very hard to shake. But if you go back to your old (high-fat) way of eating, your set point will go up. You may be able to "control" your eating, at least at first, but as you continue to eat high-fat, you will get more and more insistent signals to eat more so that you can fatten up to your new, higher set point (which your new, high-fat eating has caused). Inevitably, insidiously, the fat returns. It can happen so slowly that you don't make the connection between your newer, higher-fat eating habits and the change in the shape of your body. This is partly because it is so easy to raise the fat content of your diet dramatically by what seem like relatively minor changes. We'll talk about these high-fat habits in the next chapter.

You will remain at your new, lower, slimmer, healthier set point only as long as you continue to eat low-fat. If you start eating slightly higher-fat, you will gradually come to a new, higher set point: you will get fatter. If you start eating slightly lower-fat, you will gradually come to a new, lower set point: you will get leaner. Your body fat will faithfully follow the overall fat content of your diet.

For this reason, you must always keep in mind that you are not going on a diet, with its feelings of hunger, deprivation, and desperate longing for the light at the end of the tunnel (which is a freight train bringing you all the food your body is screaming for). You are, instead, altering the way you eat. These alterations must fit your way of living and your tastes, because they are going to be permanent. Don't force yourself to adopt an austere, pristine, saintly way of eating, even if it is low-fat. You'll experience the same feelings of deprivation you had on all your diets. Instead, make the low-fat eating fit you. From this idea, all the other principles follow.

Concentrate on Eliminating High-Fat Foods, Not on Counting Fat Grams

This is not a fat-gram-counting program. In order to understand why, we should first explain how many grams of fat you will eat daily in each phase of this program, what a gram of fat is, and where you will find fat. Then we'll explain why we don't tally our daily total of fat grams, and why you shouldn't, either.

Let's first look at what we mean when we talk about a "10-percent-fat diet," or a "40-percent-fat diet."

Fat grams and fat calories

The mythical "average American" eats about 2,000 calories a day. Ten percent of 2,000 calories is 200 calories. So, if you eat a 10-percent-fat diet, and you are an average American, you will get 200 calories a day from fat. If you eat a 20-percent-fat diet, you get 400 calories a day from fat; at 30 percent fat in the diet, you're getting 600 fat calories a day; at 40 percent fat, it's 800.

A gram of fat contains 10 calories. (It's really 9. But calling it 10 makes the arithmetic far simpler, and it's only off by a little.) So the 200 calories of fat in the 10-percent-fat diet is 20 grams of fat, the 400 calories in the 20-percent-fat diet is 40 grams, etc.

A good rule of thumb is to take the percentage of fat in the diet and multiply by two. That will give you roughly the number of fat grams in the diet.

But how much *is* a gram of fat?

A gram is a measure of weight. Let's say you're enthusiastic about the weight loss you can expect and you want to go straight to a 10-percent-fat diet. You might want to know how much the 20 grams of fat in your 10-percent-fat diet will weigh. In our workshops, we demonstrate this. We give everyone a plastic bag with seven pennies in it. A penny weighs about 3 grams, so seven pennies weigh about 20 grams. If you find seven pennies and heft them in your hand, you will probably feel the same emotions that we see on the faces of workshop participants: disappointment and dread. Twenty grams is nothing!

Everyone begins to think that this low-fat-eating thing is going to be a real chore.

But wait. That's not really a fair demonstration, because pennies are made of metal, not fat—they are much denser and take up less space. What does a gram of fat *look* like? At this point we hand everyone at the workshop a vial containing one gram of fat. You can get some idea of how much that is by pouring some oil (any type) into a quarter-teaspoon measuring spoon. You are now looking at about 1 gram of fat (oil is 100 percent fat). To get a somewhat better view, pour out one *tablespoon* of oil. You are now looking at 14 grams of fat. So, on a 10-percent-fat diet, you would get one and a half *tablespoons* of fat. On a 20-percent-fat diet, you get three tablespoons. On a 40-percent-fat diet, six tablespoons.

We've summarized these relationships in the table below.

Percent fat in the diet	Calories from fat (approximate)	Number of grams of fat	Number of tablespoons of fat
40%	800	80	6
30%	600	60	4½
20%	400	40	3
10%	200	20	1½

When people start thinking in terms of tablespoons of fat, they get much happier. You can see their eyes light up. They're thinking, "Hmmmm . . . one and a half tablespoons is a lot. If I just cut the fat off my meat, and use less butter on my bread, and maybe use a little less oil when I cook, I can get to one and a half tablespoons a day easily. This low-fat-eating thing is going to be a snap."

You can't get away from fat

The trouble with this thinking is that *almost every natural food contains fat.* A large apple, which most people think is completely fat-free, contains about a gram of fat. *Even foods that have been processed to remove fat often contain some fat;* for example, a cup of skim milk contains about half a gram of fat. You can't get away from it—nor should you, because you need a little fat in your diet (a couple of teaspoonfuls or so).

So, if you eat the most pristine low-fat diet, containing nothing but grains, legumes (beans and peas), fruits, and vegetables (an extremely healthful diet, by the way), you will still be eating about 10 percent fat *even if you add no extra fat whatsoever to anything ever.* Thus, you really don't have to worry about getting too little fat in your diet, unless you are eating a very unnatural diet, like trying to subsist on fat-free cookies and nothing else. But you know perfectly well that that sort of diet isn't nutritionally sound, and you'd run into far more severe problems than not getting enough fat.

It is because almost every food has some fat in it that we don't recommend that you try to eat a low-fat diet by setting a daily "fat-gram budget" and then trying to stick to it. You would have to keep track of every morsel you eat. You would have to know the serving size, and how many servings you had. You would have to know how much fat is in a serving. You would have to write it down, then use your calculator to add it all up. You might start to consider carrying a minicomputer and a table of fat values to keep track of everything (look on the bright side: lugging a computer around will increase your daily exercise). Your daily eating would be transformed from a pleasant experience into a scientific experiment.

Instead, the approach we take is to increase your awareness of the fat content of foods. Then you avoid or substitute for the highest-fat foods. In Phase 1, you learn to eliminate some of the foods that are 60–100 percent fat, and substitute some of the lowest-fat foods, which average 5 percent fat. That's all it takes to cut *half* the fat from your diet. If you choose to eliminate even more fat, in Phase 2, where you can come down to 10 percent calories from fat, you will learn to eliminate the foods that are 20–60 percent fat.

There really aren't all that many high-fat foods. They just happen to be very plentiful in our American diet, which is why most of us are eating 40 percent fat. Once you have awareness of the really high-fat foods, and your low-fat alternatives, and you are aware of how much weight you can lose by eating the low-fat foods, the switch to a low-fat diet is almost automatic.

Don't Allow It to Take More Time Than Your Present Way of Eating

No one has enough time in the day. The demands of careers, family, and social life keep most of us busy from the second we wake to the instant we turn out the light at night (and we usually steal a little more time by not giving ourselves enough sleep). The average American works four hours more per week now than he or she did in the 1950s. If you spend more time at work, you must spend less time somewhere else, and the place that we've cut down on is the kitchen. Americans spend an average of thirty minutes a day in the kitchen, compared with an hour a day for the Germans, and over two hours a day for the French.

So, if low-fat eating is to succeed, it must not take any more of your precious time. Low-fat eating did not start to work for us until we cut down on some of the enormously time-consuming chores that some of the early books on the subject suggested. We started using canned tomatoes instead of boiling fresh ones, peeling off the skins, and chopping them. We rarely eat homemade low-fat muffins as snacks because we rarely have the two hours it takes to prepare them. Instead, we buy low-fat bagels by the dozen, store them in our freezer in freezer bags, and microwave them for one minute when we want a snack. They'll keep for several weeks without getting mushy or hard and dry. If we eat rice with a meal, it is often white rice (which can be prepared in fifteen minutes) rather than brown rice (which takes an hour). When we do make brown rice, we prepare enough to keep in the fridge for two or three days.

Now, the beans you boil yourself may taste slightly better than the canned. And there is no doubt that brown rice is nutritionally superior to white rice. But a meal that is made with canned beans, canned tomatoes, and white rice can be delicious if you use the right recipe, and it's nutritionally far superior to a McDonald's hamburger and fries. And if you have to face the choice every night between two hours of bean-boiling and rice-cooking, and popping down to the local McDonald's and having dinner available instantly, McDonald's is going to win four nights out of five.

In Phase 1, we've made it really easy. There are no choices in Phase 1 that involve more time in cooking or shopping. Yet you can cut half the fat out of the foods you eat by following these guidelines. In Phase 2, in which you come down to 10 percent calories from fat, you'll find some guidelines that may actually *save* you time. For example, you'll substitute chicken, turkey, or fish for red meat, and these types of meat take less time to prepare. The typical fish dish takes twenty minutes to prepare, chicken forty-two minutes, and red meat seventy-five minutes. Substitute kidney beans for meat in some dishes and you cut that aspect of preparation considerably. In Phase 2 we'll also offer some commonsense suggestions for cutting your food-preparation time in general. In the recipes appendix, we've included recipes for low-fat meals that take anywhere from five to fifty minutes to prepare. We also offer some "Tips for Every Meal" in chapter 9, where we really emphasize ease of preparation, and include many options for days when you have no time whatsoever for cooking.

If you are a gourmet cook and already spend a couple of hours a day in the kitchen, most of the above may not apply. You will find our cooking guidelines in Phase 2 helpful, especially those for modifying recipes. You will also find Dean Ornish's *Eat More, Weigh Less* to be a valuable resource; Dr. Ornish asked many of the nation's top chefs to turn their attention to low-fat cooking with a gourmet flair, and the result was hundreds of unusual and intriguing recipes. Though low-fat, these recipes do take some time to prepare, often more than an hour.

Make It Fit **You** and **Your** Tastes

Whatever your style of eating now, you can fit low-fat eating into it. Don't try to fit your style to some idealized version of low-fat eating. We've provided diagnostic quizzes to help you pinpoint where in your life you can make adjustments that will lead you to lower-fat eating. If you always eat lunch in a restaurant, you can continue to do so—but you must master the art of low-fat restaurant ordering, perhaps even exploring a few restaurants until you find some that serve low-fat fare that suits your tastes. If you eat lunch at your desk but never have more than a couple of minutes in the morning to prepare it, you must learn what low-fat lunch foods to stock in your pantry so that you can grab them and go.

You should also fit low-fat eating to your tastes. Don't accept a food as part of your diet just because it's low-fat—you must also enjoy the taste. Their are hundreds, perhaps thousands of low-fat foods to choose from. Keep experimenting until you find the ones that you look forward to eating. Some of them are already part of your diet. Others may be common foods that will be new to you—we rarely ate bagels until we started eating low-fat, but now they are a staple of our diet, because they're delicious and the ones we buy are only about 5 percent fat. Other foods will be nonfat alternatives for high-fat foods you eat now. Food manufacturers have jumped on the fat-free bandwagon. Take advantage of their enthusiasm and try the new fat-free foods coming out. You will be revolted by some, delighted by others. Try different brands, because flavors, textures, and qualities vary widely. Don't give up if the first nonfat brand you try doesn't taste good; keep trying until you find one that does. Try the "new, improved" versions. Sometimes they really are.

This doesn't mean that every new low-fat food has to taste exactly like the old high-fat foods. Mark, who read one of our early workbooks and became a true "fat detective," put it this way: "I look for a brand that tastes good, not one that tastes exactly like the high-fat version. If you'll only be satisfied with the exact high-fat taste, you'll never be happy with low-fat substitutes. But if you just open your mind and look for something that tastes good to you, you'll find all sorts of low-fat treats."

Schedule Occasional "Feast Days"

The day we gave our first workshop also happened to be Eric's birthday. Naturally everyone wanted to know what low-fat fare Eric would be eating on this day.

"We're going to a Thai restaurant and loading up on the peanut sauces, the coconut concoctions, and anything else we want to feast on," replied Eric, much to the delight of our audience. "On my birthday, fat be damned!"

There are days when eating a low-fat diet is nearly impossible. Holidays, like Christmas or Thanksgiving, which have traditional, usually very high fat fare, are examples, and perhaps, you, like Eric, really like to splurge on your birthday. Rather than fighting a nearly impossible battle on these days, why not simply enjoy? You will often be with your family, and unless you are very unusual, your family will not be card-carrying members of the Fat-Free Revolution. You may well feel that you are denying yourself pleasure if you stick to your everyday fare. So don't.

We call these days "feast days." We first heard of the idea from John and Mary McDougall who have written several books about very low fat, vegetarian eating, and it immediately made sense. We incorporate feast days into our program, and suggest that you do, too. The nice thing about designating feast days is that it makes very clear the times when you are eating low-fat and when you aren't. If, instead, you allow yourself high-fat treats every once in a while during an otherwise low-fat day, the distinction becomes blurred, and you soon find yourself inching back toward a high-fat diet (and finding inches coming back onto your waistline).

There are a few things to keep in mind about feast days.

Schedule your feast days

You might want to decide right now what religious or other holidays you're going to designate as your feast days, and mark them on your calendar. If you don't do this, it's easy to slip into allowing yourself a feast day any time you feel like going to your favorite high-fat restaurant.

You can afford one, perhaps two feast days a month. One day a month probably won't raise the overall fat content of your diet more than 1 or 2 percent (for example, from 10 percent fat to 11 or 12). Your body will faithfully reflect this by carrying a couple more pounds of fat than it would if you ate a consistent 10-percent-fat diet; most people are willing to trade a couple of pounds for a day of feasting every month. But any more than that and you will be significantly raising the amount of fat in your diet, thus raising your set point. For example, if you eat a diet that is 10 percent fat six days a week, but on the seventh you eat very high fat "treat" meals all day, your overall diet can easily creep up to 15–20% fat. That's going to add pounds to your waistline, yet you may think that you're still close to eating 10 percent fat. If you schedule your days, you avoid this trap.

Even if you don't schedule feast days, try marking them on your calendar as they occur. Just write down "high-fat dinner" or "high-fat day," or whatever it was. This will go a long way toward explaining seemingly mysterious gains and losses of a few pounds of fat—if clothes are getting tighter, you can go to the calendar and be reminded that the past couple of months contained, say, eight or ten high-fat days. If clothes are getting looser, you may find that the past few months have included only one or two high-fat days. This helps reinforce the relationship between fat in your diet and fat on your body, and it keeps you from "forgetting" feast days and then being puzzled by fat gain.

Don't be surprised if your tastes, and your digestion, change as you eat a low-fat diet

That Thanksgiving feast may taste a lot greasier than it used to. For some people, in fact, it becomes downright unpleasant, and they begin to stick with the lower-fat alternatives, even on feast days. And your body, which is not used to the fat load it will be receiving, may react with indigestion or, at the very least, slow digestion.

The fullness can be quite uncomfortable, and may last for hours (you may feel full after a low-fat meal, but it is rarely uncomfortable or lasting). You may immediately notice a greasy feel, especially on your face, which may quite literally start oozing fat (oil). And you may well feel that old tired, got-a-lump-of-lard-in-my-gut, need-to-nap feeling after your feast (which is why it's a good idea to schedule feast days on holidays, because you're not going to be able to do much work after your feast).

Won't feasting make it harder
to return to low-fat eating?

Some low-fat experts insist that people lose their taste for fat quickly, but that eating high-fat foods at any time will cause the "fat tooth" to be reborn, leading to continued cravings for fatty foods.

We've found that this isn't so, as long as people limit feasts to one, or at most two, days per month and *keep track*. If you find that you're getting into trouble and craving fatty foods, then this idea is not for you. For most people, though, it offers a bit of a safety valve, especially in a society where most social occasions are marked by the consumption of enough high-fat calories to light a small city.

Don't Make This a Holy Crusade

Many people who start eating low-fat find that they experience greater energy within days, and begin losing noticeable amounts of fat within weeks or months. It can be difficult to see those closest to you continue to eat like pigs when you have discovered the One True Way. You may face the temptation to share the good news with these unenlightened folk, to point out smugly and self-righteously the error of their ways.

Resist. There is no scientific proof that eating low-fat foods increases your chances of going to heaven. But we guarantee that you can make life hell for your friends if you start preaching and moralizing about what *they* are eating.

Your friends and family may notice a change in your appearance and your energy levels. They will certainly notice a change in what you eat, and may well comment on how much you eat (it's going to be a lot more than you used to). They may be curious. They may want to make the same sort of changes. In that case, share. But it's a good idea to wait until you're asked, because then you can be certain that your audience really wants to know.

Another pitfall of seeing fat as the Devil in Food's Clothing is that it gets you back into the good-food/bad-food trap. If you eat one fatty food, you figure you've sinned for the day, so you might as well buy that gallon of ice cream and chow down. After all, you're going to hell anyway.

Fat is not evil. It just makes you fat and sluggish. This program is about choices, not about good and evil.

Start with the Easy Stuff

This is the principle that led to the two phases of low-fat eating; Phase 1 is, for most people, the easy stuff, whereas Phase 2 requires more skill. Some of the easiest, simplest changes you can make will have the biggest effect on the fat content of the foods you eat. So why not start with them? Save for later the changes that look more difficult. The diagnostic quizzes in chapters 7 and 8 will help you pinpoint exactly what changes will make the biggest dents in *your* fat consumption. Find the changes that look easiest, and begin there.

7

Phase 1 of Low-Fat Eating—

20 Percent Calories from Fat

• • • • •

You've decided to try low-fat eating as one of your weapons for weight loss. You'll start by dropping to 20 percent calories from fat and see how it goes. But you're a little nervous. Isn't that a radical change? Relax.

You can cut half the fat out of your diet—drop from 40 percent fat to 20 percent—without reading a label, giving up meat, or even noticing much change in the taste of your food.

Making simple changes in your eating habits will cause definite decreases in your body fat—you can lose fifteen or twenty pounds in a year if you are, say, fifty pounds overweight, simply by following all three of the guidelines in Phase 1. If you find that statement incredible, go back and reread chapter 5. This kind of weight loss has been seen in dozens of scientific studies.

Certain foods are so high in fat they skyrocket the fat content of your diet, even if you eat just tiny amounts of them. These foods are also common components of our diet. In this phase we talk about changes that will get rid of the highest-fat foods in your diet. Since these are so extremely high in fat, removing them automatically drops the fat content of your diet way down.

There are three simple guidelines for Phase 1:

---

1. Don't add pure fat to food.
2. Switch to nonfat dairy products and salad dressings.
3. Eat at least five fruits and/or vegetables daily.

These guidelines can be incorporated into your life in a matter of days or weeks (although you can take as long as you want).

Where's the Fat?

The following diagnostic quiz will help you see exactly how this chapter will be most useful for you. Take it before you read the rest of the chapter. Be honest and careful in your answers. There are no right or wrong answers—this quiz is simply designed to help you see how much of an effect the changes outlined in Phase 1 can have in *your* life and in the way *you* eat. Not your idealized life, the way you should be eating, but the way you really eat and live now. It will also help you zero in on which parts of this phase will give you the most dramatic results.

For each of the following statements, choose the single answer that most accurately reflects the way you eat or think. Place the letter of the answer you selected on the line in front of the question. The quiz is divided into three sections corresponding to the different guidelines for Phase 1. The page numbers following each question tell you where you will find information in this chapter about the eating habits referred to in the question.

Section 1: Do you add pure fat to your foods?

_____ 1. I eat deep-fat-fried foods (French fries, potato chips, fried chicken, etc.) (page 115)

A. less than once a week   B. once a week
C. 2–3 times a week   D. 4 or more times a week

_____ 2. I use oil (corn oil, safflower oil, olive oil, canola oil—*any* type of oil) to sauté vegetables or meat, or add oil to the water when I cook pasta so it doesn't stick together (page 113)

A. less than once a week   B. once a week
C. 2–3 times a week   D. 4 or more times a week

_____ 3. I use oil, butter, margarine, lard, or shortening in my baking (page 114)

A. less than once a week   B. once a week
C. 2–3 times a week   D. 4 or more times a week

_____ 4. I feel that margarine is a healthier choice than butter. (page 112)

A. No   B. Yes

_____ 5. I use butter or margarine (including reduced-fat or low-calorie versions) with my meals (on top of oatmeal, to butter bread, on potatoes, on vegetables, etc.) (page 115)

A. less than once a week   B. once a week
C. 2–3 times a week   D. 4 or more times a week

_____ 6. I use mayonnaise (on sandwiches, on vegetables, in dips, in casseroles, etc.) (page 116)

A. less than once a week   B. once a week
C. 2–3 times a week   D. 4 or more times a week

_____ 7. I eat peanut butter or other nut butters (page 118)

A. less than once a week   B. once a week
C. 2–3 times a week   D. 4 or more times a week

_____ 8. I eat sunflower seeds or other seeds, nuts, or trail mix (page 118)

A. less than once a week   B. once a week
C. 2–3 times a week   D. 4 or more times a week

Section 2: Do you use dairy products that are not nonfat?

_____ 9. I drink whole milk or 2-percent milk (page 119)

A. less than once a week   B. once a week
C. 2–3 times a week   D. 4 or more times a week

_____ 10. I use cream, half and half, whole milk, 2-percent milk, or nondairy creamer in my coffee. (page 121)

A. No   B. Yes

_____ 11. I drink cappuccino, latte, or café mocha made with whole or low-fat milk (this includes powdered instant brands as well as what is served at an espresso bar) (page 122)

A. less than once a week   B. once a week
C. 2–3 times a week   D. 4 or more times a week

_____ 12. I use regular, low-fat, or reduced-fat sour cream or cream cheese (page 121)

A. less than once a week   B. once a week
C. 2–3 times a week   D. 4 or more times a week

_____ 13. I eat yogurt (regular _or_ low-fat) (page 120)

A. less than once a week   B. once a week
C. 2–3 times a week   D. 4 or more times a week

_____ 14. I like to have ice cream or low-fat frozen yogurt (page 121)

A. less than once a week   B. once a week
C. 2–3 times a week   D. 4 or more times a week

_____ 15. I eat cheese (_any_ regular, low-fat, or reduced-fat cheese, even Parmesan cheese) (page 121)

A. less than once a week   B. once a week
C. 2–3 times a week   D. 4 or more times a week

_____ 16. I use regular, low-fat, or reduced-fat salad dressing on my salad (page 123)

A. less than once a week   B. once a week
C. 2–3 times a week   D. 4 or more times a week

Section 3: Are you eating your fruits and veggies?

_____ 17. I eat vegetables (one serving is a half-cup of chopped vegetable or one cup of green salad) (page 124)

A. 2 or more servings a day   B. 1 serving a day
C. 3 servings a week   D. 2 or fewer servings per week

_____ 18. I eat fruit (one serving is one piece of fruit; fruit juice doesn't count) (page 124)

A. 2 or more servings a day   B. 1 serving a day
C. 3 servings a week   D. 2 or fewer servings per week

_____ 19. I feel that drinking juice is an adequate substitute for eating fruits or vegetables. (page 124)

A. No   B. Yes

Any question with a "D" answer represents a "Hot Spot" for you. *Hot Spots are eating habits that keep you fat.* Questions with "B" or "C" answers are less urgent Hot Spots, but nevertheless areas where you can cut fat. Not until you reach an "A" have you cut all the fat from an area of your eating.

Guideline 1: Don't Add Pure Fat to Food

The highest-fat foods are those which are pure, 100 percent fat. Adding these to your food is the fastest way to balloon the fat content of your diet (and your waistline). So removing them is the fastest, easiest way to make a big dent in the amount of fat you eat, and the amount of fat you carry around.

Pure fat foods include:

- oils
- butter, margarine, and mayonnaise
- lard and shortening
- nuts and seeds

All oils

Any oil is 100 percent fat. That includes polyunsaturated oils, monounsaturated oils, megaunsaturated oils—*all oils.*

You may safely ignore the health claims for some forms of oil (mainly monounsaturated). They will not make you healthier if you eat them. They will only make you *less sick* than other forms. *Adding* olive oil to your diet will not protect your heart. *Substituting* olive oil for, say, butter, is better for your heart. But the best thing to do is not to use any added oil at all.

Just a decade ago, heart experts were exhorting us all to switch to polyunsaturated oils rather than saturated. So everyone started eating margarine instead of butter. Now it looks as if margarine may be *worse* for your heart than butter (although, to be fair, it's a different sort of fat that manufacturers sneaked in that may be the culprit). And some experts have believed all along that polyunsaturated oils increase cancer risk (could this be one reason why breast-cancer rates are rising?). Now the heart experts are touting monounsaturated oils. We wonder what evidence will emerge in the next decade showing that monounsaturates weren't quite the miracle they were cracked up to be. Or perhaps unscrupulous manufacturers will adulterate the monounsaturated oils with harmful forms of oil, as they have done for margarine.

And monounsaturated oils will make you just as fat as any other type of oil. In America, where obesity is a real health problem, perhaps we should concentrate on getting people to use less of any oil, rather than sending confusing messages that seem to imply that adding a certain type of oil to your diet will improve your health. Obesity is a major risk factor for heart disease, diabetes, and some forms of cancer.

By far the healthiest diet is one with *no* added oils—the countries that have the least heart disease and cancer are the ones where people hardly eat any oil, of any type. You get plenty of fat and oil in your food naturally. For example, corn oil, obviously, comes from corn. But it takes *fourteen* ears of corn to get *one* tablespoon of oil. Eat the corn in its natural state and you get just the right amount to keep you healthy. Eat the pure oil and you're getting a huge excess which produces disease and obesity.

The people who are able to reverse their heart disease through diet do so on a diet with no oils. People who lose the most weight do so by avoiding oils. Period.

Don't cook with oils.
The suggestions given here will almost completely eliminate oil in your cooking.

Use nonstick pans.
If you don't already have one, buy a large nonstick skillet with a lid. It can be as plain or as fancy as you like, as long as it is nonstick. *This is the single essential piece of kitchen equipment that you must have to start decreasing the fat you use in cooking.* You need add no oil whatsoever to prevent sticking. If you do a lot of baking, you must also purchase nonstick baking dishes.

Sauté food in defatted chicken, vegetable, or beef broth
(skim fat off the top of broth), water, or wine.
Use whichever is compatible with your tastes and the meal you are cooking. To defat broth use a teaspoon to skim away fat floating on the surface. Even if you run out of broth or wine, you can *always* use water as long as you cook in a nonfat skillet. Never use oil or butter. Ever. Every drop of oil is a drop of fat to be added to your fat stores.

Don't add oil when cooking beans, pasta, or grains.
It isn't necessary. Cooking in defatted chicken broth will add a lot of flavor but not a lot of fat.

Broil meat to brown it.
This eliminates the need for oil and gives a nice, even browning.

*Cut the oil, butter, margarine, lard, and shortening
used in baking in half.*
Oils, butter, margarine, shortening, and lard account for 75–90 percent of the fat in baked goods.

Some people balk at completely eliminating these from baking. If you just can't bring yourself to cut them out completely right away, simply cut the amount that the recipe calls for in half. You will never know the difference. Get used to this habit for a few months, and the transition to no oil or butter will be smooth and easy.

Because, sooner or later, all oil, butter, etc., must go. It's time to . . .

Get the last bit of extra oil or butter out.
There are many strategies that not only eliminate oil and butter but may actually enhance the flavor of baked goods, and give a nutritional bonus to boot.

Just cut it out.
In many recipes you can simply eliminate the oil and people won't even be able to tell the difference.

Substitute applesauce.
Often you do need to substitute something to give back the feel and moisture that oil provides, as well as to add some flavor. Try applesauce, used one-to-one as a substitute for oil or other 100-percent-fat items (like butter, margarine, lard, or shortening).

Substitute prune puree.
Another fat substitute that is picking up popularity is prune puree. This is not a joke. Prunes contain about 4 percent fat, yet they have a number of characteristics that make them ideal as fat substitutes in baked goods. They are high in pectin, adding volume, and sorbitol, adding moisture. They contain malic acid, a natural flavor-enhancer. They are especially good in chocolate recipes and in fruitcakes and

wheat breads. We've included a recipe for Bavarian Black
Chocolate Cake made with prune puree in the recipes appe
Give it a try!

You can use prune puree in darker baked goods and applesau
lighter ones (the prune puree would make these darker).

Substitute pectin or arrowroot.
For pasta salads and other dishes, and for marinades, which contai
oily dressings in their high-fat versions, try substituting pectin or ar
rowroot for the oil. Dissolve 1 tablespoon of pectin or arrowroot in ¼
cup hot water and use in place of oil. It coats the ingredients and helps
hold the dressing on the pasta or other components of the dish. Arrowroot is especially good for this.

Use a butter substitute.
There are several butter flavorings, such as Molly McButter, that de-
rive at least part of their flavor, but virtually no fat, from butter. If you
want the flavor of butter without the fat, try one of these. For example,
you can give mashed potatoes a distinctive buttery taste by sprinkling
in a butter substitute to taste and stirring. You can "butter" your corn
on the cob by rolling the ear in some of the substitute sprinkled on a
plate. You can "butter" your baked potato with it. You can even make
liquid "butter" by following the directions on the container. These
substitutes can't be used for frying.

Don't eat deep-fried foods.
You know how, when you walk into a fast-food restaurant, you hear
that sound like the crinkling of a giant piece of cellophane? That's the
sound of your food literally being boiled in oil. And the food soaks that
oil up like a sponge. For example, a baked potato is 1 percent fat—
a supremely healthy low-fat food. French fries, made by deep-frying
potatoes, are 50 percent fat. Almost all deep-fried foods are at leas
50–70 percent fat. Look for the crust over the food itself—that's
sure tipoff. You see it on fish sticks, Kentucky Fried Chicken, Chicke
McNuggets, doughnuts; even zucchini acquires a golden crust after it
been turned into a fat-loaded gut-buster by deep-frying. If you are
doubt, ask the waiter/waitress!

Butter, margarine, and mayonnaise

Butter and margarine are 100 percent fat. As we pointed out in the previous section, there is evidence emerging that margarine is less healthy—for your heart and in terms of cancer risk—than butter. Mayonnaise is 98–99 percent fat.

The move away from butter and margarine is a good example from our own experience of how a seemingly big change can turn out to be very easy to do.

At one point, we were eating very healthfully, with very low fat breakfasts and lunches and usually a low-fat dinner. But Eric retained one high-fat habit. He buttered his bread. Profusely. To the point where the butter on his dinner bread alone probably *doubled* the fat content of his diet, raising it from 15 percent to over 30 percent! It didn't take a cube of butter to do it, either, just a thick layer on three or four slices of bread. Then, one day, Eric decided to stop, cold turkey.

He had been dreading this day. He knew he probably couldn't do it—he liked the taste of that butter too much—but he decided to give it a try. He expected chills, the shakes. He might have to be tied to a bed for a few days. Should he do it under a doctor's supervision? Maybe he would have to join a support group of other former butter-eaters.

He stopped buttering his bread at dinner one night. It took him exactly one day to make the change, and he never noticed the difference. In precisely one day his tastes changed; he never craved butter or even thought about it. For a while he put jam on his bread, but he found he didn't really need it, and stopped. The huge, monumental change that was going to take enormous willpower, constant vigilance, and lots of support turned out to be about as difficult as changing toothpaste brands.

Lesson: Just do it. You may be surprised.

You can try substituting one of the fat-free brands of "butter-style spreads" or mayonnaises. *Only* accept "nonfat" or "fat-free." Beware of "low-calorie" mayonnaises, which often are still 98–99 percent fat. The manufacturers dilute regular mayonnaise with water, then whip it up, so a tablespoon of the diluted mayonnaise has fewer calories (because half the tablespoon is water), but it still is 98–99 percent fat. You simply have to avoid these dishonest spreads.

As with all else, try several brands. One may taste hellish to your palate, another heavenly. Choose accordingly. We have deliberately avoided recommending specific brands, because the nonfat bandwagon is rolling with such speed now that our recommendations would be superseded by far tastier versions by the time you read this book. And your tastes will, of course, differ from ours.

Also, you will find that, even though you might not find the taste appealing when you use a fat-free mayonnaise just to moisten a sandwich, if you use the mayo to make, say, tuna salad, it can become indistinguishable from the high-fat spread. You may want to try the couple of recipes in the appendix that use fat-free mayonnaise.

If you want to moisten your sandwiches, try mustard (some people love it, some hate it; there doesn't seem to be any in-between). The amount you will use on a sandwich contains very little fat. You can also try tomatoes, pickles, ketchup, canned green chilis—your imagination is the limit.

Finally, you might try plain sandwiches occasionally. They soon start to taste normal.

Cooking tips: For butter and margarine, follow the guidelines given above for oils. For mayonnaise, which is used in sandwich spreads, salads, etc., try nonfat mayonnaise brands, which often taste great in salads and spreads. You can also try substituting nonfat yogurt, the tangy taste of which many people enjoy.

Lard and shortening

Lard is just a harder form of oil, and shortening is any form of fat that is added to baked goods. They are both 100 percent fat. You may not put a dollop of lard on your evening stew, but many people do use it in baking. All the tips that we gave for cooking without oil apply to lard and shortening.

And when you see lard or shortening on a label, it means FAT. (More about reading labels in Phase 2. It's not something to worry about too much now; we just wanted to alert you to these code words for pure fat.)

Nuts and seeds

Nuts and seeds are so high in fat (over 90 percent in many cases) that we consider them "honorary pure fats." If you eat three or four handfuls of almonds while you are cooking your low-fat dinner, for example, you will raise the fat content of your diet 10 percent—you can go from 20 percent fat to 30 percent fat for the day in about five minutes. Think of eating nuts as eating handfuls of butter, because in terms of the amount of fat you're adding to your diet they are almost equivalent. Same with seeds—sunflower seeds, for example, are almost 80 percent fat!

As for oils, as for butter, so with nuts. You don't have to spend time and energy finding out which ones are lower in fat. They are all so high in fat that you should just avoid *all* of them.

This also means nut butters. Peanut butter, for instance, is usually just ground-up peanuts (sometimes with sugar, but the fat content is still sky-high). And we hate to sound like a broken record, but you can forget "reduced-fat" versions. One brand's regular peanut butter has 16 grams of fat per serving; the "reduced-fat" version has 13 grams per serving. You have to wonder why they bothered.

Guideline 2: Switch to Nonfat Dairy Products and Salad Dressings

Dairy products, such as milk, cheese, yogurt, sour cream, etc., and salad dressings aren't pure fat. But they are the highest-fat foods we eat aside from pure fats. And we eat a lot of them. So, just by switching to nonfat dairy products and salad dressings, you can cut another major source of fat from your diet.

This one is pretty much a no-brainer. When you get to the dairy section of the store, buy only nonfat products. Whatever you buy normally, buy the nonfat version. There is a nonfat version of every type of dairy product now—isn't it great to live in the nineties? If your store doesn't stock these products, ask them to, or switch stores. This sort of behavior is what keeps a free-market economy strong.

Same with salad dressings. They contain so much oil that they are essentially pure fat. But there are tons of fat-free dressings available now. Use them.

One caution. Make sure you use *only nonfat or fat-free versions.* By law, these must contain virtually no fat. *Beware of "low-fat, "reduced-fat," "low-calorie," "lean," "cholesterol-free," or other designations.* Although some of these terms have legal meaning, none means that the food is free of fat, or even that it contains little fat. To be safe, check the label. You don't have to read the whole thing. At the very top of the label you will see "Amount Per Serving," "Calories," and "Calories from Fat." The Calories from Fat should read zero. If it doesn't, don't use the product.

Nonfat dairy

All regular dairy products, even in their "low-fat" forms, are extremely high in fat, far too high to have in your diet in any amount if you want to eat 20 percent calories from fat.

Cheeses are 80–90 percent calories from fat. Sour cream is 87 percent fat. Whole milk is 50 percent fat. And don't be fooled by "2 percent milk" or "low-fat" milk. It's 2 percent milkfat by *weight*—and over 30 percent *calories* from fat. We'll go into how this kind of deception came about when we talk about label-reading in Phase 2. The only truly low-fat milk products are labeled "nonfat," "fat-free," or "skim."

Milk

Nonfat (skim) milk has been around for a while. Switch to it tomorrow. Within two weeks it will taste completely normal and even 2-percent milk will taste incredibly rich.

If you drink a glass or more of whole milk each day, the single largest fat reduction you can make may be to switch to nonfat milk. If you consume two to three cups of whole milk a day (drinking it with meals, putting it on your cereal, etc.), and you switch to nonfat, you will decrease the fat content of your diet by about 10–15 percent. You can go from 40 percent fat in your diet to 30 or even 25 percent, in one day.

If you are drinking "2-percent" milk (low-fat milk) and you don't think switching to nonfat will have much effect, think again. If you are a two-to-three-cup-a-day consumer and switch to nonfat, you will decrease the fat content of your diet by about 5 percent. You can drop from 40 percent fat to 35 percent in one day.

By the way, nonfat milk has just as much calcium as whole milk (in fact, it has a little more per serving). People may think that the opaque white color of whole milk indicates a higher calcium content, because calcium is white, like bones—isn't it? (Well, no, but that's what most people think.) What the whiteness of whole milk really indicates is that it's extremely high in *fat*.

If you just can't switch to nonfat milk overnight, come down gradually. Switch to 2-percent for a month. Then go to 1-percent (now available in most areas, or you can make your own by mixing half nonfat and half 2-percent). Then go to nonfat.

Milk provides a dramatic yet common example of how your taste for fat can change. The most common comment about changing tastes that we hear from workshop participants is, "I used to drink whole milk all the time, but since I switched to nonfat, whole milk is just too rich. Even putting 1-percent on cereal tastes the way cream used to. It's not even pleasant anymore."

Milk also clearly demonstrates the relationship between high-fat eating and after-meal napping. If you're accustomed to drinking a glass of whole milk with lunch, when you switch to nonfat you may experience a noticeable rise in your afternoon energy levels. If you are to experience the full effect, of course, the whole lunch should be low-fat. But because milk contributes so much fat to the lunch, this one change may be enough so that you can feel a difference.

Yogurt

Many brands of nonfat yogurt are now available. You can get plain or fruit and other flavors. The fruit yogurts usually contain sugar, which doesn't raise your set point but which some people like to avoid (see chapter 10 for a fuller discussion of sugar). If you want to avoid sugar, get plain yogurt and add your own fruit.

Ice cream or frozen yogurt

Nonfat versions of both are available for those who like frozen desserts. Again, they probably have sugar in them, so beware if you're trying to avoid sugar.

Cheeses

Almost every common type of cheese is now available in a nonfat version. Just about every store has at least nonfat cottage cheese and nonfat cream cheese (try it on bagels, alone or with some fruit spread). Almost all regular cheeses are 80 percent fat. Cream cheese is 90 percent fat! If you are a cheese lover, just can't live without it, try all the nonfat alternatives. Or just go cold turkey and see how quickly your tastes adjust (see the story of butter addict Eric, above). With this food you will really need to try many different brands to find the ones you like.

Cooking with cheese can be a problem. You have several options. There are some nonfat brands, and they are worth trying. Replace cottage cheese in dishes like lasagna with nonfat cottage cheese. Don't give up, and when a new brand comes out, give it a try. If nonfat cheeses are not to your taste, try cutting the cheese used in a recipe in half. Better yet, use one of the lower-fat (not nonfat, just lower-fat) varieties and cut the amount in half. You can replace the other half with nonfat cheese, or simply eliminate it. You can use sharper-tasting cheeses, such as extra-sharp cheddar, to get more cheese taste with less cheese fat. Parmesan cheese also adds a lot of flavor for relatively little fat.

All of these changes move you in the direction of using the higher-fat cheeses, which still hold the edge in flavor, as "spices" rather than as the main attraction in a dish. We'll pursue this further in Phase 2. For now, at the very least, cut the cheese in your dishes in half.

Sour cream

Several nonfat brands are now available. Tastes vary widely, so try more than one.

Coffee, tea, and espresso drinks

Coffee, tea, and espresso are examples of the impact that seemingly trivial changes can have. They show how increasing your awareness, simply in the area of dairy products, can help you lose significant amounts of weight, and avoid some high-fat traps that can sabotage your best efforts.

Straight coffee, tea, or espresso has no fat. If you drink these drinks with nothing added, you can stop here. But if you add even a little cream or milk, beware. And if you like your espresso drinks in the milk-diluted versions, you're in for a shock.

Let's say you drink two cups of coffee in a day, and you like about a tablespoon or so of cream in each. It gives the coffee a nice rich flavor, and takes away the bitterness. Unfortunately, you've just increased the fat in your diet by 3 percent. If you are about thirty pounds plumper than you'd like to be, simply stopping this habit, thus reducing the fat in your diet by 3 percent, will help you lose two to three pounds over the next year. Even the smallest changes have noticeable impact, and they all add up.

Nondairy creamers aren't much better than cream—they're *not* nonfat, they just use a different type of fat from milkfat. Switching to whole milk from cream lowers the amount of fat per tablespoon, but you tend to use more. As we've seen, "low-fat" milk is really high-fat, not a big improvement over whole milk. Skim or nonfat milk is really the only choice.

Beware of espresso drinks. Espresso, once the drink of beatniks and Marxist intellectuals plotting in dank coffeehouses, is now the favorite drink of baby boomers and Generation Xers. CPAs and students jostle to get their fixes at the espresso bars that seem to occupy every other shop in college towns. Farmers coming into small country villages can now relax over a latte.

You can unwittingly sabatoge your low-fat-eating efforts if you drink espresso drinks that contain milk. Especially beware of the mocha drinks, which contain enough fat to reverse completely any other dietary changes you might make if you drink them regularly.

The *Tufts University Diet and Nutrition Letter* analyzed espresso drinks from a number of different espresso bars. A Starbucks Cappuccino Grande contains 13 grams of fat, enough to send a 34-percent-fat diet to over 40 percent. If you drink their Cafe Mocha Grande daily, you can get a whopping 31 grams of fat. That could send a 25-percent-fat diet into orbit, increasing its fat content to over 40 percent. In a few swallows, you can completely negate months of dietary habit changes. *If you drink one of these daily, you're getting enough fat to raise your set point by ten to fifteen pounds over the course of a year.*

The alternatives made with low-fat milk aren't going to do you much good. They still contain two-thirds the fat of the whole-milk choices.

We've used Starbucks as an example of the bad news, but they are also a shining example of the good news—they are one of a growing number of espresso chains that provide skim-milk alternatives, which almost completely eliminates the fat in lattes and cappuccinos (but not in mocha, because the chocolate has an enormous amount of fat).

As usual, it boils down to a simple rule: Don't drink whole milk or "low-fat" milk. Not alone, and not mixed with other drinks. If you really want to cut fat from your diet, switch to skim milk for *all* the ways you use milk.

Nonfat dressings

You may think of your salad dressing as a minor source of fat in your diet, maybe something to put at the bottom of your list of changes to make. Think again. *The average nineteen-to-fifty-year-old woman gets more of her fat from salad dressing than from any other single food. Changing to a nonfat alternative may be the single largest change in fat you can make in your diet.*

Regular salad dressings are almost *pure fat.* Two tablespoons, a typical serving, contains up to 20 grams of fat. If you use this average serving, you increase the fat content of your diet by 10 percent. If you like to drown your salad in dressing, the increase could be even more than 10 percent. This means that if you start using a nonfat alternative you can drop that much fat from your diet—instantly.

Commercial dressings

There has truly been a fat-free revolution in the salad-dressing aisle of your supermarket. You will find a bewildering variety of choices. Narrow it down by, as always, only accepting fat-free or nonfat brands. Even then you'll find dozens to choose from. Start experimenting. One rule of thumb is to look for dressings that have ingredients you recognize, like vinegar, garlic, and spices, rather than an ingredients list that reads like something from Chemistry 101.

Make your own

We include one recipe in the recipes appendix. Many others are available in the books listed in our bibliography.

Lemon, vinegar

These are good choices in a restaurant, or even at home. Almost all restaurants have either lemon or vinegar and are usually more than happy to accommodate you.

Eat it plain

As you lose your taste for fat, a plain salad becomes appealing. Very appealing. The taste of the lettuce and other vegetables is enough. You don't *have* to go without dressing, but you might find it quite enjoyable.

Guideline 3: Eat at Least Five
Fruits and/or Vegetables Daily

This means five servings, total. It does not mean five servings of fruit and five of vegetables.

This also means actual fruits or vegetables, what you would buy at the produce section of your market. It does not mean juices. Ketchup does not count as a serving of tomato.

A banana would be one serving of fruit. So would a plum. A raw carrot would be one serving of vegetable. So would a cup of cooked vegetables. So would two cups of salad, as long as it was more than lettuce. Rule of thumb: a handful of fruit or vegetable is one serving. A double handful of salad counts as one serving.

There are only two fruits/vegetables to avoid: avocados and olives. Both are 80–99 percent fat. All other fruits and vegetables are very low fat, usually less than 5 percent fat. That's true no matter what they may feel like. For example, many people at our workshops ask us if bananas are high-fat, because they feel a little oily. But bananas are only 5 percent fat. So go wild in the produce section of your store—and prepare to change your wardrobe to smaller sizes as you lose fat.

There are three reasons to eat at least five fruits/vegetables daily, and two of them have to do with losing fat. At first glance, this may seem crazy. For most people, eating five fruits and/or vegetables per day means *adding* something to their diets—only about 9 percent of Americans now eat five fruits or vegetables a day. So 91 percent of us would have to add more food in the form of fruit or vegetables to our daily fare in order to hit this goal. How can you lose fat by *adding* to what you already eat?

Reason 1. Eating five fruits and/or vegetables will displace fat from your diet

Fruits and vegetables are among the lowest-fat foods around. If you eat five a day, you will be getting about 300–500 calories from this source. Your body is ever alert, and will detect those extra calories. If you eat 300–500 calories a day from fruit and vegetables, you will *automatically* adjust your appetite so that you eat 300–500 calories less from other sources (probably without noticing the change). *Since almost all other food sources are higher in fat than fruits and vegetables, you automatically decrease the amount of fat in your diet when you add fruits or vegetables.* Decreased fat means lower set point, which means you lose fat from your body—by *adding* foods to your diet.

This has been shown in many studies. For example, in some studies, people have been asked to eat five plain potatoes a day, in addition to the rest of their normal daily diet. That's all. They could eat whatever else they wanted, as long as they ate those five potatoes. Potatoes are about 150 calories each and have only 1 percent fat (they are a tremendously nutritious, very low fat food), so five a day means 750 calories a day with essentially no fat. The people in these studies *lost* weight, even though they were *adding* something to their diet. It's easy to see why, in terms of set point—750 nonfat calories displaced 750 high-fat calories from their normal diet, probably lowered the percentage of fat in their overall diet from 40 percent to 20–30 percent, which would result in substantial body-fat loss.

Reason 2. Fruits may decrease the desire for fat

Fruits get their sweetness from a type of sugar called fructose. In a study reported in 1990, researchers found that when people were given a dose of fructose their appetite in general and for fatty foods in particular diminished. So, if you eat fruit as snacks, you may find that it becomes easier at the next meal to avoid fat—pushing the fat content of your diet down still further.

Reason 3. *Eating five fruits and/or vegetables per day has profound effects on health and well-being*

About twenty years ago, studies were started in which thousands of people were asked in great detail what they ate in a typical day, as well as about every other aspect of their lives, from their jobs, to their smoking and drinking habits, to exercise habits, etc. Then, over the next fifteen years or so, the researchers kept track of the people's health: how many died, and from what, how many got ill, and what type of illnesses, etc. Over fifteen years, a lot of people died and a lot more got sick, and it was possible to find links between dietary habits and disease and death. The results of a number of these studies are just coming out, and they almost universally indicate that your mother was right—eat your fruits and vegetables if you want to be healthy.

Those who eat five or more servings of fruit and/or vegetables daily have *one-half* the chance of getting cancer that those who eat little or no fruit and vegetables have.

They also have about 25 percent less risk of heart attack. Above five servings daily doesn't seem to have much more protective effect (though it will certainly displace more fat from your diet).

Researchers also asked people about how they felt—not about how healthy they felt, but about their general feeling of well-being. Those who eat the most fruit and vegetables consistently report the highest feelings of well-being; they just feel good.

These results make sense in light of what is known about disease and nutrition. Many diseases may be caused by "free radicals," extremely reactive chemical compounds that are produced in our bodies all the time, and that also come at us in the form of smog, ozone, chemicals produced in skin by ultraviolet light, etc. There are anti-free-radical molecules called "antioxidants," which can eliminate free radicals from the body. Our cells make some of these on their own, but some must be supplied from the diet. Fruits and vegetables are among the richest natural sources of antioxidants, particularly ascorbate (vitamin C) and carotenoids. So it makes sense that if you eat more fruit and/or veggies you will have more protection against disease, which is exactly what appears to be the case.

And as we mentioned when discussing cancer, fruits and vegetables also contain phytochemicals, chemical compounds found in very small quantities that may have enormous protective effects against diseases. The study of phytochemicals is in its infancy, but it is one of the most exciting fields in nutrition today.

How to increase the number of fruits and/or vegetables that you eat

Eat a piece of fruit in the morning, first thing. Oranges are good—either navel or Valencia will be in season year-round. Eric slices one up and eats it over the kitchen sink about two minutes after rolling out of bed. But any type of fruit will get you going. Take three pieces of fruit and a carrot as part of your lunch and snack for the day. This may seem like a lot, but you'll often find you've finished all of it by noon. If you eat all of these, you are already at five fruits and/or veggies before you even dig into your dinner salad and vegetables. This way you're almost certain to get at least five every day, and usually more.

Also, be prepared to buy a helluva lot of fruits and veggies at the store. If you shop only for yourself, once a week, you will be buying about fifteen or twenty pieces of fruit and an equal number of vegetables. If your whole family of, say, five, starts to eat this way, you'll buy seventy-five to a hundred pieces of fruit alone each week. Fortunately, some fruits and vegetables are among the cheapest foods in the store (of course, if you insist on eating some types out of season you'll pay a lot more). Just don't strain your back carrying the groceries to the car!

The world's simplest low-fat diet

If you would like to get started on low-fat eating right now, without dropping anything from your diet or reading labels, we have a way of cutting the fat content of your diet by one-fourth to one-half.

The only skill required is the ability to count to ten. Do this: eat ten fruits and/or vegetables each day.

Do it every day and you automatically drop the fat content of your diet.

You're displacing fat calories, but on a bigger scale. Those ten fruits and vegetables have an average fat content of less than 5 percent, while adding up to about 700–1,000 calories. So, if you are a typical woman, eating, say, 1,800 calories a day, you have just made sure that about half of your daily calories are essentially nonfat. This will displace the calories that you were eating, which were probably 40 percent fat. The change happens automatically. When your body senses that you are taking in extra calories from the fruits and vegetables, it compensates by making you less hungry for the rest of the foods you eat. The net result is that the overall fat content of your diet drops from about 40 percent to about 20 percent.

It's not all that hard to eat so many fruits and vegetables, once it becomes a habit. Eat two pieces of fruit with breakfast (this may become your entire breakfast). Eat another piece of fruit or a carrot stick as part of your midmorning snack (bananas, at 100 calories and 5 percent fat, are an easily carried, easily eaten low-fat snack). Eat a portion of salad, another piece of fruit, and a carrot stick or two with lunch (make a double salad at night, save half in an airtight plastic container in the fridge and take it to work the next day for lunch). You will now have eaten six servings of fruit and vegetables by the end of lunch. The rest can come from midafternoon snacks, salad and vegetables at dinner, and a late-evening snack of fruit.

We're not saying you *have* to eat this way to eat low-fat, but it is *one* way to do it, and it is very healthful.

• • •

You can incorporate the changes suggested for Phase 1 into your life as slowly or as quickly as you want. You can stay at this level of low-fat eating for the rest of your life. Or you may find that you start to wonder what it would be like to drop the amount of fat you eat even more, to move into Phase 2.

8

Phase 2 of Low-Fat Eating—

10 Percent Calories from Fat

· · · · ·

Ten percent fat. This is the dietary fat level at which fat loss is the most rapid, improvements in health are most dramatic, and energy levels are highest. This is the level for people who want to be as lean and healthy as they can be. And this is the level that many old-school doctors and dieticians say is "radical" or "unpalatable" or "too difficult for the average person." To which we say, "Balderdash!" Don't let these patronizing know-it-alls bully you. They are being replaced by the new breed who know better, who know it's easy, it's tasty, and it's efficient to eat 10 percent calories from fat. And, given *their* diet, the new breed will be around for a vigorous century or so.

You may not want to come down to 10 percent fat. You may be perfectly happy with the weight you attain by eating 20 percent fat, especially if you are exercising a lot. If that's the case, you can just skip this chapter and the next one. But many people find that, even though they lose considerable weight by following Phase 1 guidelines for six to twelve months, they still are wearing more fat than is fashionable this season. And they don't have time to increase their exercise any more. There's only one way to go: down in the fat calories.

To make the Phase 2 transition to 10 percent calories from fat, you must learn three skills that allow you to avoid *all* high-fat foods:

SKILLS NEEDED TO
AVOID ALL HIGH-FAT FOODS

1. Judging the fat content of foods
2. Eating low-fat away from home
3. Preparing low-fat meals

Remember that to get to an eating level of 10 percent calories from fat you must follow the guidelines of both Phase 1 and Phase 2. Phase 1 cuts out the really super-high-fat foods. Phase 2 makes sure that the moderate-to-high-fat foods are also removed. What remains is 10 percent calories from fat, which, as you remember from Phase 1, is as low as you can go eating normal foods. It still allows you a huge variety of food, but skill is required to weed out the moderate-to-high-fat foods. They are the ones that nickel-and-dime you to death when you are trying to eat low-fat, so you need to put some effort into knowing what's what. But the rewards are worth it.

As with Phase 1, the easiest way to cut the remaining excess fat out of the diet is to look at foods from the standpoint of their percentage of fat. You simply *always* avoid the foods that are greater than 20 percent fat, eat moderately from those that are 10–20 percent fat, and pig out on those that are less than 10 percent fat. You will be eating 10 percent fat automatically if you do this.

Judging the fat content of foods is an obvious, necessary first step in avoiding high-fat foods. In this phase of the program, you will learn to assess the fat content of any food at a glance, whether packaged or unpackaged. It's especially important not to be intimidated by labels, which seem to get more complicated with every political tide. You'll find out that there are only two numbers, both at the very top of the label, that you need to look at to judge the fat content of food. The rest you can ignore.

After learning to judge fat content of food, you will be using your knowledge to make low-fat choices whenever and wherever you eat.

There are only two places you will be eating: outside your home, where you may have little control over how food is prepared, and inside your home, where you usually have complete control.

Eating away from home usually means either at a restaurant or as a guest in someone's home. You'll learn some simple guidelines to help you make the lowest-fat (but still-tasty) choices in these situations. We'll also give you some tips for traveling.

Eating at home usually means cooking. Low-fat cooking isn't some mystical experience, best preceded by a few hours of meditation and prayer. It's really just a modification of the way you cook now. You already learned most of what you need to know in Phase 1—now it's just a matter of applying it to recipes. In this section, we'll emphasize cutting preparation-and-cooking time while still preparing tasty, low-fat meals that you can eat on a regular basis. Preparing low-fat meals may seem like a big chore, especially if you go by the recipes in some of the fancier low-fat cook books. But let's face it: if you're not a gourmet cook now, you are unlikely to become one just to cut the fat out of your diet. Fortunately, cooking low-fat can be incorporated into your normal life and requires no extra time or effort. You just need knowledge.

As with Phase 1, before you start you'll take a diagnostic quiz. After that, we suggest that you read the entire chapter, then go back to the Hot Spots you've identified on the quiz.

Where's the Rest of the Fat?

For each of the following statements, choose the single answer that most accurately reflects the way you eat or think. Place the letter of the answer you selected on the line in front of the question. The quiz is divided into three sections corresponding to the different skills you'll learn in Phase 2. The page numbers following each question tell you where you will find information in this chapter about the eating habits referred to in the question.

You may note a little overlap with Phase 1 principles. These are areas that apply to both phases.

Section 1: Can You Accurately Judge the Fat Content of Foods?

_____ 1. I eat avocado (on salads or in other foods, such as Mexican cooking) (page 139)

A. less than once a week
C. 2–3 times a week

B. once a week
D. 4 or more times a week

_____ 2. I eat olives (as hors d'oeuvres, in pasta, or in other foods, such as Mexican cooking) (page 139)

A. less than once a week
C. 2–3 times a week

B. once a week
D. 4 or more times a week

_____ 3. Soy milk is lower in fat than cow's milk. (page 140)

A. No

D. Yes

_____ 4. Tofu is a low-fat substitute for meat. (page 140)

A. No

D. Yes

_____ 5. I eat some type of red meat at lunch (remember, hamburgers have red meat in them) (page 137)

A. less than once a week
C. 2–3 times a week

B. once a week.
D. 4 or more times a week

_____ 6. I eat some type of red meat at dinner (page 137)

A. less than once a week
C. 2–3 times a week

B. once a week
D. 4 or more times a week

_____ 7. I eat chicken thighs, drumsticks, wings, or backs (page 138)

A. less than once a week
C. 2–3 times a week

B. once a week
D. 4 or more times a week

_____ 8. I eat chicken or turkey with the skin (page 138)

A. less than once a week   B. once a week
C. 2–3 times a week   D. 4 or more times a week

_____ 9. I know which types of fish are low-fat and which are high-fat. (page 141)

A. Yes   D. No

_____ 10. I eat eggs (complete with yolks) (page 138)

A. less than once a week   B. once a week
C. 2–3 times a week   D. 4 or more times a week

_____ 11. I use eggs (complete with yolks) in my cooking (in sauces, salads, baking, sandwich spreads, etc.) (page 138)

A. less than once a week   B. once a week
C. 2–3 times a week   D. 4 or more times a week

_____ 12. I *always* read food labels on new foods that I buy, and occasionally check the labels even of foods that I buy every week. (page 142)

A. Yes   D. No
If you answered yes to question 12, then answer questions 13–15.

_____ 13. When I look at food labels, I look first for calorie content, not fat content. (page 142)

A. No   D. Yes

_____ 14. When I look at a food label, if the number of fat grams per servings is over 4, I don't eat it. (page 142)

A. No   D. Yes

_____ 15. I eat foods labeled "reduced-fat," "low-fat," "lean," "diet," "light," or "healthy" (page 147)

A. less than once a week   B. once a week
C. 2–3 times a week   D. 4 or more times a week

Section 2: Do You Know How to Eat Low-Fat Away from Home?

_____ 16. I have found several restaurants in my area that serve good-tasting, low-fat fare. (page 152)

A. Yes   D. No

_____ 17. When I eat in a restaurant, I always scan the menu for the low-fat entrees and order those. (page 154)

A. Yes   D. No

_____ 18. When I eat in a restaurant, I specify to the waiter or waitress *exactly* how I want my food, with no oil used in preparation and no high-fat sauces or other ingredients. (page 155)

A. Yes   D. No

_____ 19. If I'm going out to dinner, either to a restaurant or to friends', I skimp on eating during the day, so that I can eat more calories at dinner. (page 152)

A. No   D. Yes

_____ 20. When I eat as a guest, I eat several servings of the low-fat items, while eating only small single servings of the high-fat items. (page 157)

A. Yes   D. No

Section 3: Do You Know How to Cook Low-Fat?

_____ 22. I own a nonstick skillet. (page 113)

A. Yes   D. No

_____ 23. I use *no* oil, butter, or shortening when I cook, except occasional tiny amounts of flavored oils (like Chinese sesame oil or chili oil). (page 113)

A. Yes   D. No

_____ 24. I use high-fat cheeses in recipes as a flavoring *only,* never using more than one-fourth the amount that a recipe calls for. (page 161)

A. Yes   D. No

_____ 25. When I cook with packaged foods, I read labels to be sure that the final product will not be more than 10 percent fat. (page 168)

A. Yes   D. No

_____ 26. I use no egg yolks in my cooking. (page 161)

A. Yes   D. No

_____ 27. I use only *skinless* turkey or chicken *breast,* or low-fat fish, as meat in my recipes. (page 162)

A. Yes   D. No

_____ 28. I have a collection of low-fat recipes that have been taste-tested by me and anyone else who eats my cooking regularly. (page 165)

A. Yes   D. No

_____ 29. I know how to spot high-fat ingredients in recipes and how to modify recipes to eliminate them. (page 164)

A. Yes   D. No

_____ 30. I regularly make up a menu and a shopping list, so I'm not caught in the middle of the week with my pantry down. (page 170)

A. Yes   D. No

_____ 31. I make large batches of favorite low-fat meals and freeze them, as well as keeping available the ingredients for several quick and easy low-fat meals, for days when I have no time to cook. (page 170)

A. Yes   D. No

Any question with a "D" answer represents a "Hot Spot" for you. *Hot Spots are eating habits that keep you fat.* Questions with "B" or "C" answers are less urgent Hot Spots, but nevertheless areas where you can cut fat. Not until you reach an "A" have you cut all the fat possible from an area of your eating.

Now it's time to learn the skills that you need to become as lean and healthy as you can be.

1. Judging the Fat Content of Foods

When you go into a supermarket, with its thousands of food choices, or into a restaurant, with its dozens of choices, you can feel a bit overwhelmed. Are you going to have to learn the fat content of every one of these foods in order to eat low-fat?

No! You don't need to memorize lengthy tables of the fat contents of foods. Those thousands of foods in the supermarket break down into only two types: unlabeled and labeled. The foods in the produce section, the meats, and a few other unpackaged items don't have labels. All the rest of the foods are packaged, and have labels. So we'll divide all foods up into these two types, and talk about judging fat content of each type:

- **Unlabeled foods**
  There are only two groups, low-fat and high-fat.

- **Labeled foods**
  A couple of simple rules will tell you whether to buy it or leave it on the shelf. In ten minutes you can become a label-reading expert.

Unlabeled foods

Unlabeled foods are easily divided into two groups, high-fat and low-fat. There really isn't much middle ground here.

Unlabeled foods, high-fat

In Phase 1, you have already learned to avoid the super-high-fat foods: oils, nuts, seeds, high-fat dairy, salad dressings. These foods, *plus* two additional types of unlabeled high-fat foods, are responsible for 90 percent of the fat in your diet.

What are the other types? High-fat meats and egg yolks. That's it. The two types of food to avoid, in addition to those in Phase 1, are:

HIGH-FAT UNLABELED FOODS: AVOID

1. **All meats** except skinless white turkey breast and chicken breast, and some fish
2. **Egg yolks**

For decades, the meat industry has strived to produce meat that is ever more marbled with fat—because that was what Americans liked, and what we bought. As a result, domesticated animals have become fat, bloated caricatures of the wild game that our ancestors used to hunt. Can you imagine a herd of domestic cattle trying to avoid a natural predator, like a wolf? Half of them would keel over from heart attacks during the stampede.

Now that consumer demand has shifted toward lower-fat fare, however, the meat producers are back-pedaling at world-record pace, trying to produce meats that they can label "low-fat" or "lean." They *are* producing some leaner cuts, but as of this writing there is no form of red meat that derives less than 10 percent of its calories from fat—which would be a *true* low-fat meat.

Even the "leanest" beef, labeled "10 percent fat," such as filet mignon or New York strip, is 30–40 percent calories from fat. How do the manufacturers get away with that? This "lean" beef is 10 percent fat by weight, not calories. *You can assume that any type of meat (except skinless light chicken or turkey, and some fish) is at least 30 percent calories from fat and probably over 50 percent—no matter how it is labeled.* Don't let sleazy food industries desperate to cash in on the "low-fat craze" fool you. By the way, the meat and dairy industries are still allowed to practice this deceptive way of designating percent fat by weight because their lobbyists made sure that loopholes were inserted in current labeling laws. You can teach them a lesson by simply avoiding their products—and in the process lose weight and gain health.

Do you have to give up meat completely? No. Turkey breast and chicken breast, without skin, are moderately low-fat, as are many types of fish (as you will see in the next section).

But you must be careful. Many people think that, since they've switched to chicken or turkey, they are now eating low-fat meats. But that is true *only* for turkey or chicken breast without skin (and even the chicken is a little high, at 20 percent fat). *Turkey dark meat and chicken dark meat are high-fat*—dark turkey meat, even without skin, is 34 percent fat; chicken dark meat without skin is 43 percent fat. And *even breast of turkey or chicken must have the skin removed, because it adds half the fat.*

What about eggs? Hard-boiled eggs have long been the staple of a dieter's lunch. High in protein! Low in calories! But the yolk is loaded with fat, over 80 percent. The white has no fat. Because the yolk contributes most of the calories, the overall fat content of an egg (yolk plus white) is 64 percent. Eggs are not a diet food, at least as long as you leave the yolk in. We've been very specific here, because egg whites are still quite useful in baking and other cooking, and if you do get a dish in a restaurant with hard-boiled eggs, you can either avoid the eggs completely, or eat the whites.

Unlabeled foods, low-fat

Many unlabeled foods will be your tremendous allies, because they are so low in fat that you can eat all you want. Let's look at those foods. The first category is already familiar to you from Phase 1:

LOW-FAT UNLABELED FOODS

1. All fruits and vegetables (*except* avocado and olives)
2. All whole grains, legumes (*except* soybeans and soybean products such as tofu); grains include oats, wheat, rice, barley, corn; beans and legumes include kidney, black, red, white, pinto, peas, lentils
3. *Skinless* light turkey meat, some fish, and small amounts of skinless chicken breast

---

Fruits and vegetables

We encouraged you in Phase 1, and we encourage you again: go to the produce section of your store and go wild. Apples, bananas, grapefruits, and oranges are almost always available; other fruits are seasonal. A huge variety of vegetables is available year-round. Frozen vegetables and frozen fruits (such as berries) contain almost all the nutrients of fresh. As we cautioned in Phase 1, avoid avocados and olives (80–99 percent fat).

Beans and grains

Beans are incredibly low-fat, ranging from less than 1 percent (lentils and peas) to 4 percent (kidney beans, pinto beans). That's one reason why switching to a vegetarian diet, and substituting beans for meat, can be so helpful for weight loss and health. Grains are also quite low-fat: brown rice and whole wheat are 5 percent fat, corn is 10 percent fat, oats, the only grain above 10 percent fat, are 18 percent fat. You might also consider potatoes an "honorary grain," because, at 1 percent fat, they can be one of the staples of a low-fat, healthful diet.

If you buy dried beans and dried grains and cook them yourself, you can be sure that the fat contents remain low. You don't have to cook beans or grains from scratch, however. As discussed in Phase 1, you can buy canned beans of many different types. Many grains come as packaged, easily prepared dishes, or as dried breakfast cereals, many of which are also fine (you must read the labels, which you will learn to do in the next section). Grains, of course, are also in breads, pastas, tortillas, bagels, etc. All of these easier-to-use versions of beans and grains are perfectly acceptable *as long as you check the labels to make sure the manufacturer hasn't slipped in some fat.*

Inevitably, when the topic of beans comes up at a workshop, jokes about flatulence are not far behind. Some people are far more affected than others. The problem is that bacteria that normally live in your gut use some of the starches in beans as fuel, with intestinal gas as a byproduct. There are several approaches to minimizing the problem.

First, if you cook your own beans, cover them with water, boil for three or four minutes, then let sit for one hour. Pour out the water and use new water to cook the beans. This will get rid of some of the starches that the bacteria use.

Second, introduce beans slowly, and don't eat large amounts at any one meal.

Third, experiment. You may be affected by kidney beans but not lentils, or vice versa. Start with the types that affect you least.

Fourth, there are products that you can use prior to a bean-containing meal that will digest the starches before the bacteria can. Ask at your drugstore. One popular brand is Beano. Studies show these products really work.

Finally, be patient. As your intestinal bacterial population changes to types that thrive on your new diet, you may find that your problems disappear.

Beware of soybeans and soybean tofu. Tofu has built a reputation as a healthful meat substitute, and many people believe that tofu is a low-fat alternative to meat. *Soybeans are 40 percent fat. Soybean tofu is 52 percent calories from fat.* Though tofu is probably more healthful than meat (some studies indicate that soybean products contain cancer-fighting substances), it is simply not part of a truly low-fat diet. Some "low-fat" brands are now appearing that may be acceptable (under 20 percent fat). Check the label to make sure it really is low-fat before you use it.

Meats
As discussed, there aren't many meats that fall into the low-fat category. Turkey and chicken (*breast* only, *skinless* only) are it, and chicken

is marginal. Many stores now carry ground turkey breast (make sure it is skinless; many types aren't), which works as a substitute for other meats in an enormous variety of dishes—more on this when we talk about cooking low-fat.

Fish
A lot of people are eating less meat and more fish because they think all fish is low-fat. In fact, some fish is incredibly high in fat, as high as many red meats. These high-fat fish include herring (53 percent fat), Atlantic mackerel (62 percent), orange roughy (48 percent), salmon (45 percent fat), and shad (62 percent fat).

But there are enough truly low-fat fishes and shellfish to allow you to eat a different seafood dish every night for over two weeks, if you desire. It's especially important to know at least a few of these when ordering in restaurants, since many restaurants feature fish dishes. At least *sole and snapper, both of which are about 15 percent fat, are widely available at restaurants.* Take the time to learn the following list if you like fish.

Type of fish	Percent fat	Type of shellfish	Percent fat
Tuna, yellowfin	6%	Scallops	8%
Sole	8%	Crawfish	8%
Haddock	8%	Lobster	9%
Perch	8%	Shrimp	9%
Pike	8%	Clams	12%
Pollack	8%		
Lingcod	8%		
Cod	9%		
Red snapper	14%		
Flounder	15%		
Rockfish	15%		

Some brands of *water-packed* light tuna are only about 6 percent fat (as with all packaged food, you will have to check the label; some brands use different varieties of tuna, which are higher in fat).

Labeled foods

Reading labels

Labeled foods with nutritional breakdowns allow you to estimate the percent fat in the food, and determine whether the food is low-fat. *You* must make this decision. Do not rely on the food manufacturer or even the government to do it for you. Food manufacturers lie without hesitation to cash in on the low-fat craze. And the governmental agencies are dominated by old-school medical folk, and swayed by lobbyists from the food industry. A packaged food that the Food and Drug Administration allows to be labeled "low-fat" may be very high in fat. And even the government's "official" breakdown of the fat content of foods (the Percent Daily Value) is misleading, because it is based on a high-fat (30-percent-fat) diet.

Fortunately, labels contain some bits of truth. These nuggets are easy to find and easy to evaluate, so that you can tell in a few seconds whether a food is low-, medium-, or high-fat, without carrying your calculator with you to the store.

As of May 1994, 90 percent of processed foods are required to carry the new "Nutrition Facts" label. *You can use this label to decide instantly whether a food is going to make you fat or keep you lean.* However, although these labels are far superior to the old ones, there are still pitfalls to be aware of when dealing with packaged foods.

Let's take a look at one of the Nutrition Facts labels. This is the label for smoked cooked ham:

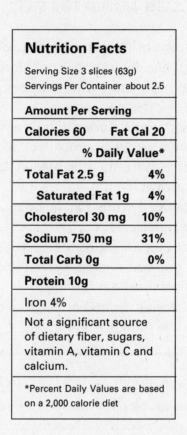

Nutrition Facts

Serving Size 3 slices (63g)
Servings Per Container about 2.5

Amount Per Serving

Calories 60	Fat Cal 20

% Daily Value*

Total Fat 2.5 g	**4%**
Saturated Fat 1g	**4%**
Cholesterol 30 mg	**10%**
Sodium 750 mg	**31%**
Total Carb 0g	**0%**
Protein 10g	
Iron 4%	

Not a significant source
of dietary fiber, sugars,
vitamin A, vitamin C and
calcium.

*Percent Daily Values are based
on a 2,000 calorie diet

*The only part of a label you need to look at to judge a food's fat con-
tent is the Amount Per Serving section.* It shows Calories, and Calories
from Fat. All the rest can actually be confusing, as we'll explain.

We teach a two-step method for estimating the percentage of fat in
a product. It requires no calculator, and very little practice. People get
the hang of it in about ten or fifteen minutes in our workshops. So
here's our:

LABEL-READING TWO-STEP:

1. **Find 10 percent of the total calories.** Under Amount Per Serving, find the number of calories. Knock off the last digit. The remaining number is 10 percent of the total calories per serving.
2. **Compare with Fat Calories.** Find the Calories from Fat. Compare it with the number you found in step 1.
   a. **If the Calories from Fat is below 10 percent: the food is LOW-FAT.**
   b. **If the Calories from Fat is below 20 percent: the food is MEDIUM-FAT.**
      (To get 20 percent of the calories, double the number you got in step 1. That is 20 percent of the total calories in a serving.)
   c. **If the Calories from Fat is above 20 percent calories, the food is HIGH-FAT.**

Let's look at a few examples from the soup aisle of our supermarket, which contains dozens of brands. We selected four that all *looked* low-fat, at least from the claims on the front of the label. But whereas three of our choices can be the centerpieces of low-fat, lean, and healthful meals, the fourth can lead you into a high-fat disaster.

Example 1: Navy Bean Soup. Sounds good; we know beans can be very low fat. What does the label say? We zero in on Nutrition Facts, Amount Per Serving, where we see:

Amount Per Serving

Calories   140   Calories from Fat   0

This soup contains no fat! You don't need to look any farther than that to know that this food is as low-fat as they come, and a perfect choice as part of a low-fat meal.

Example 2: Red Beans and Rice Soup. The Nutrition Facts are:

Amount Per Serving

Calories   190   Calories from Fat   15

There is certainly some fat in this soup. But is it still a low-fat food? Let's follow our label-reading procedure:

Step 1: The number of Calories is 190. If we knock off the last digit we have 19. So 10 percent of the total calories is 19 calories.

Step 2: The Calories from Fat is 15.

The 15 fat calories are less than the 19 calories that we found in step 1 to be 10 percent of the total calories. This soup contains less than 10 percent calories from fat, and is a good part of a lean and healthy meal.

Example 3: Chicken Noodle Soup. Chicken is a low-fat meat, isn't it? And noodles are made from grain, which is low-fat. Not only that, it says on the can "97% FAT FREE." If it's 97 percent fat-free it must be only 3 percent fat. Sounds as if we've got another winner. Let's just confirm it by checking the Nutrition Facts:

Amount Per Serving

Calories   70   Calories from Fat   30

Even if your math is a little rusty, you can see that this soup is *not* 3 percent fat. Let's follow our label-reading procedure:

Step 1: The number of Calories is 70. If we knock off the last digit we have 7. Ten percent of the total calories is 7 calories.

Step 2: The Calories from Fat is 30.

Thirty calories from fat is a lot more than the 7 calories that we found in step 1 to be 10 percent of the total calories. This soup contains more than 10 percent calories from fat.

Is it less than 20 percent calories from fat? To find what 20 percent would be, double the number of calories that we found to be 10 percent of the total (7 calories):

$$2 \times 7 = 14 \text{ calories.}$$

So 20 percent of the total calories would be 14 calories. Thirty calories from fat is a lot more than the 14 calories that represent 20 percent of the total. This soup contains more than 20 percent calories from fat. It is a high-fat food. Put it back on the shelf.

We'll explain in detail how a "97% FAT FREE" food can contain over 20 percent fat in just a minute. First let's look at a final example.

Example 4: Split Pea with Ham Soup. After our experience with Chicken Noodle Soup, we know to be skeptical about any claims concerning fat percentage. This one says it's "98% FAT FREE." Yeah, sure. It's got ham in it. It's probably a fat-fest, but let's check it out:

Amount Per Serving

Calories 170	Calories from Fat 25

Step 1: The number of Calories is 170. If we knock off the last digit we have 17. Ten percent of the total calories is 17 calories.

Step 2: The Calories from Fat is 25.

The 25 calories are more than the 17 calories that we found in step 1 to be 10 percent of the total calories. This soup is greater than 10 percent calories from fat.

Is it less than 20 percent calories from fat? To find what 20 percent of the total calories would be, double the number of calories that we found to be 10 percent of the total (17 calories):

$$2 \times 17 = 34.$$

So 20 percent of the total calories would be 34 calories. The 25 calories from fat are less than the 34 calories. This soup contains less than 20 percent calories from fat. It can be part of a low-fat diet if used in moderation.

You should practice this label-reading technique until it's second nature. *It is the single most important skill that you can learn to help you with eating 10 percent fat.* Go to your cupboard right now and get out some packaged foods. Practice the method on several items. The next time you go to the store, choose one particular food type—cereal, or bread, or yogurt, or whatever—and compare brands. You'll be amazed at the range of fat levels in different brands of the same food. And now you can choose the brands with the lowest fat.

Label pitfalls

These examples make it obvious that the only information you can trust on a label is the Nutrition Facts box—the only place where the manufacturer *must* tell the truth. Everywhere else, they will lie as much as the government allows (and it allows a lot) in order to fool you into thinking a product is something it's not. Even the Nutrition Facts can be confusing if you look at some of the other information at the bottom of the label. You can avoid label-reading pitfalls by following a few rules:

*1. Never trust a manufacturer's claim of "low-fat," "lean,"
"reduced-calorie," "reduced-fat," "light," "diet," etc.*
The Food and Drug Administration has set certain standards a food must meet if it is to display such claims, but there are exceptions and loopholes galore. For example, the FDA now says that "low-fat" means that a food can have no more than 3 grams of fat per serving. That is, unless it's an entree, which can have 3 grams of fat per every 100 grams (about three and a half ounces) of total weight. And either way, there is no limit to the percentage of calories from fat that those 3 grams could represent. The term becomes almost meaningless. The same is true for "lean." A food can be labeled "lean" if it has no more than 10 grams of fat. That's an enormous amount, about half of the total fat that you would eat in one day on a 10-percent-fat diet—all coming from one serving of one food.

And so it goes. Assume that all claims on the package are lies. Find the Nutrition Facts box and use it, and it alone, to make your decision.

2. Never trust manufacturers' claims about percentage of fat.
Manufacturers can legally claim a much lower percentage of fat than is actually in the product, and they do so for the sole purpose of deceiving you so that you will buy it.

When we teach label-reading at our workshops, this is the part that really opens people's eyes.

"I've been eating this '93% percent fat-free' lunch meat for months. Now I see that it's over 50 percent fat! No wonder I was *gaining* weight," said one participant.

Other typical comments:

"I don't believe they can get away with this."

"These are plain old lies."

"I'm really angry. I thought the government was supposed to protect consumers against this kind of deception."

Some examples: Two of the soups we analyzed in the examples claimed to be 97 percent and 98 percent fat-free, yet both contained more than 10 percent fat. The soup claiming to be 97 percent fat-free was actually *43 percent calories* from fat. You see the same sort of deception in the dairy case: milk that claims to be 2 percent fat is actually *37 percent fat.* If you walk over to the lunch meats, you'll find 96 percent fat-free meat that's really *33 percent fat.* In fact, once you realize what's going on, you'll spot dozens of examples on your next trip to the supermarket.

How can a soup say on its label that it's 97 percent fat-free yet contain 43 percent calories from fat? It's 97 percent fat-free by *weight,* not by calories. A lot of the weight in a soup, and in many other foods, comes from water. Water has no calories, nor does it contain fat. So a large proportion of the weight is "fat-free," but the actual percentage of calories from fat can be as high as 100 percent!

Let's take an example. Imagine a glass of water. It has no calories, but it weighs a substantial amount. Now imagine that you place a pat of butter in the water and blend it thoroughly. You market your product as "Butterade—the new butter-flavored drink that's 99 percent fat-free! With real butter!" It's 99 percent fat-free because butter represents only 1 percent of the weight. But butter represents *all* of the calories, and since butter is 100 percent fat, 100 percent of the calories in this drink are from fat. Drink enough "99 percent fat-free" Butterade and you will become a butterball.

The FDA has tightened up in this area, but, again, there are so many loopholes that regulation is meaningless. Much of the confusion arises because meat and dairy products are regulated by the USDA, not the FDA, and manufacturers are still allowed to make such claims of fat percentage based on weight.

Once again, your defense is the Nutrition Facts.

3. Don't worry about calories.
It's the *percent calories from fat* that's important, not the total calories. Remember, your body will regulate the amount of fat on it strictly on

the basis of the percentage of fat in your diet (and the amount of exercise you get). Pay no attention whatsoever to the number of calories in a serving. More is *not* bad. Less is *not* better.

For example, if we rank the soups we analyzed from fewest to most calories per serving, we get the following relationships (here we have calculated exact percentages of fat in the soups):

Soup	Calories per serving	Percent calories from fat
Chicken Noodle	70	43
Navy Bean	140	0
Split Pea with Ham	170	15
Red Beans and Rice	190	8

The calorie-conscious eater would choose the chicken noodle soup—and wonder why he seems to keep adding more and more chicken fat to his belly. The fat-conscious eater might choose the red beans and rice or navy bean, with at least twice the calories—and watch her fat melt away.

4. Don't be confused by the "% Daily Value" in the middle of the label.
You may find numbers that seem to refer to percentage of fat in the Nutrition Facts label, yet bear no relation to the actual percentage of fat in the food. What do these numbers mean, and why are they there?

Let's look again at our original label example for smoked cooked ham ("96% FAT FREE," shouts the front of the package), on page 143.

The first thing you see on the label is that the "96% FAT FREE" claim is the usual lie. With 20 of its 60 calories from fat, this food is really 33 percent fat, and has no place in a true low-fat diet. Yet under "% Daily Value" the label says "Total Fat . . . 4%." Is this food 33 percent fat or 4 percent fat??

It's 33 percent fat. The % Daily Value represents the percent of the maximum amount of fat that you should eat in one day that you will find in one serving of this food. It has nothing to do with the percent of calories that come from fat in that serving. To make matters even more confusing, the U.S. government has decided that the amount of fat you should strive for in one day is about 65 grams (for a 2,000-calorie diet, that's about 30 percent fat), rather than the optimal 20 grams, which would represent a 10-percent-fat diet.

If reading the last paragraph has brought back terrifying memories from high-school algebra, just remember that you don't need this information on % Daily Value for Total Fat, that it is misleading, and ignore it. You can never go wrong with the two-step label-reading for fat content, which will always steer you toward decisions based on an optimal fat content of 10 percent or less.

We'll say it again. *You can avoid all these pitfalls by going straight to the Amount Per Serving section of the Nutrition Facts, and judging the percentage of fat for yourself. This part of the label never lies.*

Labels without Nutrition Facts
Very occasionally, a label will have only a list of ingredients. If the food contains a high-fat ingredient, avoid it. Period. You know already, from Phase 1 and the first part of Phase 2, what high-fat ingredients are:

- oils of any type, including hydrogenated and partially hydrogenated oil
- shortening or lard
- nuts, seeds
- butter, margarine, mayonnaise
- any dairy products that are not specified as nonfat or skim
- meat

Ninety percent of the time, the fat in a food is oil. Read with care! When in doubt, throw it out.

"Fat-free" does not mean "nutritious"
We've emphasized fat percentage in these label-reading instructions, because this book is primarily about weight loss. And fat content is the number-one concern for those who wish to lose weight.

But we know you understand that a food is not nutritious just because it's less than 10 percent fat. You can't eat bags of fat-free cookies as the staple of your daily fare and expect to be eating a nutritious diet. Those cookies are fine as dessert, but cookies have never been a healthful main course. That's not going to change just because the fat has been removed. Empty calories are still empty calories. Fruit is still a better snack than a nonfat cake. You still should be eating a healthful entree for dinner (like the ones we have included in the recipes appendix) along with vegetables and salad. Then have the nonfat ice cream for dessert.

You knew this already. We just wanted to remind you gently.

•　•　•

That's it. You now have the information to determine whether just about any food fits into a 10-percent-fat diet. Now you need to apply your skills to the situations that you face every day. You will either be eating away from home or at home. Let's look at how to put your fat-detecting abilities to work in each of these situations.

2. Eating Low-Fat Away from Home

When you are not eating at home, you are usually eating either at a restaurant, where you have considerable control over the food you are served, or as a guest in someone's home, where you have less control over the food you are served.

Either way, there is a choice to be made. Will you eat low-fat or not? Make the choice consciously, and then enjoy. Choosing to eat high-fat for a special occasion will not ruin your life. So, if you're someone for whom eating at a restaurant is a special treat, to be indulged in once a month, and you also eat at friends' tables only once a month or so, you can eat high-fat and consider these your "feast days." It will add a couple percent to the overall fat content of your diet, which most people find acceptable. If you don't find that acceptable, follow the guidelines below carefully.

On the other hand, if you eat two meals a day at restaurants, you *must* learn how to make those healthful, low-fat eating occasions. For you, this will be a key section.

You are making a choice in these situations whether you do it consciously or not. If you decide not to bother with it, your choice, by default, is generally going to be a high-fat meal. Be aware that if that's happening more than once every couple of weeks you will not be eating low-fat and your set point will rise.

Eating at restaurants

We'll give some general rules, followed by specific suggestions for each meal.

When eating at restaurants, there are four aspects you may be able to control:

- how hungry you are when you get there
- the restaurant itself
- what you order
- how it's prepared

The choices you make in all four of these areas will determine whether you're eating a low-fat, slimming meal, or a high-fat, artery-clogging gut-buster.

Don't be ravenously hungry when you arrive at the restaurant
The first choice, and one that many people don't even realize they have, is whether to be starving or not when they arrive at the restaurant.

Many people with the dieting mentality think that they can skip breakfast and lunch, and then use those "extra" calories that they have saved to go wild at a restaurant in the evening; they eat more calories than usual at dinner, but that's okay because they saved them up from the rest of the day. *This is perhaps the single most effective way to put on fat at the highest possible rate.*

Why? Because you are so ravenously hungry when you get to the restaurant, all caution is thrown to the winds. No matter what your good intentions when you walk in the restaurant, you end up ordering the highest-fat option on the menu, because you are getting signals from your body that you need a lot of calories *now*. Then the high-fat meal nudges your set point up even higher.

Instead, if you are going out to dinner, eat your normal low-fat breakfast and lunch. Even eat a fairly large (low-fat) snack before dinner if you want. Then, when you get to the restaurant, your hunger won't overpower your better judgment. You'll be able to order a low-fat option and enjoy it. If it is a business meal, you will appreciate the fact that your thinking isn't dulled by the high-fat overload. If it's a social occasion, you'll be fueled up and ready to go for the rest of the evening, without drooping eyelids and the feeling of grease oozing from your pores. The next day, you'll wake up rested and refreshed, rather than with a high-fat hangover.

Choose a restaurant where you have a fighting chance
The second choice is the restaurant itself. If you've decided that a particular restaurant-eating occasion is going to be a feast day, then simply choose according to what suits your tastes at the moment, which may be very high fat indeed (remember, it's a feast, not everyday fare).

But if you are eating lunch at a restaurant every day, you want it to be one where you can get low-fat options that suit your palate. Many restaurants, especially in major urban areas, make a special effort to provide low-fat entrees. You can even get very low-fat meals at most fast-food restaurants. It is your job to seek out the ones in your area and to try them, finding one or more that suit you.

Such restaurants are not necessarily obvious. We'd been living in our present home for over two years before we discovered a little fast-food Mexican restaurant, six blocks from our house, where the owner uses no oil in his cooking, very little cheese, serves beans that haven't been cooked in lard. . . . It's a low-fat haven for days when we're just too rushed to cook. But there is no neon sign outside flashing LOW-FAT.

Call around and ask if the restaurant serves Pritikin dishes or other very low fat food, if they sauté their vegetables or meats in oil, and, if so, if it's possible to have them sautéed in water. Ask if they have a salad bar. Are fish or vegetarian dishes available? These won't necessarily be low-fat, but they at least have a chance of being so. Dishes in which red meat is the centerpiece can't possibly be low-fat.

Seafood restaurants, especially, will have a number of low-fat options, because so many fish are very low fat, and you can usually get them broiled or blackened, both low-fat methods of preparation. Visit several restaurants and eat at them, ordering from the menu as we will describe below. Beware of menu pitfalls, however. Remember that what a restaurant calls "low-fat" or "heart-healthy" may really be high-fat. Make a systematic effort to find the low-fat jewels for your daily eating and you will be rewarded with leanness, vitality, and health.

Order the fat to disappear

Once you've selected a restaurant, your third choice is what to order.

The Center for Science in the Public Interest periodically evaluates restaurants of different types in terms of the healthfulness of their meals and releases its results. These invariably make headlines screaming that the particular type of restaurant evaluated has nothing but high-fat horrors available to the unwary eater. Chinese, Italian, and Mexican restaurants were found to be dens of oil-laden, fat-dripping, greasy grimy gopher guts—or at least that's what the stories on the local news said. Lost in all the shouting was the fact that, in every case, the CPSI also found low-fat options—entrees below 20 percent fat, and often vegetables and salads galore.

What you often must do is follow Sherlock Holmes' dictum: "When you have eliminated the impossible, whatever is left, no matter how improbable, is the true low-fat option." (Okay, we modified it a little bit, but we feel that this is the *spirit* of what Sherlock meant.)

So first eliminate the impossible. This means using your knowledge of high-fat foods, from Phase 1 and Phase 2, to eliminate some dishes instantly. Oils, butter, red meats, and milk products (unless they are nonfat) are all items that you know have huge amounts of fat. Sometimes you can get rid of the higher-fat part of an entree by discussing it with your waiter or waitress. But sometimes entrees read like an itemized list of the highest-fat foods ever eaten by human beings. An entree that reads "Tender medallions of veal sautéed in heart-healthy olive oil and served with a cream sauce" is beyond hope. In general, high-fat red meats such as beef, pork, and lamb will add so much fat to a dish that it can't be salvaged.

Be wary of claims of "low-fat" or "heart-healthy" or "meets guidelines of the American Heart Association for reduced-fat diets." You know by now that what is truly low-fat bears little resemblance to what official agencies think is low-fat.

After the impossible is eliminated, there are usually at least a few dishes left. They generally are chicken, turkey, fish (you know now which are low-fat and which are high-fat), or vegetarian. They still may not be perfect. The usual culprit is oil. Here you will need to talk to your waiter.

There are also many items on the menu that, though not main dishes, can actually make up a delicious low-fat meal. Salads (ordered without dressing, or with oil and vinegar on the side, or with lemon), vegetables, fruits, baked potatoes (without topping), extra French bread (very low fat), extra rice at Chinese restaurants, extra corn tortillas at Mexican restaurants, etc., etc. If you're eating in a fast-food restaurant, the salad bar can be your savior. A huge salad, with lots of kidney and garbanzo beans (beware of oily marinades), together with a couple of baked potatoes (try them with ketchup, or A.1. Steak Sauce, or any other low-fat topping) and a soft drink, is a fast, healthful, low-fat meal.

"Hold the oil, please!"

The fourth and final area that you control is the instructions that you give to your waiter or waitress. Give specific instructions on how the food is to be prepared. Most servers are accommodating and friendly. (They are supposed to be serving you, remember? That is one of the pleasures of going out.)

The most common problem is that an otherwise perfectly acceptable dish is ruined by being sautéed in oil. If you're not sure, ask! No oil should be used in sautéing. Period. Common responses are "Oh well, we just use a little oil. Otherwise it sticks, you know." Or "But the oil adds flavor. Otherwise is will taste awful." Politely but firmly request that your fish, vegetables, or whatever be sautéed in water or wine. *Make no assumptions; people add fat to almost anything!* If you can get your meat or fish broiled, or grilled, so much the better (although they may still add oil to the grill to prevent sticking).

Other common fat-adders are cream sauces or cheese toppings. Ask that these be eliminated from your dish.

Order clearly and politely. Specify your instructions *for every dish* (no oil to sauté my fish; no butter on my vegetables, etc.). That way, if your vegetables come dripping with butter, you can send them back with a clear conscience. One of our friends suggests that you tell the waitperson that you will gladly talk to the chef or cook about your desires (culinary, that is). And remember, the quality of service should determine the size of the tip and whether you return to the restaurant.

You may be pleasantly surprised at how many restaurants are now prepared to accommodate low-fat requests and actually know what they are doing. Many now serve entrees that are truly low-fat. Reward these restaurants with your patronage. Tell the manager how much you appreciate the service, and tell your friends about it. If you're a regular at a restaurant, they should be willing to accommodate your requests. If they aren't, take your regularity elsewhere.

Now let's look at some specific suggestions for each meal.

Breakfast

As always, *avoid all known high-fat foods.* One of the biggest offenders at breakfast is eggs, especially in omelets with cheese or ham. Simply avoid these dishes. You will have plenty of choices left. In fact, breakfast is one of the easiest meals to eat low-fat, because restaurants almost always offer at least fresh fruit and dry cereal. Here are some options:

- low-fat cold cereal with nonfat milk or juice (beware of granola, which is high-fat)
- oatmeal (with nonfat milk and brown sugar or fruit)
- fresh fruit
- dry toast or English muffin with jam or jelly
- bagels (plain or with jam; no cream cheese)
- any juice
- pancakes or waffles (if cooked with nonstick spray) (the nonstick sprays are 100 percent fat, but because they spray a small amount covering a large area, they are much better than oil or butter) This is a last-ditch alternative. While the batter will probably be made with whole eggs and 2 percent milk, overall they are a better choice than bacon and eggs.

Beware of breakfast muffins. They are often loaded with oil.

Lunch and dinner

When ordering entrees, follow the general guidelines that we gave above. In addition, almost all restaurants offer low-fat items around which you can build part or all of your meal. These will "dilute" any higher-fat items that you happen to eat. Here are a few suggestions:

- bread without butter (especially sourdough French bread, which has little or no fat)
- salads with no salad dressing, or just vinegar or lemon (request salad without egg, cheese, or croutons)
- vegetables, steamed or sautéed in water or wine
- baked potatoes, plain or with soy sauce, Tabasco sauce, A.1. sauce, ketchup, salt and pepper, chives, onion, lemon, or whatever other low-fat topping you can imagine
- soups, if broth-based with no meat added
- pasta dishes in Italian restaurants with plain tomato sauce
- corn tortillas and salsa in Mexican restaurants (not flour tortillas, which are made with lard)
- extra rice in Mexican, Thai, or Indian restaurants (both brown and white rice are very low in fat; make them the center of the meal)

Guidelines for eating low-fat as a guest

What do you do when you're invited to a friend's home for dinner, or as a guest at a banquet or other social occasion?

Close friends usually will know about your dietary habits and try to accommodate you. You can offer to bring a (low-fat) dish yourself to help out. If you don't know your hosts well enough to ask for changes, you have a choice. You can decide that this will be a feast day, and simply eat all of everything. Or you can choose to do your best to eat low-fat at this meal, recognizing that you may not achieve perfection. If this is your choice, there are some ways to minimize the fat:

- eat a low-fat snack before you go
- eat lots of bread (especially French) without butter
- eat lots of salad and any other vegetable served; try to avoid high-fat sauces
- if the main course is very high fat, eat a small portion (the low-fat snack you ate before arriving will help)
- have coffee or tea instead of a high-fat dessert

- do your best without offending your host or hostess, and don't worry—eating a high-fat meal on occasion will not ruin you

One or two white lies won't hurt: "My doctor has put me on a low-fat diet." Or, more truthfully, "I'm eating low-fat for health reasons." Humor can be helpful. We sometimes tell people who try to push helpings of high-fat foods on us, "Gosh, I'd like to, but I'm on a strict low-fun diet." That usually gets a smile and an easing of the pressure to have "just one helping of these delicious deep-fried pig jowls."

And when you face the choice between offending your host or hostess or eating a high-fat meal, you may just have to swallow your principles along with a few ounces of grease. We were once invited to eat Sunday breakfast out with a friend. He took us to his fraternal lodge, where they served eggs, sausage, hash-browns grilled in margarine, biscuits cooked with lard, and bacon. We decided on the spot to dub that day a feast day. We ate breakfast and enjoyed our neighbor's company, then ate low-fat the rest of the day. We did not balloon, even a little bit. Retain your sense of humor and perspective.

Tips for traveling

If you travel a lot for business, you must realize that this is part of your life, and it is essential that you master the skills necessary to eat low-fat while traveling. And when you go on vacation, you can't let your low-fat eating go on vacation as well. Here are some suggestions.

First, realize that traveling usually combines restaurant eating with eating as a guest. These are skills that you may already have mastered. If not, master them.

Second, it's a good idea to bring along your own "survival kit." Even if you're traveling by air on a business trip, you can fit a dozen bagels, a package of fig bars or other low-fat cookies, or even a few low-fat candy bars in your overnight bag. These will tide you over inevitable airport delays, or that time when you've arrived in the hotel room famished and want something to eat *now,* and the minibar beckons with smoked almonds, vanilla wafers, and other high-fat horrors. Make sure you carry a few snacks onto the airplane, to substitute for the salted nuts that are the inescapable airline snack choice.

Third, as soon as you can after arriving at your destination, find a store with low-fat items, especially fresh fruit, and stock up. If you have low-fat options with you or in your room, it becomes much easier to snack often and keep hunger at bay. This is, as always, a key to restaurant restraint.

We go one step further when we travel by car on vacation. We bring our complete breakfast and lunch needs—cereal, sugar, fruit, bagels, jams, pretzels. In a small cooler we store nonfat milk, nonfat cream cheese, and vegetables like carrots that can be eaten raw. We bring a few dishes and some silverware. We keep everything in our motel room, so that it's as easy to eat low-fat breakfasts and lunches as it is at home. When we go out to dinner, either we select low-fat options or—since it's vacation—we include a couple of feast meals. By planning ahead in these ways, we make it easy to eat low-fat and rarely end up in situations where we're hungry, tired, and have minimal resistance to fat.

Do the best you can, which may not always be perfect. Carol once attended a two-week teaching conference at which all meals were served in a cafeteria whose dietary policies apparently came out of a time capsule from the 1950s. Every main course was fried in oil or dripping with cheese or cream sauce. Barbecued beef was followed by pizza, then roast beef. Hamburgers and French fries were always available. Even the good food was ruined. Chicken sandwiches were made with chicken breasts grilled in oil and covered with cheese. Carol wound up eating a lot of unconventional meals. For instance, at breakfast, ham, bacon, eggs, hash-browns, toast, and pancakes were offered. No dry cereal. A few pieces of fruit left over from the previous day's lunch. So Carol's breakfast was often six pieces of toast with jam and a couple of pieces of fruit. Her lunches and dinners were mainly rolls, bread, plain salad, and more fruit. Occasionally a side dish, such as rice or soup, wasn't too oily, and she ate it. She was careful not to go hungry, and often had to fill up her tray twice to get enough to eat. It was certainly a challenge, but in the midst of a grease-fest she ate about 10 percent calories from fat, lots of fruit, and a nutritionally balanced diet, helping to keep her body fat, not to mention her risks of heart disease and major cancers, low.

After you do this sort of thing once, your confidence in your skills will skyrocket, and you'll feel ready to go anywhere and still eat low-fat.

3. Preparing Low-Fat Meals

Many people think that low-fat eating, especially as low as 10 percent fat, will require strange new recipes and exotic cooking techniques that may take hours. But, again, eating low-fat meals at home will *not* require revamping your kitchen, shopping for obscure ingredients, or puzzling for hours over strange recipes.

You have already cut down from 40 percent fat to 20 percent fat in Phase 1. Now it's time to apply the additional skills you've learned in Phase 2 to drop the fat content of your diet from 20 to 10 percent, in a way that fits into *your* life:

If you always eat microwaved frozen dinners, you simply use your label-reading skills to find the ones in the supermarket that are low-fat. Several major brands make entrees below 10 percent fat.

If you cook, but only the simplest dishes, you can probably modify most of your recipes to be low-fat without much change in taste; you can also try some of the recipes that we have included in this book, most of which are designed to be easy, fast, and tasty.

If you are a gourmet cook and you pride yourself on your culinary skills, you're in luck—there are now several books that cater to those who wish to eat light but lively dishes. You, too, will need recipe-modifying skills, however, since many purported "low-fat" recipes are not.

Three types of advice are important in enabling you to transform your cooking to low-fat:

1. General tips for cutting fat in cooking
2. Tips for altering recipes
3. Tips for cutting cooking time

1. General tips for cutting fat in cooking

Congratulations! If you've been following Phase 1, you are well on your way to low-fat cooking. In Phase 1, you eliminated pure fats like oil and butter from sautéing and baking. You also substituted, eliminated, or reduced regular high-fat dairy products. Now, in Phase 2, it's time to learn how to get the last bit of extra fat out of your cooking. You need to learn how to:

- use high-fat cheeses as spices only, or eliminate them completely
- eliminate egg yolks from your cooking
- eliminate red meat from your recipes

If you make these final changes, you are automatically cooking low-fat.

Use high-fat cheeses as spices only, or eliminate them completely
In Phase 1, you eliminated many high-fat dairy products in your cooking—substituting skim milk for whole and evaporated skim milk for cream, and reducing the amount of cheese that you used in cooking.

But even cutting the cheese you use in half usually won't be enough to get you down to 10 percent fat in a recipe. You have to change your thinking about high-fat cheese. It is no longer an integral ingredient but, rather, a "spice"—something that's added sparingly, for flavor.

Any way that you can substitute a nonfat dairy product for a high-fat one, you should. We mentioned a few in Phase 1: using nonfat cottage cheese in place of ricotta, using nonfat cheeses (try various brands!). If you've cut the cheese in a recipe in half and nobody noticed, try cutting it in half again; you'll now be down to one-fourth the original amount, which usually puts cheese in the "spice" category. For the missing high-fat cheese substitute nonfat; this can be remarkably effective. Also try some of the "low-fat" cheeses, using your label-reading skills to determine if they really *are* low-fat. For example, some varieties of mozzarella are 20 percent fat and taste great in lasagna. Don't forget the trick of using the strongest-flavored variety of a cheese to get the most taste for the least fat.

Consider the idea of simply eliminating cheeses completely. There are thousands of recipes that require not a shred of cheddar or a pinch of Parmesan. Give them a try. Even if you feel you "can't live without cheese," you may be surprised at how easy it is to eliminate it.

Eliminate egg yolks from your cooking
Leave the yolk in the egg and you have a high-fat bomb. Take the yolk away and it's a nonfat gift. Egg dishes, such as soufflés, become a thing of

the past on a 10-percent-fat diet. But eggs can still be used in baking; simply eliminate the yolks. For every whole egg that a recipe calls for, use two whites. Packaged egg whites are available that are the real thing and save you the trouble of separating the yolks. Powdered egg whites are now also available in many supermarkets. They are indistinguishable from fresh egg whites in baked goods, cost about the same, and are easier to use.

Eliminate red meat from your recipes
This may well be the biggest change you make. But remember, it's an unusual red meat that's less than 50 percent fat, and *many are 70 percent fat or higher*. That's true even if you trim all visible fat, since most of the fat is marbled into the meat itself. Even if the rest of the foods you eat in a day are exemplary low-fat items which contain an average of 10 percent fat, adding red meat to the evening meal can more than double the fat content of your overall diet.

Some foods that you can eat instead of meat will actually *lower* the overall fat content of your diet. Low-fat varieties of fish are as low as 8 percent fat. If you start making dishes without meat at all, using beans and vegetables instead, you will be eating the lowest-fat diet, because beans and vegetables contain less than 5 percent fat. Here's a summary of these ideas:

If you eat 10% fat all day, but *one* meal a day contains a large portion* of	This food item alone contains	Your overall diet for the day will contain
Red meat	50–90% fat	18–26% fat
Chicken breast without skin	20–25% fat	12–13% fat
Turkey breast without skin	10–15% fat	10–11% fat
Fish (low-fat varieties)	5–10% fat	9–10% fat
Beans or vegetables	1–5% fat	8–9% fat

*This analysis assumes you eat 2,000 calories a day, and that the portion of meat, fish, or beans constitutes 400 calories. That's about what you'd get in a large hamburger at a fast-food chain, or a serving of fish about the size and thickness of your hand, or two cups of cooked beans.

You can see the dramatic effect that red meat has on the fat conten[t] your diet. You continued to eat it in Phase 1, because your goal there 20 percent fat, just about the range you can achieve eating one large [por]tion of red meat per day. But in Phase 2, where you are going for the [low]est fat and the greatest weight loss and health benefits, it's got to go.

If you are following all the guidelines of Phase 1, and now you s[imply] change one dish a day from a meat-containing stew to a vege[table] pasta, you can decrease the fat in your diet from about 25 perc[ent to] less than 10 percent.

Of course, you can start eating leaner cuts (there are a few be[low 15] percent fat), and you can reduce portion sizes. But that's al[l a] guessing game, and you will never find a cut of red meat as low [as] turkey breast, fish (low-fat varieties), or beans. There are better [ways to] go about eliminating red meat. Here are some suggestions:

Broil red meat to brown it, never sauté it in oil.
This won't, of course, cut down on the red meat you use, but [at] least eliminate some oil. You started doing this in Phase 1.

Start substituting ground, skinless turkey breast for ground beef.
You often can tell little difference, but ground beef is a hig[h-fat mat]ter (even extra-extra-lean is 50 percent fat), whereas grou[nd] turkey breast is less than 10 percent fat. Don't be fooled [by "ground] turkey," which includes high-fat parts of the bird. It shoul[d be] *turkey breast only.*

Start substituting recipes with skinless chicken breast or turkey breast for recipes with red meat.
And always remove the skin and any visible fat before [cooking. Skin] equals fat.

If you like fish, eat some fish dishes instead of red-meat dishes.
Don't forget that tuna is a fish, and canned white tuna [packed in water] is often very low fat, below 10 percent. We give a lo[vely Tuna] Sandwich Spread recipe in the recipes appendix.

Gradually decrease the number of meat dishes
you eat each week and substitute meatless dishes.
You don't have to give up meat by going cold turkey (skinless breast, of course). That's tough to do, because it may require that you learn several new recipes containing no meat all at once, and there are bound to be a few that don't agree with your palate. Instead, one day a week try a new meatless recipe, a dish in which the main attraction is beans or vegetables. You'll like some and loathe others. Build a repertoire. When you have several that you and those you cook for enjoy, have two meatless dishes a week. Then three. Every day you substitute one of these for a red-meat dish is a day when you probably cut your fat consumption in half (assuming you are following all the other guidelines of Phases 1 and 2). As you expand your horizons, you will shrink your waistline.

Your tastes will continue to evolve. Two years ago, we ate chicken dishes several times a week. These days, we have dishes containing chicken or turkey perhaps once every two or three weeks. Eventually, we may eliminate meat completely.

2. *Tips for altering recipes*

There are two ways to add to your low-fat-recipe arsenal: try new recipes, or modify old ones. In both cases, you must know how to modify recipes to make them truly low-fat.

Some new recipes that you try, including those in our recipes appendix, will already be truly low-fat, containing 10–15 percent calories from fat. Other authors whose books offer truly low-fat recipes are Nathan Pritikin, Robert Pritikin (Nathan Pritikin's son), Dean Ornish, John and Mary McDougall, and Neal Barnard; you can be assured that their recipes are carefully designed for a 10-percent-fat diet or lower!). But beware of other "low-fat" cookbooks. If the fat content of a recipe is not given (as *percent* fat), the recipe may be a high-fat booby trap. Inspect it for known high-fat items. If it asks you to add ⌐, egg yolks, red meat, or dairy products that are not nonfat, it is unlikely to be a a truly low-fat recipe. That doesn't mean you need to reject it, but you must modify it.

You may have some favorite recipes that you are reluctant to give

up, even though they contain enough oil to lubricate a small car. You may be able to modify these, also.

Modifying high-fat recipes is simply a matter of applying the guidelines you've been using all along in Phase 1 and Phase 2. If you've completely eliminated fat in a recipe, you may even be able to allow small amounts of high-fat items as "spices."

There are four steps in modifying a recipe:

Step 1. Identify all high-fat foods in the recipe.
You know what they are: oil, butter, dairy products, red meat, egg yolks, nuts, and seeds.

Step 2. Eliminate or substitute for every single
high-fat food in the recipe, without exception.
You know what to do: substitute for oil, no egg yolks, substitute turkey or chicken for red meat. For nuts and seeds, follow the principle of step 4.

Step 3. Try the recipe.
The proof is in the (low-fat) pudding. How does the new recipe taste? Don't expect it to be the same as the old. But *do* expect it to be good enough that you want seconds. If it is, you're done. Congratulations! You've added a recipe that is 10 percent fat to your collection. If not, don't give up on it. Proceed to step 4.

Step 4. Judiciously add back high-fat foods
as spices and try it again.
You must use your judgment here. In general, try to get down to less than one-fourth of what the original recipe called for. For example, if it calls for four cups of grated cheddar cheese, try one cup, and use extra-sharp cheddar. Some recipes call for flavored oils, such as Chinese sesame oil or chili oil. You will probably find that you need to include these, but, again, try to use about one-fourth the original amount. If a recipe calls for bacon, try bacon bits. Hormel's brand is 23 percent fat. A few go a long way.

As an example, let's compare traditional lasagna with a low-fat modification. The traditional recipe was taken straight from a package of lasagna. The modified recipe is our own, and is included in the recipes appendix:

TRADITIONAL			MODIFIED		
Ingredient	Total cals	Cals from fat	Ingredient	Total cals	Cals from fat
8 oz. lasagna	840	40	10 oz. lasagna	1,050	50
1 medium onion	40	1	1 medium onion	40	1
2 cloves garlic	10	0	2 cloves garlic	10	0
1 12-oz. can tomato paste	215	10	1 12-oz. tomato paste	215	10
1 28-oz. can tomatoes	360	4	1 28-oz. can tomatoes	360	4
1 egg	80	52	(omit egg)	0	0
2 lbs. Italian sausage	2,000	1,448	1 lb. ground skinless turkey breast	550	55
2 16-oz. containers ricotta cheese	1,920	1,440	1 16-oz. container nonfat cottage cheese	280	0
1 lb. mozzarella cheese	1,440	1,008	8 oz. Frigo brand Lite Mozzarella cheese	480	144
1 c. grated Parmesan cheese	350	210	(omit Parmesan, or use fat-free)		
herbs and spices	0	0	herbs and spices	0	0
Total	7,255	4,213	**Total**	2,985	264
PERCENT FAT = 58%			**PERCENT FAT = 9%**		

This traditional recipe contains so much grease we're surprised it doesn't burst into flames in the oven. Half-measures don't help much. For example, if you use part-skim mozzarella and halve the amount of ricotta in the traditional recipe, it still comes out to 6,119 calories and 54 percent fat. If you use part-skim mozzarella, half the ricotta, and two pounds of the leanest ground beef (labeled 10 percent fat, actually 50 percent fat) rather than the Italian sausage, you can get the traditional recipe down to 5,735 total calories and 47 percent fat.

Don't even bother. It's still a gut-buster. If you're going to serve the traditional lasagna, say on a feast day, just make it as is.

On the other hand, if you truly modify this lasagna, you can get the fat down to *one-sixth* of the traditional recipe. And the modified recipe still tastes rich and flavorful. Let's see how the recipe was changed:

Step 1. Identify all high-fat components.
You have learned to identify all of the high-fat components found in this recipe. The egg will, of course, contain an egg yolk, and the Italian sausage is red meat. All the dairy products called for—the ricotta, the mozzarella, the Parmesan—are in their high-fat versions. *All* of these high-fat items must be modified if the recipe is to have a chance of being low-fat.

Step 2. Eliminate or substitute.
We simply eliminated the egg. If this were a baked good, like a bread, you would want to substitute egg whites, because they help hold the dry ingredients together in the final product. But in this case it isn't necessary, so the egg is history. Next we substituted ground skinless turkey breast for the Italian sausage. We use a pound instead of two pounds, and increase the amount of lasagna pasta a little to compensate.

We sautéed the onion and garlic in defatted chicken broth, rather than in oil.

In our first attempt at modifying the cheeses, we simply substituted nonfat items for all the high-fat cheeses, or eliminated them: nonfat cottage cheese for the ricotta, and nonfat Parmesan for the regular Parmesan; the mozzarella, eliminated, because we couldn't find a nonfat version. Things are moving so fast that by the time you read this there will probably be several nonfat mozzarella cheeses to choose from.

Step 3. Try it.
When we tried the lasagna made this way, it was acceptable, but not mouth-wateringly good. It lacked the richness of traditional lasagna; we didn't want seconds. If you accept a recipe at this stage, you probably will begin to dislike it after making it a few more times, and eventually long for the old high-fat version. You'll think that all the "experts" are right—low-fat eating is tasteless and boring.

That's why you absolutely must *not* accept a recipe if you don't genuinely like it. It's crucial that you build a collection of recipes that you and your family truly enjoy, that you look forward to making and to eating. It doesn't have to taste like the high-fat version. But it does have to taste *good*.

*Step 4: Judiciously add back high-fat foods
as spices and try it again.*

We added back the mozzarella but used *half* what the original recipe called for, and cut the fat in half again by using a mozzarella that was 30 percent fat, compared with the original, which was 70 percent fat. In this way, we were using a high-fat food as a spice, something to add an accent of flavor.

We tried the recipe again, and now it was a tasty treat. When we serve it to family and friends, there never seems to be enough—the true sign of a successful recipe. We added it to our collection, as a special dish for us and a great one to serve when we have guests for dinner.

By the way, this lasagna can be modified further to cut the fat even more. You can use kidney beans in place of the turkey. Using six cups of canned, drained, and chopped kidney beans in place of the pound of ground turkey lowers the fat content of the recipe to 7.5 percent. It gives the dish a new flavor, which you may enjoy more than the lasagna with meat. And it's even faster to prepare, because you don't have to cook the meat—the canned beans are already cooked. Some people like spinach lasagna. We haven't tried it this way, but if you think you might like it, try it. It will be as low-fat as the lasagna made with beans.

Altering packaged food recipes

What about packaged foods that require preparation? First, read the label. If the packaged food itself is over 20 percent fat, reject it. Otherwise you're starting with two strikes against you when you try to modify its final version—no matter what, the ingredients in the package are adding a lot of fat, and there is usually nothing you can do to modify them. After that, it's a matter of applying the guidelines we've already given for any other recipe: eliminate oil and other pure fats, replace eggs with egg whites, substitute nonfat dairy products, etc. Try it and see how it is, then further modify.

3. Tips for cutting cooking time

Like it or not, we still live in a high-fat world. If you come home from work hungry and tired, and the cupboard is bare, or the only possibility for a low-fat meal involves an hour of preparing ingredients and another hour of cooking, your chances of eating a healthful low-fat dinner are low. You scramble around, and it's very easy to give up and order something to be delivered. It would be great if you could order a tasty low-fat meal delivered to your door, but for now you can't (budding entrepreneurs, take note). So you end up ordering pizza. Or you go to a restaurant, tired and hungry, and wind up eating enough blubber to float a whale.

Especially when you are just starting to eat low-fat, you will be more tempted by high-fat alternatives and less willing to wait for some low-fat food. And, of course, in the beginning is when you tend to be least familiar with the tricks and shortcuts that allow you to multiply your low-fat options so that there is *always* something tasty and tempting available.

So beginners can get caught in a vicious cycle. You do well most of the time, but there are several occasions a week where nothing low-fat is on hand for dinner, or you didn't bring anything for lunch and you're so hungry at lunchtime that you go to the nearest fast-food place. You end up eating quite a few high-fat meals per week. Because you're eating so many high-fat meals, your overall diet will probably be high in fat, so you don't really experience the benefits of low-fat eating, like the energy and the weight loss. Since you're not seeing any benefits, you have even less motivation to eat low-fat on the days when you *do* have time, and start eating high-fat even on those days. You finally give up, after deciding that low-fat eating is just too much of a hassle. And it didn't really seem to work anyway.

To avoid this vicious cycle and the feeling of failure that it generates, you want to make it easy for yourself to eat low-fat by developing your own personal low-fat, healthful food "cocoon." You can do this, and at the same time actually *save* yourself time. You need to do two things:

- plan
- cut preparation time

Some of the tips we give here are applicable to low-fat cooking only, but most are general ideas that will save *anyone* time. Here are a few cooking and organization principles that we use:

Plan

Go to the store once a week.

Make a weekly menu and shopping list. Go through your low-fat recipes (you might want to list them on a piece of paper that you keep on your refrigerator or bulletin board). Then make a menu. Just list the meals that you plan to have that week (we always count on leftovers for two or three meals). From the menu, write up a shopping list. Go to the store and you're done for the week.

This will not, of course, directly cut the fat content of your eating. But it does have indirect effects. Now when you stagger through the door at the end of a long day, you have a list of meals for the week to choose from, and you know you have all the ingredients.

You'll also be alerted to high-fat pitfalls in the immediate future. Is there a wedding that you are going to on Saturday? Make sure you have something on hand for a low-fat snack before, so that you won't be starving at the reception. Business lunch on Tuesday? Pack a couple of bagels or other snacks to eat before. Guests coming on Friday? Pick out one of your low-fat "guest" meals to serve them from your list of recipes.

Also, having the right sorts of food in the house will help you live up to your good intentions. If you intend to eat five fruits or vegetables each day, you need to have some on hand each day to eat. Which, as we mentioned in Phase 1, means that your weekly shopping cart will be full to overflowing with fruit and veggies. If you've decided to eat completely low-fat snacks, you need to have some on your shelves.

The once-weekly planning and shopping also saves you time in the long run, no matter what the fat content of the foods you eat. If you are racing to the store three times a week, that's three times the amount of driving, standing in line, loading the groceries, unloading the groceries, etc.

Make double or triple recipes.

It takes little additional time to double or triple a recipe. You can use the extra food in two ways. You can save some of tonight's dinner in an airtight plastic container for tomorrow's lunch. That way you already have your low-fat lunch almost complete—add a couple of pieces of

French bread, some carrots, a few pieces of fruit, and you're set for the day at work. Or you can freeze some of the extra. This is a real life-saver on nights when you have almost no time to prepare dinner. Thaw some spaghetti sauce while you boil the spaghetti and make a quick salad, and you have a delicious low-fat dinner in less than fifteen minutes. Or thaw some of the Mexican beans you prepared a few weeks ago, slice up a tomato and some green pepper, and make yourself a few tacos or burritos. The possibilities are limited only by your imagination and the size of your freezer. Make sure you have enough Tupperware-type containers on hand to handle lots of leftovers, so you always have something to put tomorrow's lunch or next week's dinner in.

Have a few "emergency" meals on hand.
After reading the preceding sections, you may think that we're the sort of people who plan our lives so completely that we store our cereal boxes in alphabetical order. But there are plenty of weeks when we can't do all of our weekly shopping at once, or are simply so pressed for time that meal preparation must be kept to the absolute minimum. For these times, we keep some "emergency" foods around. These aren't necessarily what we would like to eat every week, but they get us through the really rushed times with a low-fat, nutritious diet.

First, remember the frozen meals. These can be either your own recipes that you have frozen, or a few of the low-fat entrees available in supermarkets. Frozen vegetables will also do quite well to round out a dinner. We keep plenty of carrots on hand so that we can always have *some* vegetable, no matter how rushed we are—it takes about fifteen seconds to wash a couple of carrots. There are a variety of soups available that require no more than heating. These, plus bread and perhaps a salad, make a quick, tasty, and nutritious meal. We also keep cans of refried beans on our shelves (now available in many brands as nonfat; we mix nonfat with 20-percent-fat vegetarian to get a tasty 10-percent-fat mix). These, on low-fat tortillas, provide a quick, easy dinner. We have even, in particularly frenetic moments, eaten cold cereal for dinner. It's not nutritionally perfect, but it beats a fast-food hamburger.

Cut preparation time

Use canned or bottled beans, tomatoes, etc.,
and dried spices where you can.
Using canned foods is as quick as opening the can.

Frozen vegetables are as nutritious as fresh; they're even more nutritious than the "fresh" that are out of season and have been shipped great distances.

Many people make them a nightly staple. Here you must rely on your taste, as well as your label-reading ability to check that the food processors haven't added butter or other high-fat booby traps to these otherwise supremely low-fat foods.

If a recipe calls for fresh herbs or spices, use dried. Most recipes will have directions for using either fresh or dried. It's not going to change the flavor much, if at all.

White rice is faster than brown rice.

And so on.

Now, please don't get the idea that we are saying you should switch to the quicker alternatives if you are now using the ones that take more time. Or that we think these quick alternatives are nutritionally superior to their more leisurely counterparts. If you already grow your own vegetables and serve them fresh from the garden, by all means continue! But if you, like most of the rest of this overworked, overstressed nation, don't have the time to grow anything but weary, these alternatives at least give you a fighting chance at a nutritious, low-fat meal.

Find quick recipes.
Some of our favorite low-fat meals take less than half an hour to prepare. You may have some favorite recipes that are quick and tasty; many of these may be modifiable to low-fat status without sacrificing taste. The more such recipes you have to choose from, the less likely it is that you will be stuck for something to prepare on a night when you have twenty minutes to make and eat dinner, three cans in the cupboard, and a refrigerator that contains only one low-fat item—the light bulb.

9

You Can Do It Fast,

or You Can Do It Slow

· · · · ·

This chapter is mainly for those who want to start eating 10 percent fat *now.* Those who decide only to drop to 20 percent fat generally don't require specific transitional instructions of the sort you'll find in this chapter (although they may certainly find some useful tips). But a large percentage of the people that we teach in our workshops want to go to the lowest level of fat, and they want to do it *immediately.* That's great! Before telling them where they can stock up on the bagels and rice cakes, however, we offer a cautionary tale.

In his early days of experimenting with a low-fat diet, Eric at one point decided that he was going to follow the principles laid out by Nathan Pritikin in his books. Pritikin encouraged people to try a complete, abrupt changeover to a 10-percent-fat, high-fiber diet, and he offered some very impressive testimonials from people who had experienced dramatic improvements in health. Even more impressive to Eric were the hundreds of scientific studies that supported Pritikin's claims. Despite the backlash of some members of the medical community against Pritikin (oddly reminiscent of the present backlash against low-fat eating for weight loss), the scientific evidence was so much in Pritikin's favor that Eric decided to give the low-fat diet a try.

So Eric switched completely to a low-fat, whole-grain-based diet—

literally overnight. One day he was eating pizza and burgers, the next it was pasta and bagels. At the time, he was on a swim team. Before the switch to the low-fat diet, he found that he often ran out of gas before the end of his morning workout; his muscles just seemed to be out of fuel. And he was more tired during the rest of the day than he felt he should be. Within days of making the switch, Eric was able to complete his workouts with fuel to spare, and noticed a definite improvement in energy levels. Switching to a low-fat, high-carbohydrate diet allowed his muscles to store much more glycogen, the fuel for intense exercise, so he could swim longer. And without the fat from meals circulating in his blood vessels, he no longer felt tired in the afternoons. This way of eating was great!

But after a few days, Eric noticed something happening. Or, rather, something *not* happening. A lot of food was going in one end, but nothing was happening at the other. He hadn't read anything about this. His diet was much higher in fiber, which should promote regularity, not constipation. His abdomen started to get bloated, and he felt uncomfortable all day long. Running out of gas was no longer a problem, but now it wasn't the kind of gas that you really want in excess. These were clearly effects of the diet, but he had no idea what to do about them, except to switch back to his pre-Pritikin, high-fat diet, which he did. Within days, his digestive tract was back to normal. But, of course, all the benefits disappeared, too. Disappointed, he gave up on low-fat eating for a while.

Eric had taken what we now call the "Just Do It" approach to eating 10 percent fat, an abrupt, overnight transition. It works for many people, whose digestions adapt smoothly. It didn't work for Eric. No one had told him of the possible pitfalls, only the benefits, so he wasn't prepared when his greater energy was accompanied by painful digestive problems. And since no one had suggested any other way of making the transition, Eric had no Plan B to fall back on. It was all-or-nothing.

Today, Eric eats 10 percent fat with no digestive problems whatsoever. By trial and error, we discovered that the way to switch to a 10-percent-fat diet that worked *for us* was what we now call the "Gently Do It" approach. This is a more gradual shift (for us it took more than a year). It's a Plan B.

Which will work for you, Just Doing It, or Gently Doing It? Only you can say. We've had people attend our workshops who successfully shifted to eating 10 percent fat the next day, and who reported no problems of any sort. Others tried the abrupt shift and found it didn't work, but made the gradual transition easily. Still others knew from the start that a gentle, gradual approach was right for them.

You'll learn in this chapter the advantages and disadvantages of each approach, and you'll also receive step-by-step instructions for each. There is no "right way" to do it, and there is no such thing as failure. Eric came away from his first low-fat-eating experience with the certain knowledge that if he *could* make the transition he would experience tremendous vitality and energy. That knowledge motivated him to keep trying, and eventually to succeed in eating 10 percent fat. You can, too, but you will have the advantage of learning from our experience and that of hundreds of others.

The "Just Do It" Approach

No doubt about it, an abrupt shift to eating 10 percent fat offers the greatest advantages. But it also may lead to the biggest pitfalls for you, and requires the most preparation.

Advantages of Just Doing It

Most rapid fat loss
The all-out change will cause the most rapid fat loss, as you would expect. People who are greatly overweight—say, more than seventy or eighty pounds—often experience losses of two to five pounds of fat a week. People who are less overweight—say twenty or thirty pounds—often lose two to five pounds of fat a *month*. Many studies report initial weight losses that are much greater than these estimates (see chapter 5), but we think that this may be due to the subjects' not eating enough when they switch to lower-fat foods. It can be difficult, especially at first, to believe the amount of food that you must eat to keep from going hungry when you are eating a low-fat diet. So people tend to eat less than they really need. We recommend that you resist this tendency,

because you're more likely to continue with the new way of eating if you're eating until you're satisfied.

Most rapid improvement in health

Many conditions begin to improve within days, and adjustments in medication for diabetes or high blood pressure often have to be made in a matter of weeks as these conditions improve.

The taste for fat is lost within weeks

Fat has a definite taste and feel; if you eat a lot of it, you become addicted to this taste and feel. People who switch completely to low-fat foods report initial cravings for fat, which disappear in one to two weeks. If you eat fat substitutes, you will retain your taste for fat (See chapter 10 for more about fat substitutes).

Energy increases within a week

You might want to go back to chapter 3 and look at why energy increases on a low-fat diet. Remember that one reason is immediate—you no longer eat high-fat meals, so you no longer have fat clogging up your blood vessels after meals. The other effect, on brain neurotransmitters, may take longer (although in several studies it's been shown to happen after a single high-carbohydrate meal). Most people report more energy within a week. Everyone should feel an effect within a month.

Disadvantages of Just Doing It

As Eric discovered, there can be disadvantages to a rapid changeover. Some of these are physical, and may require that you try a more gradual approach. Others are psychological, and can be avoided if you know about them in advance.

Possible digestive upset

You may experience gas, diarrhea, or constipation if you switch suddenly from a high-fat, low-fiber diet to a low-fat, high-fiber diet. The gas may be partly due to beans (see page 140 for suggestions on how to reduce it). Everyone has bacteria living in the intestinal tract, and these bacteria are used to a high-fat, low-fiber diet. As your intestinal flora changes to species better able to handle the new diet, the gas disappears. The diarrhea or constipation is often a reaction to the greater fiber that is usually part of a low-fat diet—high-fat foods, like meats, have no fiber, whereas low-fat foods, like grains, beans, fruits, and vegetables, have lots of fiber. The fiber is good for you, helping to prevent colon cancer and to lower blood cholesterol, but your gut may not get the message at first—it may react by moving things through too fast, or by stopping completely. If you decide to gut it out (sorry about that), be prepared to wait. You will come back to normal, but it will take time, weeks to months. Let your digestion readjust naturally. Don't resort to laxatives or other medications.

Difficulty making so many changes

It can be overwhelming to keep so many changes in mind at once. Some books try to overcome this by giving people strict menus, with recipes, to follow for the first month or so. This may be helpful for you (try *The Pritikin Promise*; see bibliography).

Eventually, however, this program must be integrated into *your* life, the way *you* eat. If the way you now prepare your meals is to boil water and pop things into the microwave, or if you eat two meals a day in restaurants, it's unrealistic to plunge into complicated low-fat recipes and expect to be able to handle it. We have found that people get the best results if they stick to the way they normally eat, modifying it to low-fat. But this will take attention and perseverance. It can be too much to handle if you also have other demands on your attention, such as family or career.

The solution, of course, is to prepare, which we will discuss in a moment.

Tendency to take all-or-nothing attitude

If you do get overwhelmed, it's easy just to throw up your hands and say the whole thing's impossible and go back to your high-fat ways. Or you may continue with the low-fat eating without really integrating it into your life, perhaps eating meals that don't appeal to you because you haven't learned any that you like. Even though you can lose weight and gain health benefits this way, you are as doomed to failure as if you were on a low-calorie diet. You force yourself to continue until you just can't take it any more, then switch back to a high-fat eating style. You feel disappointed and angry.

Don't despair. Remember, this is *not* a temporary diet. It's a way of eating, and if you have been eating one way for several decades, it may be unrealistic to expect to switch to a brand-new way in several days. If you just can't make all the changes, eat high-fat for a few days, then try the Gently Do It approach.

If you are on medication, you must be under a doctor's supervision

We will repeat the only medical caution for this program:

If you are taking medication for high blood pressure or diabetes, or if you take any other medication regularly, **make sure your doctor knows you are going on this program and monitors your condition carefully.** You may get too healthy to take the dangerous drugs your doctor prescribes.

Preparing

If you want to make the change to eating 10 percent fat overnight, you still must take the time to prepare. Read over both Phase 1 and Phase 2 very carefully. Study them. Here are some areas to which you will want to pay special attention:

Use the diagnostic quizzes to see where your dietary Hot Spots are, and read the relevant sections of each phase very carefully. You must follow the guidelines for *both* phases to drop to 10 percent calories from fat, and it may be quite a switch from your present way of eating, so you have to have the guidelines clearly in mind. The results of your diagnostic quizzes may lead you to any or all of the following changes:

Make a clean sweep of your kitchen if you can, tossing (or giving away) all high-fat foods, so that there will be no "mistakes." If you will

be cooking, get a big (the bigger the better), sturdy, high-quality non-stick frying pan. Get lots of airtight plastic containers for storing left-overs to simplify and speed up your meal preparation. If you bake a lot, get nonstick baking pans and have the ingredients on hand for substituting for oil and butter in recipes.

Make a shopping expedition and stock up on low-fat foods

Expect the first few times you shop for low-fat foods to take longer than your usual shopping, as you learn which foods are to be your new staples. You must know how to identify high- and low-fat foods that are unlabeled. (Quick, what are the only fruits and vegetables high in fat? Right—avocados and olives.) For labeled foods, you must know how to read labels—make sure you understand how, and practice on a few items from your shelves, as well as on every labeled item you buy at the supermarket. Do not assume that any packaged item is low-fat, no matter what the label claims. You must go straight to the Nutrition Facts part of the label and determine for yourself whether the food is really low-fat. You will find yourself buying an enormous amount of fruit and veggies in order to eat a minimum of five servings a day.

Get to know several low-fat meals you like

If you cook, you must have several recipes that you know you like before you start. You can build your repertoire to include as many as you want, but you must start with a few tried-and-true winners. If you are completely new to low-fat cooking, try some of the recipes we include in this book. They're simple, and most people like them.

Also become aware of the dozens of simple low-fat options for meals that require little or no cooking (like cereals for breakfast, soups for lunch, etc.). And make sure that you have found several low-fat snacks that you enjoy. See "Tips for Every Meal," later in this chapter, for some suggestions.

Become a restaurant expert

If you eat in restaurants more than once every couple of weeks, you must become familiar with the guidelines for restaurant ordering. It's not a bad idea to go out to eat a few times to some of your favorite spots and practice your low-fat ordering. Read the low-fat-ordering section of

Phase 2 before you go, and look at the menu carefully. When you order, make sure you clearly request exactly the modifications you desire. Assertiveness gets easier with practice. As with shopping, expect your first few restaurant ordering experiences to take longer than usual, as you get used to studying the menu. You may be in for some pleasant surprises as you try new dishes and new restaurants.

Assess your environment
You must also anticipate how your dietary changes will affect those around you. In terms of living situations, there are three possibilities.

First, if you live alone, it's easy in one sense, because you are free to eat exactly as you please, but harder in another, because there's no immediate support. Consider switching to low-fat with a friend or group of friends (make sure they understand the program clearly and are as enthusiastic as you are).

Second, if you live with others who share your enthusiasm for this change, you are in the easiest situation in many ways, because everyone can help.

Third, if you live with others who aren't interested, control what you can. Almost any situation allows you to control most or all of your breakfasts, lunches, and snacks, which can be three-quarters of your total caloric intake. So at least these components can be pristine. At dinner, if you are the cook, you might consider switching to some moderate-fat recipes (*Jane Brody's Good Food Book* is a tremendous source; see bibliography) or even throwing in a true low-fat recipe and seeing if anyone can tell the difference. It's not a good idea to proselytize and force people to eat dishes they don't really want to eat. If you're not the cook, see if you can at least get a few moderate-to-low-fat choices. At any rate, you can stop buttering your bread, potatoes, etc., stop putting dressing on your salad or switch to nonfat dressing, and eat smaller portions of high-fat entrees (make up for it with low-fat snacks—don't go hungry!). If you keep a sense of humor and don't get self-righteous, people usually become interested and often get enthusiastic.

Gently Do It

If you decide to go on a low-fat diet gradually, there are many different approaches. We suggest a few below, or you may want to do it your own, completely unique way. There is no single right way, and there is no right level of fat in the diet to attain. The *optimum* level is 10 percent calories from fat, but that may not be the level you wish to be at, at least for now. Any change downward will reset set point downward and give health benefits. Small changes give small benefits, large changes give large benefits, but it's completely up to you. This life-style is a matter of choice.

Advantages of Gently Do It

Digestion adjusts smoothly
The nice thing about the gradual approach is that your gut adjusts gradually, too. Any time you experience digestive upset (such as gas or bloating), just back off a bit, perhaps eating more processed foods for a while (such as switching from whole-grain cereal to bagels and non-fat cream cheese for breakfast). Your gut will adapt slowly, with little complaint.

Integrates more easily into your life
You make the changes at whatever pace allows you to integrate them fully into your life. If one particular aspect is troublesome, and you find yourself unable to follow a particular guideline, try another.

First steps are very easy
One thing that is probably clear by now is that there are many sources of fat in your diet, so eliminate the easy ones first. It's not always obvious what will be easy and what will be hard until you actually try it. But *anybody* can find at least a few guidelines in Phase 1 or Phase 2 that fit effortlessly into his or her life. Then you can build on those. Changes start to have a snowball effect. As you notice that you are feeling better, perhaps losing a little fat, it becomes easier to make the more difficult changes.

More relaxed attitude

You're less likely to be tense about your eating choices when you only make one change at a time, because you have less to keep track of. Also, slow changes lead to less self-righteousness and proselytizing, which your friends will surely appreciate.

Disadvantages of Gently Do It

Slower fat loss

Obviously, if you are not at the lowest fat level in your diet, your body will not seek its lowest fat level.

If you really want to lose fat *now,* but you just couldn't handle the complete changeover to a 10-percent-fat diet, just make a couple of changes in diet and meanwhile use the other weapon in your arsenal—exercise. Increase your exercise and you will lose fat just as surely as if you eat a low-fat diet. To learn how to increase the amount of exercise in your day, often without doing a single workout, see part four, beginning on page 229. An increase in exercise of about half an hour a day, coupled with a decrease in dietary fat from 40 to 30 percent, will probably cause enough fat loss so that your clothes will start to get downright baggy. And, of course, as soon as you've adjusted to 30 percent you can drop further, so you keep getting more and more benefit from your low-fat eating.

More gradual health gains

As with fat, so with health. The benefits come more slowly. No matter how gradually you're doing this, however, make sure your doctor knows what you are doing if you are using any prescription medication.

You may retain your taste for fat

Some people find this to be true, some don't. After our early Just Do It approaches failed, we took the gradual approach and Eric never craved fat for a second, but Carol did sometimes feel a strong urge to binge on high-fat foods. If you find yourself craving fat, you might try eating more fruit, since fructose, the sugar in fruit, cuts fat appetite. You might also want to drop the fat content of your diet *lower,* paradoxical as that may sound, because the *less* fat in your diet the faster you lose your appetite for it. And remember, don't use fat substitutes: they will cause you to retain your taste for fat.

Approaches to Gently Doing It

One way to make a slow change is to start with the first guideline of Phase 1 (don't add pure fat to food) and incorporate that into your life over a period of days, weeks, or months, whatever is comfortable for you. Then move to the second guideline, then the third. Or do them in any order you want. When these changes are no longer changes, but just part of your life, move to Phase 2. Again, you move into Phase 2 all at once or gradually.

Another approach is to change one meal at a time. See the next section for specific suggestions. You might go low-fat for breakfast this month, add lunch next month, throw in totally low-fat snacks the third month, and tackle dinner in month four. Or you might want to do it in a matter of weeks, or over a longer period.

And remember: *there is no such thing as "cheating" in this program; there are only choices.* Just make your choices with your eyes open.

Tips for Every Meal

Whether you have decided on Just Do It or Gently Do It, you may be impatient at this point to get going, to start eating truly low-fat meals. But it will take time to master the skills presented in these chapters, and to get comfortable with applying the principles outlined here to your life. To help you make the transition, we've consolidated some tips for very quick breakfasts, lunches, dinners, and snacks, some of which you've already seen in these pages. These, together with the recipes in the appendix, should help you get a good start as you learn the techniques to make the program work for you.

Breakfast

You may be very close to eating a low-fat breakfast already. Some people like to eat the same thing every day; others like variety. You can suit your tastes by choosing from the following list, which is really just a bunch of very familiar foods. And, of course, there is no reason why you can't eat a meal that is really a "lunch" or "dinner" for breakfast.

Fruit

Any variety and any quantity. Fruit is absolutely the healthiest way to start your day, not only because it is so low in fat, but because many fruits contain abundant vitamin C. If you usually don't feel like eating much in the morning, you can make your entire breakfast from a couple of pieces of fruit. It's better to eat the whole fruit rather than juice, because you get more filling fiber that way. But in a pinch, a glass of fruit juice is better than nothing at all. The sweetness of many fruits, such as bananas and strawberries, makes them ideal sugar substitutes for those who wish to avoid sugar.

Cold or hot cereal

If you eat a cold cereal already for breakfast, chances are very good that it is low-fat, since most cold cereals are surprisingly low in fat (with the exception of granola). It may be that the only change you need to make is to switch to nonfat milk. The more nutritious cereals, like shredded wheat, are made from whole grains and contain no added sugar. Check the label. A sliced banana on your cereal, together with another piece of fruit before breakfast, puts you at two pieces of fruit before you even step out the door. And it tastes delicious.

Toast

Find a low-fat bread. As with the cereals, there is a large variety to choose from; whole-grain breads are the most healthful, but we often eat toasted French bread. A dab of jam on top can complete the picture. If you prefer not to eat the sugar in jam, fruit spreads are available. They are made with no added sugar, and their taste is indistinguishable from jams made with sugar (an example is Smucker's Simply Fruit brand). These spreads still contain high amounts of fruit sugar, however. Best is something like apple butter, which usually contains only apples and cinnamon (check the label to be sure).

Bagels
A sliced bagel, plain or toasted, with nonfat cream cheese and jam on top, seems almost sinful—but it is a nutritious combination that is less than 5 percent fat. We'll have a lot to say about bagels in the snacks section.

Nonfat yogurt and fruit or nonfat granola
If you're tired of the same old cereal for breakfast but still want something fast, try nonfat yogurt with fruit or nonfat granola mixed in. It's a different taste, tangy and refreshing. For those concerned about calcium intake, this is a good source. You can get plain nonfat yogurts and mix your own fruit in. If you get premixed nonfat yogurts with fruit, be aware that you will be getting a big shot of sugar along with it (and not much fruit in many brands).

Nonfat pancakes, waffles, or French toast
On weekends or other days when you have a bit of time, you may enjoy these old favorites. You can make them in nonfat versions (see recipes) and serve them with fruit toppings (frozen fruit, especially strawberries, thawed in the microwave, is excellent) or with syrup.

Lunch

Lunch is the most variable meal. Some people never eat it; some take one or two hours for a huge meal. What we suggest here are some options for quick meals, lunches that can be eaten sitting with friends, or divided into snacks throughout the day.

Bagels and fruit
This is probably the "lunch" that we most frequently grab in the morning, when we have perhaps thirty seconds to prepare the meal. We keep several dozen bagels in our freezer, and always try to have a variety of fruits on hand. Just grab two or three of the frozen bagels and a few pieces of fruit and run out the door. The bagels thaw in a couple of hours (they can be helped along by thirty seconds in a microwave) and are available for snacks or a sit-down lunch. Just make sure you take a lot more than you think you'll need, because you don't want to run out

of food early—that leads to extreme hunger in the afternoon, and the tendency to succumb to any high-fat snacks in the vicinity. Better to have too much and bring home a few bagels and pieces of fruit, which can be used in the next day's lunch.

Vegetables, plain or with nonfat dip

A surprising variety of vegetables taste delicious when eaten raw. They are a great choice to munch on when you are not particularly hungry but just want to chew on something. Carrots and celery are the old standbys. If you like carrots, get in the habit of making one, two, three, or more peeled carrots part of your lunch—they are a potent source of carotenoids (like beta carotene) and other natural chemicals that combat cancer and heart disease. Try broccoli or cauliflower raw. The taste grows on you, and these, too, are potent sources of natural anti-carcinogens. Raw veggies also are a nice breath freshener after lunch.

If you don't particularly like the taste of plain raw vegetables, try bringing some dip. We describe one in the recipes appendix that has proved quite popular—and fat-free.

Salads

One step beyond raw vegetables is a salad. You may not have time to make one in the morning—so make a big one at night and store part of it (without dressing) in an airtight plastic container in the fridge. It's ready the next morning to be taken to work, or to be pulled out at lunchtime at home. If you want dressing, bring it in a tightly sealed container. If you have a refrigerator where you eat lunch, consider keeping one or two bottles of your favorite dressings on hand.

Instant soups and pastas

There are now dozens and dozens of delicious low-fat soups and pastas on the market. Most require only hot water. *Read labels carefully,* however, to be sure that your choice is truly low-fat, since impostors abound.

Add some French bread or other low-fat bread, and a couple of pieces of fruit or veggies, and you have a tasty, nutritious lunch that is probably less than 5 percent fat.

Frozen microwave entrees
If you have a microwave available where you eat lunch, the possibilities multiply. Try some low-fat frozen entrees.

Leftovers from dinner
Always make more than you can eat at dinner and save the leftovers. You can eat them the next day for lunch, or later on for an easy dinner.

Sandwiches
If you *must* have your sandwich at lunch, convert it to a low-fat variety. First, make sure the bread is low-fat. Here in the San Francisco Bay Area we are lucky to have available many types of sourdough French bread—which is not only low-fat but delicious—and it's our first choice for sandwiches. But, of course, any variety you like that you know from label scrutiny to be low-fat is fine. Next, the filling must be low-fat. A good choice is turkey breast (if you get the meat at a deli, make sure it has not been basted with butter). Tuna is an old favorite. There are also many, many low-fat luncheon meats appearing on the market. You're bound to find something here that appeals. Some books, such as *The Pritikin Promise*, provide recipes for bean spreads that may strike your fancy. To moisten the sandwich, try nonfat mayo (remember to try various brands), mustard, ketchup, tomatoes, lettuce. You can probably create a sandwich that tastes as good as or better than your favorite high-fat variety.

Rice and beans, plain or with salsa
This is a very simple meal that is surprisingly good. Just scoop some rice into a plastic container, and cover with beans. (You can make enough rice to last several days and store it in the fridge.) For added spice, pour some salsa over the top. Snap on a tight lid and you're ready to go. Try this for lunch a couple of times and you may be hooked. An added bonus, especially with brown rice, is that the complex carbohydrates of the rice and beans are digested slowly and evenly, providing you with smooth energy throughout the afternoon.

Dinner

These suggestions are for the times when you must keep the preparation time to an absolute minimum. When you have more time, of course, you can cook very elaborate meals.

Cereal

Why not? Many nights we have had time for nothing more. Nutritionally, a dinner of whole-grain cereal with fruit on top and nonfat milk beats a pizza—and it's faster than even the fastest food.

Frozen dinners

Keep several low-fat selections in your freezer. Just a few minutes in the microwave and it's ready. Add some French bread, some frozen vegetables prepared on the stove while the dinner is microwaving, and you're set.

Leftovers

Make it a habit to cook double or triple recipes and freeze the leftovers. Dinner can be prepared in the time it takes you to thaw them in the microwave. The taste of these "homemade frozen dinners" is almost always superior to the store-bought variety (and they are much, much less expensive).

Low-fat soup, crusty French bread, fresh fruit

Those same soups that you keep on hand for lunch make terrific quick dinners, as well. Add bread, vegetables, and fruit.

Pasta with low-fat prepared spaghetti sauce

In addition to the frozen dinners in your freezer, keep some low-fat spaghetti sauce in your pantry and pasta on your shelf. The pasta takes less than ten minutes to prepare; the sauce can be heated in less than five. Microwave some vegetables, put out some bread, and dinner is served.

Tacos or burritos

Keep a package or two of low-fat tortillas in the fridge. Low-fat and fat-free refried beans are now available. The tortillas and beans, both heated in the microwave, are the main ingredients of burritos or tacos. Add tomatoes, lettuce, green pepper—we've even tried shredded cabbage and carrots—along with some nonfat sour cream, if you desire. Top with salsa. A complete meal in itself.

Barbecued skinless chicken or turkey breast, with baked potatoes and steamed fresh or frozen vegetables

Okay, the total preparation time for this meal is not minutes, it's more like an hour and a half. But the actual time you need to be involved is just a few minutes, and the result is a delicious light supper for spring or summer. First, wash the potatoes and put them in the oven to bake (350 degrees for an hour to an hour and a half). Then prepare the coals and lay the chicken or turkey on the grill to barbecue. You can jazz it up with a barbecue sauce. While the chicken or turkey is barbecuing, make a simple vegetable, either frozen or fresh. If you time it right, the potatoes, poultry, and vegetables all are done at the same time, ready to serve.

Baked fish with potatoes

Again, this is a very simple meal whose total preparation time is more than an hour, but that requires only a few minutes from you. The potato takes about forty-five minutes, so if you serve the fish with bread instead of potatoes, you can cut the time to less than forty-five minutes. The cooking time for most fish steaks and fillets is less than half an hour.

Snacks

Snacks are important, more important than any single meal you will eat during the day. When you eat fatty meals that may provide you with over a thousand calories before you even start to feel full, you are taking in so much fuel that your body may not send you hunger signals again for hours. By contrast, a low-fat meal containing only several hundred calories may leave you feeling comfortably full, satisfied, and energetic, but you will probably need refueling in two hours or less. Your stomach simply can't hold enough low-fat foods to provide you with energy for longer than that. So you're going to be snacking during the day, probably two, three, or even four times. You want to be sure that you anticipate this, and have plenty of low-fat snack foods available, or you may find yourself ravenous at three in the afternoon with nothing but the lunchroom candy machine, stuffed with high-fat monstrosities, as your source of food. Hunger almost always wins out over good intentions under these circumstances.

Children, especially active children, seem to need feeding every hour or so. It's especially important to establish some low-fat snacks that they enjoy. When they start asking for a particular snack, you know you have a winner (more on dealing with children in chapter 10).

So we have provided a fairly extensive list of snacks that people have found to be effective during the day. These are easy to carry, easy to eat, low-fat, and, for the most part, nutritious. We've also included a few not-so-nutritious choices, because everyone needs a treat now and then. They're not intended to be the mainstay of your diet, but they allow you to be a little sinful without paying for it by putting on extra pounds.

Fruit
It gets our number-one billing. It's natural, packed with nutrition, easy to carry, easy to eat (at least most types are), and extremely low in fat. Bananas are about the easiest snack fruit, nature's own candy bar, available year-round. Just peel and eat. Apples are another easy choice that are available most of the year. Other fruits are more seasonal. Check your produce aisle and pack your lunch bag or briefcase.

One word of caution: Any fruit that is potentially squishable, even bananas, should be in a plastic bag if it's put in a briefcase or knapsack, to avoid getting goo on important papers. Or even unimportant papers.

A second caution: The energy from one or even two pieces of fruit will probably not last more than about an hour. Be prepared to snack again.

Vegetables and nonfat dip or dressing
The same ideas that you can use for lunches apply for snacks also. As with fruit, don't expect the energy to last more than an hour or so.

optimum for health by the overwhelming
studies, the only fat level that has been scien-
everse heart disease. At this fat level, almost
ces dramatic fat loss over time. We call this

lly an inaccurate term. To our bodies, a 10-percent-
normal-fat" diet, a 20-percent-fat diet is a "moder-
" and a 40-percent-fat diet is an "extremely high fat
eaten on the face of the earth."

2. Can I eat too little fat?

workshops often worry that if they cut out too much fat
unhealthy, maybe even fatal. Shouldn't we be making sure
at least a little fat, perhaps by taking a spoonful of veg-
each day (as some "experts" recommend)?

require "essential fatty acids," components of fats and oils
can't manufacture ourselves, necessary for a number of body
ns. If you get just two of these essential fatty acids—linoleic
nd linolenic acid—in your diet, your body can make all the rest.
how much do you need of these two?

hat is a matter of some debate. Prisoners have been fed diets with
than 1 percent calories from essential fatty acids for six months
and remained healthy; developing children were fed the same diet for
thity months and grew rapidly. Some experts think that the daily re-
qurement for essential fatty acids may be as low as 0.55 percent of the
total daily calories.

Not all the fat in food is made out of essential fatty acids. But, especially in plant foods, a large portion is—often half or more. So it is virtually impossible, eating normal foods in normal combinations, not to
eat at *least* the minimum requirement of essential fatty acids—as we've
emphasized earlier, it's almost impossible to eat less than 10 percent
total calories from fat, which will provide you with a big margin of extra fat. You can probably go as low as 5 percent safely, as long as you
eat natural, mostly vegetarian foods.

Even foods that are the lowest in fat, such as fruits and vegetables,

fattiest ice cream for richness and flavor. You can also find it in most
supermarkets, but don't let yourself get confused by the bewildering
variety of regular, "low-fat," and nonfat frozen yogurts: make sure you
get one that is truly nonfat.

Air-popped popcorn sprayed with soy sauce or nonfat butter spray

The only way to make truly low-fat popcorn is with an air popper. You
may want to invest in one to prepare treats for video nights or just general munching. Instead of salt, try spraying the popcorn with soy sauce.
Pour the soy sauce in a sprayer like the ones you use to spray plants
(reserve this sprayer only for soy sauce; do not fill it with plant products). Spray the popcorn. Eric's daughter Monica loves popcorn this
way. Another possibility is to use nonfat butter spray.

Cereal or bananas with nonfat milk

Not only do we eat cereal at breakfast and for the occasional dinner,
we also snack on it when we want something substantial—for example,
to carry us for two or three hours until a late dinner.

Dried fruit of any kind

Raisins, apricots, prunes, apples, etc.—they are a more concentrated
form of energy than fresh fruit, so a handful will probably last you two
or three hours. Fresh fruit is nutritionally preferable; but dried fruit
now and then makes a welcome change.

Nonfat muffins and breads

Make sure that they are nonfat, or at least low-fat.

10

Twenty Questions

· · · · ·

Workshop participants, friends, and others have asked us hundreds of questions, mostly concerning the low-fat-eating part of the program. Although we inevitably talk about exercise in the answers to these questions, because exercise is a second key element of any weight-control program, you will find more detailed explanations of some of the misconceptions about exercise in chapter 11.

Many of these questions have to do with integrating low-fat eating and exercise with your family, so we'll devote a special section of this chapter to that aspect of the program.

General Questions

*1. What does "low-fat" mean, anyway—
is there a definition that everyone agrees on?*

No, and this leads to a lot of confusion. The phrase "low-fat" has about as much meaning these days as the word "organic" used to—it seems to mean anything that any huckster wants it to mean.

Broadly speaking, a "low-fat diet" is a diet that contains less fat than you now eat. But there are many different levels within that definition. So let's look at some dietary levels of fat, and point out some areas of confusion.

- **40 percent calories in**
  This is the typical Ame
  forms of cancer, diabetes
  but it is not natural.

- **30 percent calories from fat**
  This is the official recommendat
  government and of the American
  benefits are minimal, and you wor the
  level, either. As Dr. Dean Ornish p e h
  worst of both worlds, where you make at
  get few benefits.

  In news reports about scientific studie
  themselves, a diet of 30 percent fat is often
  ing to many reports of minimal or no benefi le
  diet. Keep this in mind when listening to news
  find out what the actual fat level used in the stu
  above 20 percent fat, the study is virtually useless
  the effects of a true low-fat diet.

  To make matters worse, this level of dietary fat has
  officially adopted by the FDA as the "daily value" th
  should shoot for, and fat percentages on food labels are ca
  from it. This can make reading labels confusing if you are
  trying to cut fat.

- **20 percent calories from fat**
  This is the level of fat in the diet that the American Heart Assc
  ation recommends for people with heart disease. It is the low
  level that most commercial diet programs get to, and many d
  even get this far (Nutri/System, for example, is 30 percent fat)

  At 20 percent calories from fat, you will experience s
  health benefits and noticeable weight loss. This much fat is
  more than our bodies evolved to use, but it is far superior
  40-percent-fat diet.

- **10 percent calories from fat**
  This is the level of fat in the diet that our bodies evolved to

contain enough fat to cover your requirements (for example, an apple is about 6 percent fat, a banana 5 percent, a carrot 3 percent, a sweet potato about 3 percent). In our program, Phase 1 will get you down to 20 percent calories from fat; at this level, your only worry is that you are still getting too *much* fat. In Phase 2, 10 percent calories from fat, you'll be getting about *three to ten times* the minimum level of essential fatty acids.

What about taking a tablespoon or two a day of vegetable oil, just as "insurance," when you get down to really low fat levels? This has been recommended by some authors, who claim that ordinary foods don't contain enough essential fatty acids, or that they have been "processed away." They even claim that some essential fatty acids will cause weight loss. There are several problems with this.

First, even at the lowest levels of fat consumption, as we just pointed out, the practice is unnecessary, since your fatty-acid needs are amply met.

Second, why eat the pure oil? Eat the vegetable or grain itself (for example, corn instead of corn oil). Our hunter-gatherer ancestors didn't press the plants they found and eat only the extracted oils. They ate the whole damn plant.

Third, if you *add* oil to your diet, you can kiss any fat loss goodbye. Two tablespoons of oil is 28 grams of fat, enough to raise a 15-percent-fat diet to about the 30-percent level. Will this make a difference to your set point?

Eric tested it with an experiment. He adjusted his diet, normally about 10 percent fat, in one way: he started eating two tablespoons of vegetable oil per day. This brought him to about 25 percent total fat in his diet, over double what he had been eating. It probably also doubled his essential-fatty-acid intake. According to our set-point concept, his set point should have become higher, and he should have started depositing fat. Sure enough, over the course of two months he watched his waistline expand an inch, the equivalent of a fat gain of about five pounds— despite his somewhat *increasing* levels of exercise during this time. At this point Eric decided to stop the experiment, rather than see just how far his navel would migrate away from his spine as he reached his new, higher set point. When he stopped taking the extra oil, the fat disappeared, again over about two months. It was an insidious demonstration of a basic principle: fat makes you fat. And the extra essential fatty acids in the oil made no difference to his state of health; once you are eating the minimum, the rest is only stored as fat.

It's also ironic that some misinformed "authorities" are voicing concerns about people's getting too little fat, now that the fat-free revolution is on. Our emergency rooms and cemeteries are crowded with people dying or dead before their time because we eat five to eight times more fat in our diet than our bodies are designed to handle. About a million people each year die in America from diseases caused, in large part, by our high-fat diet and sedentary life-style, and millions more live at far below optimum health and energy levels. Tens of millions are overweight. The problem is not, and will never be, too *little* fat.

3. But I've read that some heart experts say that your "good" cholesterol goes down when you eat low-fat, and you may actually increase your risk of heart attack. I don't want to do that. Shouldn't I just stick with exercise?

No. There is no evidence that a diet of 10 percent calories from fat is harmful to your heart or anything else. The evidence overwhelmingly supports a protective role. So why the dire warnings?

The warnings are theoretical. You have two types of cholesterol, LDL-cholesterol—the "bad" cholesterol, which is deposited in artery walls—and HDL-cholesterol—the "good cholesterol, which may actually remove fatty deposits in artery walls. Low-fat diets appear to lower the blood levels of *both* types of cholesterol. So some scientists, such as Dr. Frank Sacks at Harvard, have said that eating low-fat won't do any good, and may even be harmful, because you might lose too much of your good HDL-cholesterol and lose your protection against heart attack.

By this theory, you would predict that populations that eat low-fat diets would have lots of heart disease. But the opposite is the case: they have very low levels of heart disease. Figure 1 in chapter 3, a graph of the rates of heart disease in various countries and how they vary with fat content of the diet, makes this vividly clear. Strike one against the theory.

You can also see this for groups of people, such as the Tarahumara Indians, who have extremely low cholesterol levels, because of a combination of low-fat diet (10–12 percent calories from fat) and high levels of exercise. The average total cholesterol level is 133, the average HDL is 25, making the total cholesterol-to-HDL ratio 133/25, or 5.3. In other words, less than one in five cholesterol particles in their blood is the "good cholesterol." This ratio is considered unhealthy, with dangerously little good cholesterol in the blood; heart disease should be prevalent in a population with such a ratio. Yet heart disease is very rare among the Tarahumara. Strike two against the theory.

You might think that heart patients on a true low-fat diet (10 percent calories from fat) could be in danger. The low-fat diet might actually increase the rate at which their heart disease progresses, for it lowers amounts of protective HDL. At least this theory predicts that it would. But Dean Ornish has shown that, in patients with pre-existing heart disease, switching to a 10-percent-fat diet and practicing stress-reduction techniques and moderate exercise can lead to a reversal of coronary blockage, to a greater degree than even drugs can achieve. This reality check so completely contradicts Dr. Sacks' theorizing that we can call strike three. His theory is outta here.

But what can we offer in its place? How about this? At cholesterol levels below about 160, the amount of "good cholesterol" and "bad cholesterol" is no longer important. There is so little cholesterol of *any* type that your arteries are safe. In the Framingham study that we mentioned in chapter 3, researchers found that, in this town of thousands of people, *no one with a blood cholesterol under 150 had a heart attack in over thirty-five years of the study.* Not a single person. It made absolutely no difference what the total-cholesterol/HDL ratio was. So just shoot for a low-level cholesterol by eating low-fat.

Finally, two of the few ways that you can *raise* HDL-cholesterol are by losing weight and exercising. So, if you also choose the exercise portion of the program, you get to hedge your bets. As your cholesterol is dropping into the guaranteed safe range, you can enjoy elevated, protective HDL.

4. Will I get enough protein if I eat low-fat?

The situation with protein is much like that with fat: we require small amounts to live, it is very hard to become deficient, even the most stringent low-fat diet provides more than adequate amounts, and too much is harmful.

Protein provides the building blocks (amino acids) that we use to re-build muscle and other tissues that are lost during the normal wear and maintenance of everyday life. It's an essential nutrient. The Recom-mended Dietary Allowance (RDA) for protein is 0.8 gram per kilo-gram of bodyweight per day. For a 165-pound man, that's about 60 grams a day; for a 140-pound woman, about 50 grams a day.

How much protein will you get if you adopt the eating styles we rec-ommend? Phase 1 of the program probably won't change your protein consumption much—which means, if you are eating typical American fare, you are consuming close to *100 grams* a day. In Phase 2, you make additional changes that may lower the amount of protein in your diet, but by no more than about one-third. You will still be getting far above the RDA for protein.

As an example of the level of protein intake you can expect, let's look at Carol's typical breakfast. She usually has shredded wheat, per-haps with half a banana on top, along with skim milk. Her cereal bowl holds two cups of cereal—two "servings," according to the package (you will find that, when you eat low-fat, your actual serving sizes make a mockery of the official servings), containing a total of 10 grams of pro-tein. She uses about a cup and a half of nonfat milk. Another 13 grams of protein. Even the half-banana contributes a gram. Before Carol is out the door in the morning, she's eaten 24 grams of protein, about half of her daily requirement. And all this just from a couple of bowls of cereal with fruit and milk.

But what if you don't drink milk, or use any other "high-protein" sources? Won't you be dangerously close to deficiency? No. As with fat, almost every natural food contains *some* protein. A large banana contains 2 grams, a large apple .5 gram, a baked potato 4 grams. Grains are rich in protein, and beans are an especially good source. Of course, meat and most dairy products are very high in protein—perhaps ex-cessively high, as we'll see in a minute.

But don't we have to be careful about combining vegetable proteins to make sure that we get "complete" protein? No. The idea that all the essential amino acids must be present in exactly the right combination in a given meal or the protein is unusable was popularized by Frances Moore Lappé in her otherwise excellent book *Diet for a Small Planet.* It's since been found that our bodies are far more flexible in their abilities to use protein of all sorts.

Protein deficiency rarely occurs if there are adequate calories in the diet. When calories are inadequate, the first priority becomes simply fueling the body, and everything eaten, including protein, is burned as fuel. As a result, protein deficiency can develop. There is only one way the average American ever experiences inadequate calories—by cutting calories in order to lose weight. If you are worried about protein deficiency, never diet again. And never go hungry. Eat the calories your body asks you to eat. The protein will take care of itself.

Actually, from a health point of view, a better question is "Is there too *much* protein in my diet?" A great deal of research indicates that most Americans get far *too much* protein. It can lead to such conditions as osteoporosis. Your blood becomes acidic when you eat too much protein, especially animal protein, and your bones are literally dissolved to neutralize the excess acid. Too much protein can also worsen kidney disease (because part of protein is poisonous and must be flushed out of the body through the kidneys, which can become damaged if they are overloaded due to excess protein consumption). One effective treatment for existing kidney disease is to place patients on a low-protein diet so as not to stress these organs further.

Worried about cancer? Experiments conducted at Cornell University indicate that it's not just fat that we should be cutting down on. Animals were given a cancer-causing chemical, then fed diets that were low-, medium-, or high-protein. The more protein in the diet, the earlier and faster the tumors developed. Other studies show the same results. Fat *and* protein both appear to promote cancer.

Rural Chinese eat only 6–7 percent of their calories as protein and not only survive but thrive, avoiding most of the chronic degenerative diseases that we Americans face. Here in America, we eat 14–18 percent of our calories from protein, *double* what the Chinese have shown is completely adequate. Are we in the danger zone for protein consumption? Our burgeoning rates of cancer, osteoporosis, kidney disease, and other chronic ailments that have been linked to protein indicate that we may well be. To lower your protein consumption, shift from animal to vegetable products.

5. Don't I need to become a vegetarian to eat really low-fat?

No! A few of the best low-fat-eating programs around, those of Dean Ornish, M.D., Neal Barnard, M.D., and John McDougall, M.D., and Mary McDougall, recommend a vegetarian diet (Ornish allows some milk products). Because of their popularity, people seem to be confused about whether it's possible to eat any meat at all on a low-fat diet.

If you just want to drop to 20 percent fat in your diet (Phase 1), you need not give up any meat, as long as you keep it within reasonable limits. The changes in Phase 1 focus on nonmeat aspects of the diet partly because many people are attached to their carnivorous ways. As long as you don't add *more* meat to your diet in this phase, you can reach 20 percent fat in the diet fairly easily.

As we showed in chapter 8, if you want to drop to 10 percent fat, you will have to forgo many types of meat, because most commercial meat is over 50 percent fat. But you can still eat turkey and chicken breast, and many types of fish.

Of course, there are moral arguments for becoming a vegetarian. And some evidence suggests that protein from vegetarian sources is more healthful than that from animal sources. Because of one or both of these arguments, many people find themselves, over months or years, eating more and more of a vegetarian diet on this program. But it's not essential. You'll get all of the weight-loss benefits and the vast majority of the health benefits if you continue to eat meat within our guidelines.

6. Doesn't low-fat eating cost more than eating the way I do now?

A young mother once asked at a workshop, "This low-fat eating all sounds great, but my husband and I are on a tight budget, and with the

groups had lost weight, an average of about four and a half pounds. The nonfat eaters now rated fatty foods as less tasty than before the study. The artificial-fat eaters liked fat as much as ever. The nonfat eaters had changed their tastes in only twelve weeks, so that, wherever they went, fat was less of a temptation. They were on their way to a diet that would work for them anywhere. The artificial-fat eaters still had the same craving for fat, and they couldn't count on their artificial-fat products always to be there when they wanted a fix.

Give yourself a break and avoid fat substitutes.

9. Alcohol makes you fat, but isn't it healthy for your heart?

There is some evidence that moderate alcohol use has effects that may raise set point. On the other hand, heavy drinkers actually weigh *less* than normal drinkers, mainly because of malnutrition, so the exact situation regarding alcohol and set point isn't clear. It is clear, however, that overweight people *do* eat more fat than normal-weight people. So, purely from the vantage of set point, worry about your fat intake, not your alcohol intake. The only problem here is that alcohol certainly has the effect of releasing inhibitions (the reason most people use it in the first place), which makes you more likely to eat high-fat foods in the beginning, when you are still adjusting to a low-fat diet.

Much has been made of the supposed health benefits of a glass or two of red wine every day. This makes good newspaper stories, but it tells only part of the truth. There may be some decrease in the risk of heart disease in people who drink up to, but *no more than,* two glasses of wine a day. This effect is marginal and is far smaller than that achieved by switching to low-fat eating. Balance against it the increase in cancer risk (of the esophagus, stomach, colon, and other organs). *Any* amount of alcohol increases this risk. Women who drink even *one drink a day* have up to a 50-percent-increased risk of breast cancer. Also, for most people, two glasses of wine measurably impairs driving ability. Finally, getting in the habit of drinking daily may be okay for most people, but for a substantial minority of the population it tends to lead to alcoholism.

So popular perceptions of alcohol are just the reverse of the true situation. In moderation it will not cause weight gain, and in excess it causes weight loss. And its use, even in moderation, is not an overall health benefit.

10. What about "fat genes"? Is being fat just genetic?

In 1994, scientists discovered a gene that was abnormal in a certain strain of mice. These mice are enormously obese, growing to over three times the weight of normal mice. What made the discovery so exciting was that evidence for a similar gene was also found in humans.

The natural reaction from many people was, "I knew it. It's all genetic. My mother was fat, my father was fat, now I'm fat, and there's nothing I can do. I've got the fat gene."

But when you understand what the gene actually does, you'll see that this isn't so. Even if there is a genetic predisposition to obesity in your family, the situation is actually quite hopeful.

One puzzling aspect of set point is the question of how your brain, where the bodystat is, knows how much fat is on your body. There must be some way that fat cells "talk" to the brain, letting it know just how big (or small) the body's fat stores are getting. But, up until this discovery, it wasn't known how this was done.

The "fat gene" is the answer. It is the genetic blueprint for a messenger molecule that is sent out from the fat cells and goes, via the bloodstream, to the brain. The more fat in the fat cells, the more of these molecular messengers are sent out. So the brain can tell very precisely how big or how small the fat stores are, by "counting" the number of messages that it's getting.

In the obese strain of mice, the fat gene is mutated—the mutated genetic blueprint directs the production of damaged molecular messengers in the fat cells. These damaged messengers can't communicate with the brain anymore. The brain, receiving no messages from the fat stores, thinks that fat stores have dropped to zero. So the bodystats in these mice are getting continual signals that fat stores are far below set point, causing the mice to be constantly, ravenously hungry. They eat all the time, and are never satisfied. Their fat stores grow larger and larger, but the brain never gets the message.

You have to keep in mind that the obese mice have a *mutation,* a very rare event. Human beings who are fat don't have this mutation (except possibly in extremely rare cases, which would be people who weigh over five hundred pounds). Everyone has the normal gene, which is doing its normal job—telling the brain how big the fat stores are. The reason the fat stores are big in most overweight humans is that the set point *in the brain itself* has been raised—by high-fat eating and by inactivity.

Certainly, some people are more predisposed to getting fat than others. But the genetic component probably has to do with how sensitive their set points are to environmental influences. People who are very sensitive to changes in activity levels will get fat easily if they are inactive. People who are very sensitive to changes in fat levels in the diet will get fat easily if they eat a high-fat diet. And, of course, these sensitive people will also *lose* fat easily if they become more active or eat a low-fat diet. That's why studies have shown that, the more overweight you are, the more fat you lose in response to either exercise or low-fat eating. Genetics works *against* people with sensitive set points when they eat high-fat and are inactive. But genetics works *for* them when they eat low-fat and exercise, because their set points respond more dramatically and quickly to any change, whether it's one that raises the set point or lowers it.

So don't blame your genes if you're fat. Instead, take advantage of them to make yourself lean.

11. *What do you two eat in a typical day? What kind of exercise do you do?*

Our diet varies as we go through food-preference cycles. We'll eat lots of oatmeal for breakfast, then it's raisin bran, or corn flakes, or pancakes. We might eat bagels as snacks, then switch to baked potatoes. Soups might dominate dinners one week, to be superseded by stews the next. The only constant is a fat level that averages about 10 percent. But since we are often asked *exactly* what we eat, and what exercise we do, we kept track of our food intake and exercise for a couple of consecutive days.

DAY 1

	Carol	Eric
Food	2 c. oatmeal	3 c. oatmeal with 1½ T.
	3 c. decaf coffee	brown sugar
	3 peaches	1 orange
	4 apples	2 bananas
	1 plum	2 c. spaghetti with garbanzo-
	½ c. blackberries	bean sauce
	8 Jolly Rancher hard	3 SnackWell's low-fat
	candies	chocolate sandwich
	2 c. spaghetti with garbanzo-	cookies
	bean sauce	2 peaches
	1 banana	2 burritos (corn tortillas
	2 tostadas (open-faced tortilla	and homemade beans,
	with beans, green pepper,	red and green peppers,
	onions, tomatoes)	and salsa)
	2 corn tortillas with salsa	¾ c. corn
	1 c. rice	2 c. mixed green salad
	2 c. salad	
	1 c. nonfat ice cream	
Exercise	Ride exercycle for one hour while talking on the phone, 90 stomach crunches	Walk 20 minutes to and from train to work, two 15-minute walking breaks at work (total for day, 70 minutes of walking), 20 stomach crunches

DAY 2

Food	1 c. oatmeal	3½ c. oatmeal with 2 T.
	1 banana	brown sugar
	½ c. blackberries	1 orange
	1 peach	2 bananas
	2 c. decaf coffee with	3 tuna-fish sandwiches
	skim milk	(tuna salad made with
	2 corn tortillas with salsa	fat-free mayonnaise)
	2 tostadas	7 Entenmann's fat-free
	6 large (huge) pretzels	chocolate-chip cookies
	1 c. corn	3 oranges

So George not only did not cut fat from his diet, he actually added fat. His effort was real, but he lacked the tools to make it work.

Even if he *had* cut the fat in, say, his weekday lunches (while leaving his breakfasts and dinners as they were, and eating as usual on weekends), such a change would lower the overall fat content of his diet from 40 percent to, perhaps, 35 percent. That kind of change would produce results. George might lose two to five pounds over the course of a year (depending on how overweight he was to begin with). But the half-pound to pound of fat that he lost in the first two months would not even show up against the day-to-day fluctuations in his weight (throw away your scale!). Again, George could weigh himself at two months, not see a noticeable change, and give up.

If you *truly* cut the fat from your diet, you will lose fat. But you must have the tools to make a true effort, and you must give it a real chance to work. And if you want to see dramatic losses, you must make dramatic changes.

13. How can I lose fifteen pounds in the next month for my wedding (or a big date, or a vacation at the beach)?

This kind of "deadline" tempts you to use the calorie-cutting approach. And let's be honest, the fastest way to lose weight is through extreme calorie-cutting, so the temptation is strong. Let's compare that approach with low-fat eating and exercise. You have a big event coming in six weeks: your wedding. You *must* lose ten or fifteen pounds in that time.

Let's say you choose to lose weight for your wedding by eating 800 calories a day for six weeks before the ceremony. The first week is pretty easy, and you notice changes right away. But it gets harder as you go on. Just at the time when you need added composure and calm to deal with the seemingless endless details, you find yourself tired, irritable, moody, depressed. By the day of the wedding, you've lost your fifteen pounds. About five pounds will be fat, perhaps five will be water, and the last five will come from muscle. Still, people tell you how great you look (you'd enjoy their comments more if you weren't about to faint from hunger). But what happens after the wedding? You can be sure that six weeks

---

¼ c. beans	1 baked potato with salt and
1 c. rice	pepper
2 c. green salad	3 c. tuna-and-pasta salad
1 medium nonfat-frozen-yogurt cone	½ c. corn and peas
	8 carrot sticks
5 pieces red licorice	¼ c. blackberries
1 banana	1 c. mashed potatos

Exercise	Ride exercycle 40 minutes while reading, then ½ hour of very light weight training, 90 stomach crunches	Walk 45 minutes

Please don't think you have to eat exactly as we do. Don't look at this two-day snapshot of our eating habits and say, "My God, they ate a lot of oatmeal. Well, I hate oatmeal. I couldn't possibly eat the way they do. Oh, and look, Carol ate a plum on day 1. I despise plums. No wonder they stay thin—they eat foods I hate." To tell you the truth, we're kind of sick of oatmeal now, and have switched to cold cereal for a while. So look at the principles illustrated by these two days, not at the exact foods.

The first principle is that we don't go hungry. We eat a lot. We also don't get fat. We do *not* belong to the group of people who can eat whatever we want and not get fat. We have both been unhappily plump for periods in our lives. But by eating the way we do, we can consume a lot of food, food we like, and stay lean. We *do* belong to the group of people who will stay naturally lean on a low-fat, moderate-exercise program. So do you, if you belong to the human race.

A second principle illustrated here is that the foods we ate were *all* low-fat. We don't play the game of counting fat grams and "saving" them up for high-fat treats. If you do that, you find yourself having more and more treats, until your diet is all treats. Plus, it gives us a headache even to think about counting fat grams at every meal, then adding them up. It's a pain in the butt to balance our checkbook every month. We're supposed to balance our fat book every day? Instead, we simply eat low-fat *all the time.* When we want a "guilty pleasure," we eat a nonfat version. There are so many nonfat products out there, you're bound to find some that taste so good you'll be sure you're "cheating" if you eat them. Carol had a bowl of nonfat ice cream and a nonfat frozen-yogurt cone in these two days; Eric had a total of ten cookies (seven in one day!).

A third principle is that we snack whenever we want. That's important, because we never let ourselves get really hungry. It's tough for anyone except a few fat-free saints to pass up a doughnut shop when he or she hasn't eaten for eight or ten hours. We'd all feel ourselves being pulled in by the vacuum created by deep-fat frying. But anyone can be a hero when he or she is well fed. Give yourself a chance to resist temptation by not allowing it to become tempting. Don't go hungry!

A fourth principle is that we don't insist on perfection. Our major imperfection is that we eat sugar. On these particular days, we ate more than we usually do, but we eat sugar on a regular basis. We like it. We like the way it makes our cereal taste, and we like it in cookies and ice cream. We know that if we were perfect we wouldn't eat it—sugar, again, has no nutritional value and rots your teeth. We know some people think it's evil, the devil's candy. But it makes many foods taste good, and it doesn't affect our set points. Maybe we'll give it up in the next lifetime.

A fifth principle is that we eat lots of fruits and vegetables. Despite all our talk about sugar and cookies, the huge majority of our snacks are fruits, and we eat a lot of vegetables with meals. In these two days, Carol had nineteen servings of fruits and vegetables. Eric had eighteen. So we averaged about nine servings each, per day. We make a conscious effort to do this. We pack fruit and vegetables in our lunch. We make a huge salad with dinner. We each eat a piece of fruit with breakfast, usually the first thing we have each day. These are all habits we have consciously cultivated.

A final principle is that, although we exercise a lot, we get a lot of our exercise as opportunistic exercise. We'll explain this concept more thoroughly in chapter 12, but it boils down to simply taking advantage of exercise opportunities. Carol doesn't just ride the exercycle. She uses the time to talk on the phone with her friends, or to read. You might want to watch TV if you ride an exercycle (if you watch anyway, it takes no more time to ride the bike while you're doing it). You may wonder how Carol can talk on the phone while she is riding, and the answer is that she exercises at a pace that allows conversation. All her

friends are used to her doing this. It's another habit. In fact, arranges to talk with a friend in Seattle during her *friend's* time. Eric got quite a bit of his exercise by walking to the work. Those are our solutions, based on our situation. We gu that you can fit *at least* as much exercise into your day.

12. I tried eating low-fat once and I didn't lose any weight at all. Are you sure this approach works?

Are you sure you were eating low-fat? And how long did you try it

Consider the curious case of George, who sincerely thought he cutting fat from his diet when he decided to eat low-fat lunches. started making his sandwiches with turkey lunch meat labeled "93 fat-free," put between two slices of "low-fat" bread, and moistene with mayonnaise that contains "half the fat per serving of the regula brand." He replaced his usual lunchtime banana (they have kind of greasy feel, and he'd heard they were high-fat) with a cup of "2-percent fat" milk. He was sure he had just slashed the fat in his lunch. The pounds should start coming off now.

Two months later, George had *gained* a pound. He was disgusted and discouraged. Then he read a newspaper story in which scientists said that obesity may be largely genetic. No wonder the low-fat approach didn't work; he was probably just genetically programmed to be fat; it obviously didn't matter how little fat he ate, he would still gain weight.

George's approach to "low-fat eating" is a composite of beliefs that we've heard from workshop participants and others over the years. His "low-fat lunch" is actually about 50–60 percent fat, by calories—a *very high fat* lunch indeed. The meat is 50 percent fat, the mayonnaise 99 percent, and the milk 40 percent. George only read the front of the food labels, where all the lies are; he didn't bother to learn how to read the Nutrition Facts box on the back of the labels for the true fat content of foods. The banana that George thought was a fatty food is actually very low in fat, about 5 percent. George didn't know the value of fruits and vegetables in a low-fat diet.

after the ceremony the honeymoon will really be over. Your weight will be skyrocketing, seemingly out of control. You'll be bingeing regularly, maybe secretly, feeling terribly guilty about it (even though it's your body's natural response to the end of the prewedding "famine"). The stage is set for the vicious diet-regain cycle, whereby you diet, lose weight, stop the diet, gain the weight back, feel terrible about the extra weight, diet again, lose less weight, stop the diet, gain it back. . . . Even worse, the extreme stress and failure at weight control create a perfect psychological and physiological setup for eating disorders.

Compare this with an approach to the big day through low-fat eating and exercise. You take a look at the studies in chapter 5, on really low-fat eating (10 percent calories from fat) and see the truly incredible weight loss that people can experience. The exercise studies show that even more weight loss is possible if you add exercise. Using as your motivation the big event coming up, you decide to start eating 10 percent fat and increase your exercise. You read both the low-fat-eating and the exercise sections of this book carefully, go buy yourself a nonstick frying pan, and assiduously cut every gram of fat from your diet, reaching a level of 10 percent. You add exercise to your day in as many ways as possible, as we will describe in the chapters on exercise. You're careful to eat as much as you want, eating three meals a day and snacking two, three, or even four times during the day. Within days, you notice a new kind of energy, a smooth flow that takes you through days filled with hours of wedding preparations, with energy to spare. It's still stressful, but not overwhelming. Sometimes you find yourself still going strong after fourteen or fifteen hours. After three weeks, you notice your clothes are getting looser. By the day of the wedding, you've lost six pounds, and people are commenting on how good you look. You reply that you're *feeling* even better. Okay, you didn't lose the ten or fifteen pounds you *had* to lose. But you feel better than you ever have—*and* you're losing weight. You keep right on with the life-style after the wedding—perhaps your new spouse is intrigued by your seemingly effortless weight loss and joins you. Six weeks after the wedding, you've lost another four pounds. You look and feel terrific, and you know that you will continue to drop toward your natural, lean set point. For you, the honeymoon is just beginning.

Guess which approach we recommend?

14. *What about chromium? Or thigh creams?* *Or whatever the latest weight-loss "aid" is?*

Our general advice about the latest "miracle" weight-loss schemes is to be very, very skeptical. Some are pure scams. Some may "work," but with unknown and possibly devastating consequences for your health.

Some substances, though probably not harmful (at least in the recommended doses), are hyped on the basis of unsubstantiated claims. Their main danger is that they will make you lose focus on what really works (low-fat eating and exercise, remember?) and start looking for the quick fix.

An example is chromium. The headline of a typical newspaper article about chromium shouted "New Star in the Diet World: Chromium for Weight Loss." A smaller head in the body of the article whispered, "Mainstream physicians are cautious about these products," but everyone knows those stodgy old mainstream physicians are always the last to catch on. The article started with claims from companies who manufactured chromium-containing products, claims such as " 'Chromium picolinate . . . a natural substance that helps dieters lose the fat but keep the muscle.' " Later on in the piece, those picky old doctors and scientists are quoted as saying the claims are hogwash (our paraphrase), but once you've read the first few paragraphs of the article it doesn't matter—you want to run out and buy four bottles of the stuff.

Eric went to a large biomedical database and looked up scientific papers on chromium and weight loss. He found only one careful study. Men and women were given either a placebo or pills containing chromium picolinate. Neither they nor the researchers knew who was getting the real stuff and who was getting the placebo (until the end of the experiment, of course, when the researchers "broke the blind" to find out who had what). This is the "placebo-controlled double-blind protocol," the gold standard of experimental designs for testing any drug, nutrient, or treatment. The men and women went on a twelve-week weight-training program. At the end of that period, the group taking the chromium picolinate had lost significant amounts of body fat—but the placebo group had lost just as much fat! In other words, there was no effect on fat loss from the chromium, just from the weight training. But if you're a company manufacturing chromium picolinate, you can say, with perfect honesty, that in a twelve-week study people taking chromium picolinate lost significant body fat. You can see why you should treat every such claim with extreme suspicion.

Claims about thigh creams have some more troubling aspects. These products came on the scene with the usual blaring headlines: "New Cream Shrinks Women's Thighs, Researchers Say." The research was conducted in part by a "distinguished obesity researcher" and involved the "application of about a teaspoon of cream a day [which] seems to have taken the fat away from women's thighs." The scientific jury is still out on this one (as of this writing, we find no controlled studies in the medical literature to support the initial work by the researchers).

But consider this: Two of the researchers hold a patent on the cream. They spoke of marketing it as a cosmetic, because, " 'If you make cosmetic claims, you could market it as a cosmetic,' without going through the lengthy and expensive drug approval process. . . ." Yes, it's such an inconvenience to go through those persnickety drug-approval procedures, in which you have to prove that your product won't make people drop dead, or give them cancer, or cause them to give birth to deformed children. Why bother, if you can call it a cosmetic? There's a ton of money to be made. Another of the researchers bragged that he was also working on a breast-enlargement cream. Can a penis-lengthening cream be far behind? Which do you think these researchers are more interested in, making a fast buck or helping you lose fat healthfully and permanently?

That's not to say that some weight-loss products don't work. But at what price? We'd like to tell you about a purely natural product that's known to promote weight loss. It has been used by native peoples for thousands of years, its basic ingredient is completely organic, and studies have shown that people who use it lose weight, usually ten to thirty pounds. As a bonus, it makes you feel energetic and sharpens your mental processes. Interested? We've just sold you a pack of cigarettes.

Nicotine is a drug that lowers the set point. Smokers are leaner than nonsmokers, yet consume more calories. If they quit, they gain an average of twelve pounds. A major reason that women give for smoking is that it helps them in weight control. It really works. The weight-control aspects of smoking were touted in ad campaigns over fifty years ago: "Reach for a Lucky instead of a sweet." Women started to get the message, and the numbers of women smokers increased. Now women are dying of lung cancer in numbers that match those for men—a few years ago, lung cancer took over first place as the number-one cancer killer of women, a position it has held for decades among men. Smoking is estimated to be the number-one controllable health hazard in the United States, causing about *half a million* deaths a year. Not to mention the damage to fetuses—forty-six hundred fetal deaths each year are due to smoking, and smoking accounts for perhaps 30 percent of the low-birth-weight babies born each year, but about 25 percent of pregnant American women continue to smoke during pregnancy—and the suffering that smokers endure before they die. Some of the damage from smoking is reversed on quitting, and some is not. The effect on set point ceases immediately when you quit, as is true with any other "diet drug."

So other diet aids that come on the market may work, just as tobacco works. And they may be organic, herbal preparations—just like tobacco. They will be promoted by people who may sincerely believe that, since they are natural, since they have been used for centuries, they must be safe. There is no guarantee that they are, however. There is a good chance that they are deadly in the long run.

And we do guarantee that when you stop using them you will gain back every ounce you lost. Any method that resets set point works only as long as you continue to use the method. That's true for smoking, for diet pills, and for low-fat eating and exercise. If you simply want to lose weight, any of these approaches is effective. But smoking and diet pills will kill you. Low-fat eating and exercise will revitalize you and energize you for a long, full life. Take your choice.

Questions About Integrating Low-Fat Eating and Exercise with Your Family

15. *What if I'm the only one in my family who wants to go on this program?*

One woman at a workshop commented that she could apply the program to her life if it included "husband replacement"; she was married to a man who managed to stay slim despite drinking extra-rich milk, putting quarter-inch-thick butter on his bread, and eating sausages for breakfast. Even though there was a strong history of heart disease in his family, he had not the slightest interest in a low-fat eating program. What do you do if you're in such a situation?

First, take care of yourself. Even if you are the person who prepares all of your family's breakfasts, lunches, and dinners, you don't eat all these meals with them, and certainly don't have to eat the same food. As discussed, there are many *very* low fat alternatives for breakfast, lunches, and snacks. Dinner is the meal that you generally eat with the rest of the family. If you want to lower the fat content of the main course but you're worried that your family will object, we recommend: well . . . just do it. If you are doing the cooking, it's really up to you to determine what the eaters eat. As long as you keep their tastes in mind, you have every right to experiment with lower-fat meals for the entire family. There are some very simple ways to cut at least half, and often three-quarters, of the fat out of almost any recipe (see suggestions in chapters 7 and 8), with practically no change in taste (in fact, many recipes taste *better* with less fat). You can also introduce an occasional true low-fat main course; when you find one that everyone likes, add it to your arsenal. Go slowly, respect your family's tastes, but insist on your right to eat healthfully.

As you make the transition to lower-fat meals, you will still be serving many higher-fat favorites. But you don't have to give up on your low-fat goals each time you serve such a main course—*you* can cut your portion by two-thirds, and make up the difference with lots of French bread, vegetables, potatoes, etc. This kind of strategy, combined with eating very low-fat the rest of the day, can keep you at under 15 percent calories from fat in your daily diet, without having to prepare two sets of meals.

16. It seems as if I didn't start to have problems with my weight until I got pregnant. Does pregnancy make you permanently fatter?

Many women gain weight during pregnancy, sometimes an alarming amount, and most of it just seems to stay on afterward. When you see it happen to yourself and all your friends, you begin to believe that it's just the natural order of things—have babies, get fat.

But in primitive societies, though women gain fat during pregnancy and remain somewhat fatter for the next year or so, most do not become permanently fatter from having children. Why, then, is that pattern the norm in affluent societies?

First, most women know that it's not okay to diet during pregnancy. Many women embrace the fact that they must eat, for the sake of the baby. For a woman who has been always staying a little hungry, always staying ten to twenty pounds below her set point, this may be the first time her body has had a chance to come to set point. The result is a weight gain during pregnancy of fifty or more pounds, thirty or more of which may be fat (about twelve pounds of fat gain is average, though it varies widely). That sort of weight is not easily lost.

Second, pregnancy leads to a decrease in activity levels, probably causing some further gain as the set point increases. And, as any parent will tell you, the first six months of a baby's life are not conducive to an active exercise program on the part of Mom or Dad. So the stage is set for getting out of exercise habits and not getting back into them—permanently raising set point.

Third, many women do not breast-feed their babies. The extra fat during pregnancy appeared for specifically that purpose, and disappears within about a year if the baby is breast-fed (and if you return to normal activity levels).

So, even though it may appear "normal" for women to get fatter as they have children, a lot of the gain results from our abnormal way of life. Women's bodies just aren't adapted to dieting all our lives, stopping suddenly when we're pregnant, becoming inactive, and not breast-feeding.

17. Is it safe to eat low-fat during pregnancy?

From one point of view, the answer to this question is simple: we wouldn't be here if low-fat eating and exercise weren't safe for pregnant and lactating women, because our ancestors had no choice but to live that way. Indeed, in areas of the world where the population consumes diets consisting of 10–20 percent fat, birth weights are the same as they are in the United States, as long as the mother is consuming enough calories. So, as long as you are not cutting calories or going hungry during pregnancy, a low-fat diet is probably optimum.

But that's a crucial point—if there is one time when you must not go on a diet, or go hungry, it is when you are building another human being. A woman who loses weight during pregnancy, even an overweight woman, runs an increased risk of having a low-birth-weight baby, which has a lower chance of surviving. Occasionally, women have trouble eating enough food to satisfy their hunger on a low-fat diet because of the bulk of the food; if that is true for you, supplement your diet with higher-fat foods such as nuts, which contain lots of calories in very little space.

So the main concern in pregnancy is not the fat level of your diet, but that you eat when you are hungry, and continue to eat until you are satisfied. You will increase the number of calories that you are eating automatically to compensate for your increased energy needs. Along with those increased calories will come protein and fat, because almost all natural foods contain them. It's mainly a matter of common sense. As long as you stick to the grains, legumes, fruits, and vegetables, and follow your hunger, you're fine. On the other hand, if you eat a diet that is mainly soda crackers and jam, you might worry about nutritional deficiencies, just as you would at any other time. If you are really worried about protein, small extra portions of lean turkey or fish are low-fat and very high in protein.

The second concern during pregnancy, as long as you are getting enough calories, has to do with vitamins and minerals. Folic acid, calcium, and iron are the most important. Deficiency of folic acid is associated with birth defects, and the defect occurs right after the time of conception, before a woman even knows she is pregnant. So the U.S. Public Health Service recommends that all women of childbearing age get at least 400 micrograms per day of folic acid. Most women take in about half that amount. Among the richest sources are dark-green leafy vegetables. You may want to consider taking a B-complex vitamin as insurance. Leafy dark-green vegetables, such as kale, also contain calcium, another requirement during pregnancy. Of course, so does milk, and skim milk can be part of a low-fat diet. The jury is still out on iron; some feel that, on balance, most women should take a supplement during pregnancy, but others feel there is some evidence that excess iron may cause slightly higher rates of complications. You're best off consulting your doctor, who may want to order tests at various times during your pregnancy.

18. *What about nursing?*

Experts agree that there are no detrimental effects of low-fat diets during lactation as long as the woman eats enough calories (don't diet!).

Beyond the countless health reasons for breast-feeding as opposed to formula-feeding, there are two more reasons to breast-feed, both having to do with fat.

As we mentioned, during pregnancy, as long as you don't diet, you will put on excess fat, enough to fuel about one-third of your baby's energy needs for the first three months or so of its life. You are designed to draw on this fat, plus the rest of your natural fat, to produce the fats in your milk. It would make sense that women who breast-feed would lose more weight after pregnancy than those who don't, because breast-feeding is what that extra fat is intended for. Yet studies of breast-feeding and weight loss were inconsistent: some showed more weight loss with breast-feeding, some less.

Then researchers at the University of California at Davis did a very careful and thorough experiment. They studied weight loss in women who breast-fed compared with those who didn't, and they made one important restriction on who could be in the study: *they excluded dieters.* That's crucial, because women who don't breast-feed tend to diet more than those who do (the breast-feeding women are afraid that dieting will affect the quality of their milk). So, if you don't exclude the dieters (and earlier studies hadn't), you may find that non-breast-feeders lose more weight, in the short term (because more of them are deliberately cutting calories to lose weight). Of course, they gain it all back, but most studies don't continue long enough to see that effect. In the Davis study, the breast-feeders lost about ten pounds in the year after birth, compared with about five pounds for the non-breast-feeders. But you must breast-feed for a period of six months or so to get the big effects. There was little difference between the two groups up to three months, but by six months the breast-feeding group had lost about four more pounds than the non-breast-feeding group, and by one year the difference was five pounds. The researchers concluded, ". . . the patterns shown herein provide another argument for encouraging overweight women to breast-feed for as long as possible during the first year postpartum."

The second argument for breast-feeding has to do with the fat that your baby is eating in the first few months of its life. There is only one time during our lives when we are designed to eat high-fat animal products. That is when we are infants, and the high-fat animal product we are designed to eat is mother's milk. The fat content of human milk varies, but it averages about 40 percent. This fat is, of course, derived from the mother (now you can see why breast-feeders lose so much more weight).

The fat in breast milk seems to be specially "formulated" to meet the needs of the developing infant. As we mentioned in the answer to question 2, adult humans require two essential fatty acids, from which we can make all the rest of the fatty acids that we need. It appears that infants may not be able to use these two essential fatty acids to manufacture the rest of the fatty acids they need as easily as adults do. They may do better if they get the other fatty acids pre-made, from an animal source—their mother, whose milk contains high concentrations of these fatty acids, which seem to be especially important in the development of the nervous system, especially the brain.

What does this have to do with breast-feeding? Infant formula is made with enough fat to supply calories, but it contains only the two essential fatty acids. Infants fed with formula may suffer a lack of the other fatty acids that they would normally receive in mother's milk. Whether this is a problem with full-term infants is not known. But at least one study shows that pre-term formula-fed infants were less intelligent than pre-term breast-fed infants. The moral of all this is that, besides all the other health benefits for your baby if it is breast-fed, there may also be the benefit of optimizing intellectual development, especially if the baby is pre-term.

What should you eat during breast-feeding? The most healthful diet possible, a low-fat diet rich in fruits and vegetables.

In terms of exercise, there is no need to curtail your exercise program during breast-feeding, and if you would like to begin an exercise program, go right ahead. Studies show no significant difference in the milk of regular exercisers compared with sedentary women, or in the milk of women starting an exercise program. In fact, the only difference found in the study of the regular exercisers was that they produced a larger volume of milk. Well, there was one other difference: the women who engaged in vigorous exercise on a regular basis ate more than those who just sat around . . . but carried about *ten pounds less fat.*

19. *What about children? Is this program safe for them, and, if so, how do I get them to eat well and adopt an exercise program?*

Children up to six months of age should be breast-fed, if at all possible. Surprisingly little is known about the fat requirements of infants from six to twelve months. A recent scientific reviewer stated: "Almost no data exist to permit assessment of the optimal fat content in the diet of the 6- to 12-month-old infant." Some say that children at this age should be started on the same low-fat diet as their parents. We disagree. In primitive cultures, infants breast-feed up to the age of two years. And breast milk is high-fat—again, about 40 percent. So it makes sense that that is what children up to the age of two are designed for. Now, you may not want to breast-feed your child until he or she reaches the age of two, but if you are introducing the child to solid foods, they should be higher in fat than the ones you eat— 2-percent or whole milk instead of skim, peanut butter, etc., to bring the fat content of the diet to about 40 percent. Once the child is beyond the age of two, you can start to lower the fat in his or her diet down to the same level that you eat. If you're not convinced that this is safe, or if you'd just like to find out more about low-fat eating for kids, read *Dr. Attwood's Low-Fat Prescription for Kids*, by Charles R. Attwood, M.D. (New York: Viking, 1995). This book makes a thorough, scientific case for instilling low-fat eating habits in your children, and has a wealth of practical tips.

As for how to get children to adopt healthy eating and exercise habits, perhaps our own experience will be useful. We're helping to raise two children—Eric's daughters, Alison and Monica, who live with us for portions of the year. We don't have complete control over their diet and, frankly, we don't make an issue of it. We have found that the most effective strategy is to identify the most healthful foods that they enjoy (not the ones we *think* they should enjoy), then always to have these foods available as snacks.

Alison and Monica have typical tastes for a nine-year-old and seven-year-old, respectively. They like almost all fruit. They like only certain vegetables (raw carrots dipped in salad dressing are a particular favorite). They like nonfat pretzels, soda crackers, and low-fat bagels. So these are the snacks they have. They are allowed unlimited snacks. We don't worry about "ruining their appetite," since we feel that an apple half an hour before dinner is just as healthful as, and probably more so than, the portion of dinner it may displace. By encouraging the low-fat, healthful snacks that they like, we're getting them in the habit of thinking of these foods as simply some of their favorite foods, not the "good" food that they must eat instead of the "bad" fatty food. And they probably get about a third of their calories each day from foods that are 5 percent fat.

Regular meals are also low-fat, but not fanatically so. Dry cereal for breakfast with skim milk and fruit (they are allowed to put sugar on their cereal; after all, Daddy does). Burritos for lunch made with low-fat refried beans and tortillas. Dinners are usually the lowest-fat compatible with their tastes. But we also have high-fat treats on occasion.

Our main goal is to lead by example. Unfortunately, Alison and Monica already talk about fat on their bodies, despite being extremely lean. But we're confident that they will see us and the way we eat and live, and realize that they have a choice. Children learn far more from what you do than from what you say. If you eat a low-fat diet and lead an active life, so will your children.

A second aspect of the program is, of course, exercise. There is no need to design an exercise "program" for your child. Left to themselves, kids exercise—they run, jump, dance, swing, play tag, climb trees, play hide and go seek . . . from dawn to dusk, if you will allow them. But you need to give them the opportunity.

The first action to consider is unplugging your TV. The average American watches four hours a day (and that doesn't include time watching videos or playing computer games). TV is mesmerizing. Watch your kids watching it sometime. They may respond by facial expression.

But are they moving their limbs? Running around? They sit passively, transfixed. People may actually burn fewer calories while watching TV than they do while lying in bed. It's no accident that people who watch the most TV have been found to be the fattest. And to make matters worse, the constant barrage of advertisements for pizza, hamburger joints, the latest gimmicky junk food, can undermine your best efforts to get your children to eat even a few healthful snacks.

Without TV to babysit them, your children may come to you asking what they can do. The time-honored response is "Go outside and play." Try it! You will probably find that no other "workout program" is ever necessary. And you may be surprised at how quickly your children adjust.

20. How about teenagers? My kids are in high school and insist on a diet from the four food groups: cheeseburgers, ketchup, French fries, and Coke. How can I get them to eat a healthy diet and to exercise?

With teenagers, you have adolescent rebellion working against you, and obsession with body image working for you.

When it comes to overcoming adolescent rebellion, we again advise leading by example. Have you noticed how, as you get older, all those stodgy things your parents did that seemed so boring at the time (like saving money, or cooking good meals) begin to make more and more sense? Give your children the same sort of example. Even if it doesn't appear to make a dent now, you will get your revenge later, as your children turn into you.

And you can use the natural changes that occur at puberty to nudge your teenagers toward healthful, lifelong habits. Before puberty, boys and girls are fairly similar in terms of fat and muscle mass. But during puberty, girls gain fat while boys gain muscle. This is natural and leads to the naturally higher levels of fat in women. Another natural development is an interest in the opposite sex, and the desire to be attractive. Attractive, in our society, means less fat for women, and more muscle for men. This is reflected in statistics showing that a large proportion of women want to lose weight, but none want to gain, whereas large numbers of men *are* interested in gaining weight (muscle).

Now, you may be angry that our society imposes a body ideal that seems impossible, especially for women. No one can be as slim as the models in the ads. You may rage that your daughter is starting to succumb. And you have every right to do so.

We agree that women are exposed to a frighteningly thin ideal. But you should also realize that both men and women are naturally lean, and that most women who come down to their natural set point are satisfied with their appearance (even if they don't become model-thin stick figures).

We suggest a bit of psychological judo. Instead of trying to meet head-on the huge juggernaut of thin female images that just keep appearing on every magazine cover, in every TV show, and in every movie, maybe you can use this momentum to your advantage. Use the motivation that media images create to propel your daughters, especially, toward knowledge about set point, and how low-fat eating and exercise will work to make them slimmer.

For boys, the pressure is not so intense. But most boys want to be more muscular, to be bigger but leaner. How do you do that? Through exercise, especially weight training, and low-fat eating.

Looked at this way, the teenage years become the perfect time to instill habits of eating and exercise. Your children will be motivated. They are old enough to understand all the arguments we make in this book about what really works in becoming lean. They have large blocks of time in their day during which they can exercise, and many options for team sports or individual exercise. They can learn about the techniques for low-fat eating from you, in the home—and that type of eating will forever be associated with the comfort of home.

Sounds great in theory. But you know by now that we don't believe anything unless it's been tested by experiment. Carol performs such an experiment every year.

Carol teaches high-school biology and chemistry. As part of each class, she teaches about nutrition: she teaches a capsule summary of the principles in this book.

Now, the usual picture of the American high-school student would have him grabbing a doughnut for breakfast, a Twinkie for lunch, and a burger with fries for dinner, while turning a deaf ear to anyone who nags about good nutrition. Carol has found that this picture of their eating habits is pretty accurate. But the idea that they won't listen to nutrition information is completely false. They simply have never heard the truth about nutrition. The students in Carol's classes listen with rapt attention. The nutrition units generate more discussion and questions than anything else they study during the year—students fire questions at Carol until the bell rings, and beyond. For most, it's the first time that they have had the connection between fat and disease, and fat and weight, explained to them.

They're not solely interested in the weight aspects, either. They have dozens of questions about the connections between diet and health. Unfortunately, in many cases the curiosity is due to watching a parent with diet-related illness, such as heart disease. Carol expected the girls to be interested, because of the connection between diet and body fat. But she was surprised to find that boys are just as interested. Both boys and girls clamor to know more about their own diets.

And they find out. The students evaluate their own eating habits by keeping a food diary for two days. Then they learn how to read labels and to classify foods as high-, medium-, or low-fat. Then comes the shocker. They go back to their food diaries and, using tables of nutritional values, calculate the amount of fat in their own diets, to classify them as high-, medium-, or low-fat. Most of the students are in the high-fat category, and they are flabbergasted to find how much fat they've been eating—one boy had eaten a diet that was 80 percent fat in the two days listed in his food diary, yet he had had no idea until he analyzed his diet.

Such eye-opening exercises change thinking and behavior. One girl told Carol, "Now I go home and look at all those things that I have been eating and I don't want to eat them anymore." Students bring fruit and vegetables to class: "This is my third fruit of the day!" They even analyze labels for their parents. One student was referred to Carol by the basketball coach, who had been through our program. The player had injured his back, was unable to practice, and had gained weight. Carol spent three afternoons with him outlining the principles of low-fat eating. The boy, motivated by his desire to get back to his playing weight, took the program to heart and within two months had lost all the weight he'd gained while injured.

So the picture of the teenager who is blind to the connection between diet, health, and weight is mainly a myth. Given the right information, they can get very excited about the control that they have over their bodies and their health. Given the wrong information—thousands of TV commercials extolling the virtues of Domino's Pizza, Jack-in-the-Box, Burger King, Wendy's, McDonald's, Taco Bell, Snickers bars, Coke, Pepsi—they'll eat junk. What else can we expect? Carol's unit on nutrition probably represents less than .1 percent of the information that these kids have heard about food during their lives. But it's the truth. Given just a taste of the truth, they change their behavior in a hurry.

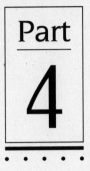

Part

4

Exercise
Your Right to
a Fat-Free Body

11

Don't Make a Myth-Guided

Attempt at Exercise

• • • • •

xercise is the second method for lowering set point. Some people choose to use exercise alone as a means of weight loss; others combine it with low-fat eating for a doubly effective approach. But anyone who chooses to add more activity to his or her day will probably start with some misconceptions, misconceptions that may have caused previous attempts at fitness to fizzle after just a few weeks. It's essential that these myths be dispelled before you consider an exercise program of any sort.

There was a "fitness revolution" in the 1970s—or so we were told. You couldn't open a newspaper during that decade without seeing a photograph of 140,000 people jammed together at the starting line of the Omaha Marathon. You were told that you needed a different shoe for everything—running, walking, aerobics, tennis, basketball, racketball. . . . There are now shoes for surfing and for river running. Feeding on the downpour of media hype, health clubs sprang up like mushrooms. And "fitness experts" multiplied like steroid-crazed rabbits.

The result? Several hundred books of conflicting advice, thousands of magazine articles, millions of sports injuries . . . and most Americans now exercise less than ever. What used to be as simple as lacing up a pair of sneakers and going out for a jog has become a nightmare of target heart rates, antipronation shoes, the latest fitness fashionwear, health clubs that cost more than food for a family of four, personal trainers who charge more than brain surgeons, pills guaranteed to protect you against the damaging effects of exercise, and dozens of other fitness "aids" marketed on the basis of our belief that exercise is now too complicated to leave to the common folk.

Now, don't get us wrong. We love exercise and have participated in sports ranging from high-school basketball to intercollegiate rowing. In our living room we have a cross-country-ski machine, a stationary bicycle, a step machine, a weight bench, and a complete set of dumbbells. And we even consult with a personal trainer on occasion (he does brain surgery on the side). One of us (Eric) completed his Ph.D. with one of the most respected exercise physiologists in the world, making him, we guess, one of those damned "experts."

But the main knowledge we have gained in about forty years of combined experience is that *exercise is simple.* And this is what we want to convey to you.

Let's look at some of the exercise myths that grew out of all the hype, hysteria, and hucksterism of the past two decades. You'll learn in this chapter why you can forget about target heart rates, choosing the "right" form of exercise, rigid exercise programs, and other gospels of the exercise elite. This time, when you start an exercise program, you won't be making a myth-guided attempt.

Myth: Exercise Is Something That Makes You Sweat and Breathe Hard, and It Hurts

If we say that we are going to recommend an exercise program to you, what is the first image that forms in your mind? Think about it for a few moments before you read on. Close your eyes and actually picture what you'll be doing.

For most people, the image that comes to mind is something like a jogger in a sweatsuit, puffing along with a look of sheer misery on his face. Or it may be an image of a woman in a Lycra bodysuit, gyrating to some impossible aerobics routine, gasping and sweating as she tries to keep up. The common denominators in these images are sweat, effort, and pain. Is this the kind of image you formed? It's not surprising.

The experiences you have had with "exercise" have probably been guided by people who also thought that sweat, effort, and pain were vital ingredients. "No pain, no gain!" your high-school coach may have yelled at you. "Feel the burn!" exhorted the aerobics mavens of the 1980s. "You must exercise at an intensity that causes you to breathe harder to attain any benefit!" command the hundreds of fitness books. The myth of exercise gets perpetuated. Exercise is: something that you must put on special clothes for (because it's going to make you sweat), something that you must mentally brace yourself for (because it's going to hurt), and something that's going to leave you exhausted (because it's a tremendous effort).

Well, erase that image from your head. That's *not* what exercise is. In fact, you are exercising right now, as you read this.

Exercise is anything that involves muscle contraction. Muscle contraction simply means using a muscle; it can be quite gentle—in fact, not even noticeable. You're exercising as you read this, because you exercise just to stay alive. Your diaphragm muscle rhythmically contracts and relaxes to move air in and out of your lungs; your heart muscle rhythmically contracts to move blood through your blood vessels; muscles surrounding your intestines rhythmically contract and relax to move food through your digestive system. Even people in a coma are exercising. They are at one extreme of the exercise continuum, the bare minimum, but they are still exercising.

If you decide actually to get out of bed in the morning, you increase that level of exercise through simply performing your daily activities, because everything you do involves muscle contraction. Rising from bed, brushing your teeth, walking to the car, etc., all require that your muscles work. Not much, admittedly, and we seem fixated on reducing it to the bare minimum, but it's still exercise. Even the most dedicated couch potato must expend about 500 calories a week going about the business of living. This person has moved up from the bare minimum of the patient in a coma, just a little.

Your body is keeping track of how much exercise you are doing, and adjusting your level of body fat accordingly. If you are doing the bare minimum—staying seated most of the time, driving when you have to travel more than 100 feet, sitting on the couch watching TV—your body adjusts its set point upward (adds more fat) to its "famine" position, because that is what it thinks is going on. Remember, the only time our ancestors were as inactive as we are was during a famine; otherwise, they had to move to get food—they had no choice. You're not moving, food must be scarce; when you do get some food, you're going to store as much of it as possible as fat.

If you exercise a little more, your body will lower the set point a little (reduce the fat on your body). If you exercise a lot more, your body will lower the set point a lot. When you look at exercise this way, you realize that *any exercise you do above the bare minimum is going to lower your set point.* You don't have to get your exercise in a workout. You don't even have to get it all at once. Anything you do that involves activity—*anything*—is exercise and will contribute to lowering the set point.

Of course, if you only do a little, you only experience a small effect. But we'll show you in chapter 12 how relatively minor alterations in your daily routine, most of which won't require any more time at all from your day, can make big changes in your activity level, and correspondingly large changes in your set point. You can make these alterations without joining a health club, wearing special clothes, sweating, or grimacing in pain. Your body doesn't care about that. All it's keeping track of is how often, each day, you are contracting your muscles.

Of course, workouts where you sweat, grunt, and groan will also be interpreted by your body as exercise. They can be added to the increases you make in your daily activities, if you want, to increase overall exercise levels even more. That will be the subject of chapter 13. But it's important to realize that even these workouts don't have to be painful or grim to be effective; in fact, just the opposite is true, as you will see.

Myth: You Lose Weight When You Go on an Exercise Program Because the Exercise Burns Calories, Which Must Come from Your Fat Stores

The conventional explanation for why people lose weight when they exercise is that they have increased their activity levels, so they are burning more calories than they eat, so of course they will lose weight (fat). But when you think about it, this explanation doesn't make much sense, at least not in the long run.

We talked about this a bit in chapter 1. The example we gave was that, if you walked two miles a day, burning 200 extra calories a day, by the end of a few years you would have burned enough extra calories so that your body would have had to consume every ounce of fat, muscle, and other parts of itself—and you would have disappeared. Why is it that instead you only lose five or ten pounds from this two-mile-a-day walking, then stop losing, even if you continue walking on a daily basis?

Set-point theory answers these questions beautifully. *Your bodystat is always keeping track of the calories you use each day. It never misses a single calorie that you use in exercise of any type, and it adjusts body-fat levels accordingly.* Ultra-low levels of activity (the norm, unfortunately, in late-twentieth-century America), lead to ultra-*high* body-fat stores. Medium levels of activity (achievable by simply moving around more each day) lead to lower fat stores. Very high levels of activity (if you work out, which your body interprets as the work necessary to gather lots of food) lead to very *low* fat stores. *Your body will adjust to the appropriate fat level automatically, and stay there, as long as your activity remains at that level.*

This explains why you don't disappear after several years on an exercise program.

It also leads to a caution. Many books and programs have charts that show the number of calories burned in various activities. With a little math, you can calculate how many calories you burn in the particular types of exercise that you choose, and how fast you "should" lose fat. You will almost surely be disappointed if you do this. First, the rate appears so slow as not to be worth it. Second, it leads you to think that you will lose weight forever if you continue with the same level of exercise. In reality, you can't predict the rate at which you will lose initially, and even if you continue the exercise program, at some point you hit a plateau. For some people, whose set points respond very quickly to exercise, the weight loss can be far more rapid than mere calorie-burning can account for. For others, far slower. And all people stop losing as they hit their new set points. If you're not satisfied with your weight at that point, you can cut the fat in your diet more, or you can exercise more.

Myth: Exercise Suppresses Appetite

Actually, this is only a half-myth. Low to moderate levels of exercise may, indeed, suppress your appetite, at least for a while. That's how your body gets your fat level to a new, lower set point: it signals you to eat less. But when you have reached your new, low fat level, it's quite likely that your appetite will now increase to compensate for the extra calories you expend in your exercise, so that you no longer lose weight, but remain at your new, lower weight. It's nothing to be alarmed about. Just eat as your body tells you to. It will keep you at your lower fat level automatically.

As you move to higher and higher activity levels, usually meaning that you start doing workouts, you find that your appetite increases, sometimes dramatically, yet your weight remains quite low. An example is our friend Ian, man of steel. Several years ago, he trained for and competed in the Ironman competition. That's the race where the competitors swim more than two miles in the ocean, bike more than a hundred miles, then top it off by running a relaxing marathon through the lava fields of the Kona Coast of Hawaii—all in one day. When Ian was training for this event, it wasn't unusual for him to exercise four, five, or even six hours a day. Going out to dinner with him was an adventure. On one particularly memorable occasion at a Mexican restaurant, Ian ate two entire meals while the rest of us barely finished our single meals, then complained that he was still hungry. Yet he was far leaner than anyone else at the table.

If, as often happens, you find that you enjoy exercise, and start doing more and more, you may have a similar experience. Though your appetite may increase, you continue to lose weight. Relax and enjoy it. You are built to eat exactly as much as your body signals you need.

Myth: Low-Intensity "Fat-Burner" Exercise Is the Best Way to Lose Fat

This myth got started because it makes perfect sense—in theory. But when the theory is tested against reality, it doesn't hold up. And, as usual, when you replace the old theory with set-point theory, things start to make sense.

The old theory is that when you exercise you *lose* what you *use* as fuel. There are only two major types of fuel for exercise, fat and carbohydrate. Slow, easy exercise, like walking at a brisk pace, is fueled mostly by fat, which requires oxygen to burn. Fast, intense exercise, like sprinting, is fueled mostly, often entirely, by carbohydrate, which can burn without oxygen. So (the theory goes) you want to do the slow exercise, which will burn up your fat, and stay away from the intense exercise, which won't call on your fat stores at all. It's a very appealing picture, the fat literally being burned up as you walk, or jog, or ride the stationary bike, at just the right, "fat-burning" pace. Usually you're told to exercise at a pace that will allow conversation. That way you know your muscles are getting enough oxygen, so you're burning fat. Really, the picture is almost irresistible.

This theory is easily tested. It predicts that people who do slower, mild exercise should lose fat, whereas people who do more intense, harder exercise should not lose fat. Slow, "fat-burning" exercise would include walking, jogging, and cycling at an easy pace. On the other hand, the most intense exercise you can do, which relies entirely on carbohydrate fuel, is weight training, which is so intense that the supply of oxygen-carrying blood to the exercising muscles is completely shut off as they are contracted (that's why weight training very quickly produces a burning sensation from lactic acid, a byproduct of anaerobic carbohydrate-burning). The theory predicts quite clearly that only the walkers, joggers, and bike riders should lose fat; weight lifters should not lose any.

But when people who lift weights are compared with people who walk, jog, or cycle, *both groups are found to lose fat at almost exactly the same rate.* This has been shown over and over again, in dozens of studies. *Intense exercise, which burns exclusively carbohydrate, is just as effective for long-term fat loss as mild exercise, which burns exclusively fat.* We must conclude that the theory is utterly, completely wrong. *You can do any sort of exercise and you will lose fat.*

Just like myths for dieting, however, this one persists, mainly because there really hasn't been any better way to explain fat loss from exercise.

Until you consider set point, and why it might be lowered by exercise. To your ten-thousand-year-old genes, programmed in the days when humans were hunter-gatherers, exercise is the signal that food is plentiful, that there is no need to keep extra fat stored on your body. The more exercise you get, the lower your set point will be set, and fat-burning mechanisms are activated to help you lose fat to get to your lower set point, automatically. Those mechanisms will not just be activated during your workout. They'll be going day and night, twenty-four hours a day. The major way you will lose fat is simply through appetite adjustment, as your body signals you to eat fewer calories than you use up, so that it can reach its new, lower set point.

What sort of activities were our hunter-gatherer ancestors doing when food was plentiful?

- They were walking to food-gathering areas.
- When they gathered food, they dug for roots, reached for berries, stripped leaves from bushes.
- When they stalked prey, they walked slowly, perhaps jogging occasionally.
- But when the time came for the kill, there could be intense sprinting, followed by a spear thrust with all the power of the hunter behind it.
- Often hunters chased animals over a cliff. To carry the carcasses to the top of the cliff often required that each member of a team move more than *four hundred pounds* uphill.
- Carrying game or gathered food back to the camp required walking, perhaps miles, with a heavy load (perhaps over a hundred pounds for the hunters).

You can see that our ancestors were the first "cross-trainers." Without ever going on a scientifically designed exercise program, both men and women got a mix of exercise that would rival the training program of the most dedicated Olympic athlete.

And these are the kinds of activities that signal your set point that food is plentiful, that it need not be carried as fat on your body. When you go out for a walk, your body is thinking "walking to the food-gathering sites" or "stalking game." When you garden, your body is thinking "gathering food." When you lift weights, your body is thinking "killing game" or "hauling game to butchering site." If you hike with a pack on your back, your body is thinking "carrying game or food back to campsite."

Set-point theory fits very nicely with the results of exercise experiments. *Any type of exercise represents plentiful food to your set point, and will allow you to carry less fat.* So the most intense weight lifting should produce the same fat loss as gentle jogging—and that's exactly what exercise scientists have seen.

Myth: You Must Exercise at Your "Target Heart Rate" to Burn Fat

Quick, what's your heart rate at this instant? Can you measure it?

Most people can't.

It's tricky to find exactly the right spot, either on your wrist or your neck, to place your fingers so that you can feel your heart beat. Then you have to count the beats for an exact period of time, and multiply to get the number of beats in a minute. If you can do all that while sitting quietly, you're unusual. If you can do it accurately while engaged in a strenuous activity, you're amazing.

But wait, there's more. Were you within your "target-heart-rate range?" This is the range of heart rates that the "experts" tell us we must be within to get any health benefits, the range in which we will burn fat most effectively. It's usually considered to be 60–80 percent of your maximum heart rate. which you get by subtracting your age from 220. Got it? No? Well, just get out your calculator and calculate it right now, if you want to get any benefits from your next workout.

Is it really true that you need to keep track of your heart rate as you exercise, making sure it's not too slow or too fast? If you get outside the optimum range, will you stop losing fat?

No. As we showed in the previous section, *any* intensity of exercise will promote fat loss. It's true that the low-intensity exercises must be done longer. On the other hand, a low-intensity exercise like walking through the park is so enjoyable that you will probably want to do it for longer than, say, running wind sprints. You certainly don't have to take your pulse.

For example, one study compared women walking at different paces. They all walked three miles a day, five days a week. But one group walked at five miles an hour (the researchers called this group the "aerobic walkers"), one at four miles an hour (the "brisk walkers"), and one at three miles an hour (the "strollers"). After six months, the strollers had lost more fat than the other two groups! Yet they were exercising so slowly that their heart rates didn't even approach the standard 60–80 percent of maximum.

How could the exercise physiologists have gotten it so wrong? Exercise physiology started out as the study of athletes and their training, and was focused on performance, not on health. One of the best indicators of your ability to exercise at high levels is *maximal oxygen consumption,* the maximum amount of oxygen that you can use in a given time.

Maximal oxygen consumption can be very easily and precisely measured, and training raises it. So maximal oxygen consumption became the focus of training studies. If a particular training routine raised an athlete's maximal oxygen consumption, it was effective. If it didn't, it wasn't. From these very narrowly focused studies emerged the guidelines about heart rates, duration, etc., for exercise. The target heart rates are the ones that will increase maximal oxygen consumption most effectively.

But when the exercise physiologists first made recommendations for the general public, they forgot to broaden their focus. The average person is not interested in becoming an Olympic athlete. He or she is interested in becoming healthier and more attractive. And as it turns out, exercise at levels far below target heart rates, and occurring in short bursts throughout the day, is just as effective, in achieving those goals as is exercise performed according to rigidly established guidelines, perhaps more so.

For example, in the study of the "aerobic walkers," "brisk walkers," and "strollers," the "aerobic walkers" achieved an increase in their maximal oxygen uptake that was over three times what the "strollers" achieved. By the old standards, they got three times more benefit. But the strollers lost more fat than the aerobic walkers. Not only that, all the groups showed similar changes in their blood chemistry, which indicated that their risk for heart attack had decreased by about the same amount. The "aerobic walkers" were no more protected than the "strollers."

So, unless you are an athlete in training, you don't need to worry about your heart rate. If you increase the amount of exercise in your day, and your heart keeps beating, you will lose fat and gain health benefits.

Myth: You Must Exercise for a Certain Duration Before You Start to Burn Fat

This was another part of those exercise prescriptions that we've all heard. "Exercise at your target heart rate at least three times a week for a minimum of twenty minutes each time. Otherwise don't even bother." So that ten-minute walk to the bus to work in the morning, and the ten-minute walk back in the evening, don't count. Might as well just drive.

This myth also grew out of exercise physiologists' prescribing what they knew, which was how to make athletes fitter. To do that, you *do* need to exercise continuously for a solid chunk of time, fifteen to twenty minutes. So this advice got carried over, blindly, to people who just wanted to get healthier, or lose a little weight.

But the truth of the matter is that *small bursts of activity—walking down the block to pick up a quart of milk, or playing catch with your child, or doing laundry—are just as effective for health and weight loss as the long bouts.* Six ten-minute walks, or twelve five-minute walks, are just as effective as one hour-long walk. And they are much easier to fit into your day.

An example of this principle is Bryant Stamford, Ph.D., co-author with Porter Shimer of the book *Fitness Without Exercise*, which was the first to explode many of the exercise myths of the 1970s and '80s. A self-confessed "exercise addict," Dr. Stamford exercised at least forty-five minutes a day, at least five days a week, for over twenty years. But one day he was struck by the absurdity of it all, not to mention that it was turning him into a virtual cripple, and quit his exercise program, cold turkey. "[Quitting] was murder," he writes, "a lot more grueling than any workout. I experienced anxiety, depression, self-doubt, and guilt. I was irritable and short-tempered. I would pass joggers on the road and feel resentful that they could enjoy what I could not." But he persevered, and eventually found himself freed from the compulsion to sweat.

But what happened to his weight? It was his exercise routine that had enabled Stamford to transform himself from a plump boy to a lean adult, and one of his major worries when he stopped his regular workouts was that he would again become fat. "I saw myself turning from Arnold Schwarzenegger to Rodney Dangerfield overnight, losing a good deal of respect along the way." Yet it never happened. Several years after he quit his grueling workouts, he weighed *less* than when he was exercising daily, and his cholesterol was about a hundred points lower. He had gone on a moderately low fat diet (about 20 percent calories from fat, the equivalent of our Phase 1).

But he credits much of his ability to maintain his leanness to the fact that he still exercises—he just doesn't work out anymore. Instead of one big, intense workout, which required enormous expenditures of physical and psychic energy and left him exhausted, disheartened, and unwilling to help with household chores, he now happily pitches in— cutting grass, stacking firewood, pruning trees, carrying groceries. And he regularly takes breaks at work to climb a flight or two of stairs. None of these activities requires more than a few minutes, but over the course of a day they add up to almost as much exercise as his old workout. And he is leaner than ever. "The point is that I try to keep moving, and preferably in ways that are as enjoyable as possible."

The fact that you don't have to worry about what type of exercise you do, or target heart rates, or minimum durations, is great news, because it opens up limitless exercise opportunities to you. You don't have to be restricted to only those activities that "burn fat." We'll show you in the next chapter how you might take advantage of these opportunities.

Myth: Only People Who Train Like Athletes Get the Health Benefits of Exercise

If you are interested in exercise mainly because of what it can do for your health, you might still be feeling discouraged. After all, the only people who get much healthier are those who jog every day, right?

Wrong again. Regular physical exercise will certainly make you healthier, and that jogger is getting some very impressive protection against diseases such as heart disease and cancer (but if you think it makes you immune to other bad habits, read the next section). Once again, however, there is confusion over what "regular physical exercise" means.

Studies by epidemiologists have shown that people who are more active tend to live longer than those who are less active. And as soon as the exercise physiologists heard the epidemiologists mention the phrase "physical activity," they started giving exercise prescriptions for all exercisers, as if they were athletes in training. Once again, these physiologists confused their concept of exercise, mainly based on what makes athletes better performers, with the epidemiologists' ideas of physical activity, which can be quite different. Consider these results from studies of large numbers of people:

- People who regularly engage in walking, stair climbing, and light sports are significantly more protected against heart disease than those who don't.
- Ticket takers in England's double-decker buses experienced less heart disease than the drivers.
- Longshoremen suffer less heart disease than sedentary workers.
- A study of 13,334 men and women showed that modest amounts of exercise can markedly reduce the risks of heart disease and colon cancer, but greater amounts of exercise offered no further protection from heart disease.

These studies all show the protective effect of regular physical activity. But they do *not* show that the activity has to come from exercise performed as a workout. They include all sorts of physical activity. The ticket takers in the English buses weren't pedaling stationary bikes in the back of the bus for thirty minutes each day; they were walking around the bus and up and down the stairs. The longshoremen weren't taking aerobics classes at their lunch breaks; they were toting heavy loads. And the final study shows that increasing the amount of exercise beyond a certain level (the equivalent, in this study, of simply walking between thirty and sixty minutes a day) doesn't increase health benefits.

To be fair to the exercise physiologists, they are now re-evaluating these old studies in the light of the new concept of activity, and coming to the conclusion that moderate amounts of physical activity, the types you can get without ever buying a pulse monitor, will give you about all the health benefits from exercise you'll ever get. That moderate level appears to be the equivalent of briskly walking two to three miles a day. Anything beyond that will give minimal increases in health (although it will lower your set point even more). And that equivalent of two to three miles of walking can be any form of moderate-to-brisk exercise, at any time of the day, broken into as many chunks as it takes to fit it into your schedule.

Myth: If You Exercise Regularly, You Are Immune to the Health Effects of Bad Eating Habits

We all know people who exercise a lot but have atrocious eating habits. They subscribe to the "blast-furnace" theory of exercise: if you exercise enough, your body becomes able to consume any fuel, no matter how greasy, because it needs it to fuel the muscles, which become like blast furnaces and burn anything fed to them. Physicians such as Dr. Thomas Bassler helped establish this myth. Bassler claimed, in the late 1970s, that marathon runners who didn't smoke were immune to heart attack. The documented heart-attack deaths of dozens of nonsmoking marathon runners, many of whom died while jogging, dampened enthusiasm for Bassler's theories, but the myth persists.

Regular physical exercise certainly has protective effects. It will change your blood chemistry, raising the levels of HDL-cholesterol (the "good" cholesterol), which is somewhat protective against heart disease. It also probably protects against some forms of cancer, such as breast and colon cancer. But expecting exercise to protect you from the hazards of a high-fat diet is like expecting your car to run better on kerosene because you put a bigger engine in it. It's still going to clog up and die.

The most dramatic example of this is the case of Jim Fixx. He, more than anyone else, embodied the running revolution of the early seventies. He jogged regularly. He wrote the best-selling book *The Complete Book of Running.* He took no special care with his diet—he even said that "Running provides at least partial refuge from the dietary pressure . . . to eat wisely." And he died of a heart attack, while jogging, at the age of fifty-two.

Fixx's case dramatically shows that exercise won't offer you *complete* protection from disease. Unfortunately, this was misinterpreted in many commentaries to mean that exercise offers *no* protection from disease. But that's not true. There was a family history of heart disease in Fixx's family; his father had died of it even younger. Fixx probably shared his father's proclivity to develop heart disease, yet he managed to live several years longer. Did his running prolong his life? There is no way to be certain, but it probably did.

Another point which was almost completely overlooked is that Jim Fixx might well be alive today if he had also changed his *diet.* There is little evidence that exercise alone can reverse heart disease, which is caused by blockage of the arteries that bring blood to the heart itself. But several studies show that a low-fat diet, alone or combined with drugs or stress reduction, can retard or even *reverse* heart disease by *unblocking* those arteries. If Fixx had been more open to such changes in life-style, his heart disease might never have troubled him.

Indeed, he might have followed the footsteps of another man, Nathan Pritikin, who was diagnosed with severe heart disease at the age of forty, in 1957. Rather than follow the standard medical advice of the time (rest and drugs), Pritikin scoured the medical literature and came up with his now-famous Pritikin Program of low-fat eating and exercise. He began eating the healthful diet that he later taught to others, and his blood cholesterol plummeted and all traces of his heart disease disappeared. After his death in 1985 from unrelated causes (leukemia), an autopsy revealed that his coronary arteries were completely clear—the *New England Journal of Medicine* reported, "... in a man 69 years old, the near absence of atherosclerosis [hardening of the arteries] and the complete absence of its effects are remarkable."

And lest you think his death from leukemia was related to his "crazy" way of eating, you should be aware that the leukemia was probably the result of a medical treatment (X rays) he was given for a skin condition. He managed to survive twenty-eight productive and energetic years despite his heart condition, and many feel that this incredible survival time was largely due to his dietary habits.

12

Opportunistic Exercise

• • • • •

In America, and in other industrialized societies, we tend to become fatter as we get older. At the same time, we lose muscle and other lean body mass. This pattern is ubiquitous, and we have come to accept it. You look around when you're in high school and you see a few obese people, but they are the exception, not the norm. But when you look around at your twenty-five-year high-school reunion, everyone seems to have put on ten, twenty, or thirty pounds. Now it's the lean people who are the exception. The pattern is so entrenched that health authorities seem to have become resigned to our getting fat as we get older. Some voices in the medical community are starting to soothe us about this weight gain, to assure us that it's natural and not harmful.

Such weight gain is not natural, however. It is the product of our unnatural life-style, of our diet and our exercise patterns. Studies have shown that, in the few remaining primitive societies in the world, obesity is *unknown* among middle-aged and older men, and very rare among women. In fact, studies of existing traditional societies show that body weight remains constant from age twenty to forty, then very gradually *declines*. At no time in adulthood is it natural for human beings to gain weight. These primitive societies generally eat low-fat diets, ranging from 5 to 15 percent calories from fat. But there are exceptions. The Masai, an East African nomadic cattle-herding tribe, eat a diet that is 66 percent fat(!) yet are an extremely lean people. The

247

major factor keeping the Masai and all other primitive people lean into middle age and beyond is exercise.

You Don't Have to Sweat to Reset

Oddly enough, health clubs are unknown among the primitive tribes that remain lean throughout their lives. These people don't use stationary bicycles, StairMasters, rowing machines, neatly groomed tracks, or other "fitness necessities." They may go weeks at a time without reaching their target heart rates. For them, of course, physical exertion is the norm, and periods of inactivity are the exception.

"But what does that have to do with me?" you say. "I don't have time to exercise the way those people do. They may walk ten miles a day during their daily food-gathering, but I don't have three hours to spare for such activities."

True, but consider this: In the past ten years, Americans have gained weight. *On average, eighteen-to-thirty-year-olds are ten pounds heavier today than they were a decade ago.* This weight gain is not due to our eating more (we actually eat fewer calories than we used to) but to our doing less. It's not that fewer people are jogging, or doing other forms of structured exercise, than a decade ago. Those numbers are actually increasing, from five million several years ago to about ten million today. But the rest of the population, the ones who aren't out there jogging, exercise even *less* in their everyday lives than they used to. And they, the vast majority, are becoming real lardbutts.

We have let our labor-saving devices save us so much labor that we are almost at the activity levels of bed-ridden invalids. We have remote controls for our TVs and even our stereos. In our cars, we push buttons to roll down the windows and open the garage door. More and more restaurants and hotels are offering valet parking, which used to be the exclusive privilege of the rich and snobbish. We wouldn't be surprised if some of the classier restaurants start wheeling their customers from their car to the table in wheelchairs, so that they can avoid the unpleasant exertion of walking those two or three hundred steps.

None of these "improvements" in our lives has saved us any significant time. They have simply robbed us of effort. But if you turn this view around a bit, it's quite hopeful. If we have managed to gain ten pounds through relatively trivial changes in life-style, we can lose ten pounds through reversing those changes. *Many of us are at such a low level of activity that even small changes, if pursued regularly, can make a big difference in weight.* In going from complete inactivity to even moderate activity, you get the biggest weight-loss benefits. And if you go a bit further, and actively seek out opportunities for exercise, you can lose even more.

- You don't have to change your clothes to take advantage of the exercise opportunities around you.
- You don't have to buy special equipment.
- You don't have to make time in your day; you just use some of your time in new ways.
- You can get your exercise in bursts while pursuing your normal life.
- *You don't have to sweat to reset.*

This everyday kind of exercise is called "opportunistic exercise." Opportunistic exercise is exercise that you don't think of as exercise— walking from the car to the store, climbing a flight of stairs, gardening, etc. As far as your set point is concerned, your body doesn't know whether you're wearing a Lycra workout suit or a wool business suit, whether you're on a StairMaster or on a flight of stairs. You can probably fit an additional ten minutes to half an hour of exercise into each day with a little creative thought and with no extra expenditure of time. For most people, that additional exercise results in an additional five to ten pounds of fat loss over the course of a year.

It's analogous to saving your change. You accumulate change each day in your purse or in your pockets. If you took that change out every night and put it in a jar, you would never miss it. But by the end of a month you might have thirty or forty dollars, and by the end of the year you could save several hundred dollars, painlessly. Not only is that a substantial, real savings, but it would encourage you to start saving money systematically in other ways.

So it is with opportunistic exercise. You can painlessly accumulate a penny's worth of exercise here, a nickel's worth there. It seems like nothing at the time. It certainly can't be exercise, because it's not painful and it's not making you sweat. Yet at the end of a few months you may notice that you're a few pounds lighter, your clothes a bit looser. That sort of experience can encourage you to try more systematic exercise. You may find yourself starting to change your routines so that you can get in an extra ten minutes of walking in the morning, or you may begin to toy with the idea of joining a health club. Slowly, without even noticing it, you can nudge your genetic program for leanness back into operation full-time.

We're going to make some suggestions, but it's important to remember that opportunistic exercise is the result of a new awareness that you apply to every aspect of your life. If you can fit activity in, do it! You'll be amazed at how quickly it becomes a habit. In fact, you may be surprised at how little bits of activity, spaced throughout the day, start to make you crave more.

First, take this quiz to see where you stand (or, better yet, walk or run) now.

When Opportunity Knocks, Do You Answer?

For each of the following statements, choose the single answer that most accurately reflects the ways in which you are active or inactive on a daily basis. Be honest and careful in your answers. There are no right and wrong answers—this quiz is simply designed to help you see how much of an effect opportunistic exercise can have in *your* life. Place the letter for the answer you selected on the line in front of the question.

_____ 1. When I am watching television, during the ads I

    A. Remain seated, watching the commercial or channel-surfing.
    B. Get up once or twice an hour to adjust the color.
    C. Get up once or twice an hour to do minor chores.
    D. Get up at every single commercial to do chores.

_____ 2. I have an automatic garage-door opener, which I use to open the garage door

    A. Every time I drive.
    B. Don't own one.
    C. Don't own a car.

_____ 3. When I drive my car to go shopping

    A. I will circle the block or the parking lot until a space opens up right in front of the store.
    B. I will park in a space within fifty yards of the store, but no farther away.
    C. I will park in any space in the parking lot that is free.
    D. I make it a point always to park in the space farthest from the store.

_____ 4. When I drive my car (or take a cab) to a restaurant or a movie

    A. I use valet parking.
    B. I wait for a parking space to open up right in front, or have the cab drop me right in front.
    C. I'm willing to park (or be dropped off) within a block, but no farther away.
    D. I make it a point to park (or be dropped off) several blocks away.

_____ 5. I climb _____ flights of stairs each day.

    A. 0. That's what elevators and escalators are for.
    B. 1–5
    C. 6–10
    D. 11 or more

Note: In questions 6–8, "work" means whatever you do all day, including being a student, or taking care of children.

_____ 6. In getting to and from work I

    A. Walk less than one block.
    B. Walk a quarter of a mile to half a mile.
    C. Walk half a mile to a mile.
    D. Walk at least a mile or use an alternative human-powered vehicle, such as a bicycle.

_____ 7. My job requires me to

    A. Sit all day at a desk or in a vehicle (example: office worker, bus driver).
    B. Stand most of the day, and walk for short distances (example: teacher, grocery checker).
    C. Walk or perform light activity for at least one-third of my working hours (examples: nurse, waiter or waitress, caregiver for young child).
    D. Walk most of the day or perform manual labor (example: mail deliverer, carpenter).

_____ 8. During my workday, the total time that I spend on breaks that include exercise, such as walking or stair climbing, is

    A. Less than one minute.
    B. 1–20 minutes.
    C. 20–40 minutes.
    D. 40–60 minutes or more.

_____ 9. I spend _____ minutes a week on yard work.

    A. less than one
    B. 1–60
    C. 60–120
    D. 120–180 or more

_____ 10. I spend _____ minutes a week on vigorous housework such as dusting, vacuuming, sweeping, and mopping floors.

    A. less than one
    B. 1–60
    C. 60–120
    D. 120–180 or more

_____ 11. If I'm early for an appointment I

    A. Sit and wait.

    B. Walk around the halls or outside.

    C. Walk around the halls or outside and climb up and down several flights of stairs.

_____ 12. When I use an airport I

    A. Hire a redcap to take my luggage and sit and wait at the terminal for my flight.

    B. Use a luggage cart to get my luggage to the ticket counter, then sit and wait at the terminal for my flight.

    C. Carry my luggage to the ticket counter.

    D. Carry my luggage to the ticket counter, and walk around the airport while waiting for my flight.

_____ 13. As a parent I (or I would)

    A. Allow my children to watch TV or play video games as their major recreational activity.

    B. Encourage my children to be active in sports or other active endeavors, and attend their games.

    C. Encourage my children to be active in sports or other active endeavors, and help coach their teams.

    D. Encourage my children to be active in sports or other active endeavors, and participate with them (running, playing tennis, basketball, etc.).

For every A answer, give yourself 1 point; for every B answer, 2 points; C, 3 points; and D, 4 points. Total your score.

If you scored:

- **40–48 points:** You're extremely active during your daily activities. You are already getting enough exercise in your day to keep your set point very low, as well as to reap almost all the health benefits exercise has to offer. Additional exercise (such as from a workout) will lower your set point further, but will probably not significantly improve your health.

- **32–40 points:** You're much more active than most Americans, and you may be satisfied with your activity levels as they are. However, there are probably a number of opportunities for exercise in your day that you are not taking advantage of, and if you wish to lower your set point further, you can focus on these areas of your everyday life.
- **20–32 points:** You are active enough to receive most of the health benefits that exercise can offer, and to lower your set point a little. However, you can probably double your daily exercise without spending much extra time.
- **Less than 20 points:** You are dangerously close to couch-potato territory. Exercise opportunities abound in your day that you are not taking advantage of. You can probably triple or quadruple the amount of exercise that you get each day by seeking out these opportunities.

Any question with an "A" answer represents a potential exercise opportunity. Of course, some aspects of your life are easier to change than others. You may not want to quit your executive job to become a fitness instructor just because it offers more exercise (although one of our friends evaluates potential careers largely on the basis of how much time he will be able to spend outdoors, exercising). But as "A"s change to "B"s, "C"s, and "D"s, you should begin to see your waistline shrink.

Exercise Opportunities

Throw away your remote controls

As a first step, you might seriously consider throwing away your TV remote control. This is more than just a symbolic gesture. When you can't mute the volume on commercials, there is more of an incentive to get up and do something else until the commercial is over. If you watch the American average of three to four hours of television a day, you are probably sitting through half an hour to forty-five minutes of commercials. Literally *sitting* through them. If, instead, you have no remote control with which to mute or change channels, you tend to look for something else to do. How about cleaning up the house a bit? You can make headway on housework and at the same time get some exercise—standing up from your chair, walking around the room, bending over to pick up anything on the floor, reaching up to put away items on shelves, walking quickly (perhaps even jogging!) to other rooms to put things away in them before the commercial is over—just as a lot of people used to do before we had remote controls. And the sound of the commercial tells you how much time you have left, so you're back in your chair before your show starts again. You can probably keep your house much neater, and get over half an hour of exercise in the bargain. All without missing your TV shows or taking any additional time.

This can become a habit, so that you find it difficult to sit for more than fifteen or twenty minutes without feeling the urge to get up and do something—which is exactly the sort of habit you want to get into. These little one- or two-minute bursts of activity add up to weight loss of pounds over the course of a year.

What about other remote controls. Do you really need your garage-door opener? Except for the few days during the year on which it is actually raining or snowing when you get to your garage, probably not. In broad daylight, you don't really need the "security" of not having to get out of your car, either (how much security does a garage-door opener really provide, anyway?). All it does for you on most days is rob you of another minute of activity.

Use your car less

Parking

Have you ever driven into a parking lot—say, at a shopping mall—and seen the people endlessly circling in their cars, waiting for the spot within ten feet of the mall entrance to become available? When the drivers get out of their cars, you probably notice that they are not paragons of leanness. Are you one of them?

Save yourself the stress of fighting for parking and instead park in the first available space. This is often a time-saver, because the "best" spaces (those closest to the store, or the movie theater, or wherever you are going) are usually taken, so you circle the block a few times until one comes free (ignoring the spaces all around the block that are already free because they aren't close enough). If you park in the first available space, even if it's a quarter-mile away, it will take you less than five minutes to walk that distance, which is probably less time than you would need to find a space nearer. At the grocery store, park in the vast expanse of the lot that is farthest from the store. If you have only a couple of bags of groceries, *carry* them to the car instead of pushing the cart. It will make you feel like a true hunter-gatherer.

You may find this habit so enjoyable that you start to park some distance away from your destination deliberately in order to get in a small walk. For example, if you take the train to work, you can park half a mile away from the station rather than in the station parking lot, giving yourself a ten-minute walk to and from the train each day.

Use a human-powered alternative
Every time you use your car, there is an alternative way to get to your destination under your own power. That's true for the trip to the corner grocery store, and for the cross-country trip you plan in the summer. For many trips, you may well decide that the car is simply the only practical way. But get in the habit of always considering the alternatives, which include walking, bicycle riding, horseback riding, hang-gliding, skate-boarding, rollerskating, rollerblading, cross-country skiing. . . .

In the simplest case, the next time you're going to drive a quarter-mile to the store to get a quart of milk, don't. Walk to the store instead. Total walking time will be ten minutes, just a few more than it would take you to find your keys, find a space in the parking lot, etc. Do that every day and you have reset your set point down about a pound or two.

A big opportunity here is commuting. Most people who work commute to work, and for most of those people that means driving. Yet there are usually alternatives that may take little or no more time and may have unexpected bonuses. As we mentioned earlier, Eric walks to the train that takes him to work, getting twenty minutes of exercise in the morning and twenty minutes in the evening (he also climbs the sixty stairs to the train platform rather than taking the escalator). On many days, the walks to the train station plus walking during two fifteen-minute work breaks is the only exercise he gets each day. But it all adds up to more than an hour of walking.

How much time does he spend compared with driving? Walking from home to the train, riding the train, and walking from the train to work take fifty minutes one way. Commuting by car (and fighting rush-hour traffic take about forty minutes each way. So Eric spends extra time, compared with commuting by car, on his walking—an additional ten minutes each way, or twenty minutes total.

But that doesn't really give the whole picture. The train ride takes thirty minutes each way, which is time that Eric can spend on reading related to his work (so he doesn't have to bring it home). That saves him an hour of time at home. Each day that he walks to the train rather than driving, he actually saves about forty minutes that would otherwise be spent on work. Over the course of a month, that's about ten hours.

There's even a monetary payoff. The round-trip commute is thirty miles. According to the IRS, each mile you drive your car costs you about $0.27, so the drive each day costs over $8.00. Parking at the university where Eric works costs over $600 a year (!), or about $2.00 per workday. Total cost of each trip by car is thus $10.00. The round-trip train fare is $2.70. Each day that Eric walks to the train instead of commuting by car, he saves forty minutes in time and $7.50 in money. In a month of five-day work weeks, that's over ten hours and $150 saved! And in that same month, Eric will have walked an additional fourteen hours.

It's like belonging to a health club where they pay *you* $150 a month to work out and also give you ten hours off from work each month.

For you, the possibility may be cycling to work. Or perhaps you want to continue to drive your car to the train, but park five minutes away from the station rather than right next to it. You can take this as far as you want, and the further you take it the leaner you become.

Stairs

The reason step machines are such popular indoor exercise equipment is that they mimic stair climbing, which is one of the most powerful forms of exercise that you can do. These machines are great, but you can get the same effect without joining a gym, getting into your workout clothes, doing a fifteen-minute warmup, and taking a shower afterward. Just climb stairs whenever you find them. And you'll find them everywhere, especially in cities. The total elevation you can climb in the stairwells of the high-rises in a single city block probably equals a trip halfway up Mount Everest.

Make it a policy never to take the elevator or the escalator. At airports, department stores, office buildings, anywhere you find an escalator or an elevator, there is also a flight of stairs. Find those stairs and climb them to your destination, or at least partway there.

If you don't climb stairs at all now, please start slowly. You will be surprised by two things. First, in the beginning climbing stairs will be an incredible effort. Start with just one or two flights a day—and expect your legs will be sore from even that effort. The second surprise is how quickly you will adapt. Within even the first week, your legs get stronger, and you feel less winded. The single flight of stairs that used to daunt you is now merely the warmup for the next several flights. For example, if you work on the twentieth floor of an office building, for the first week of your stair climbing, take the elevator to the nineteenth floor, then walk up the last flight. Next week, get off at the eighteenth floor. After a few weeks, you'll probably start climbing two more floors each week as your legs get stronger.

Stair climbing also has the advantage of being almost completely adjustable to your level of fitness. If you haven't lifted anything heavier than a doughnut in the past twenty years, you may pause literally on every stair to catch your breath. At the other extreme, super-fit oarsmen and oarswomen use stair running as a way to push themselves to their absolute limits. Go at the pace that is comfortable for you.

You also get a health-and-longevity bonus. Stair climbing is an incredibly efficient form of exercise. Two doctors from Johns Hopkins Medical School calculated that, if you simply climb stairs for six minutes a day, without doing anything else special in the way of exercise, you will extend your life by two years. For obsessive types, that works out to four seconds of life gained per stair.

It's not just the going up that gives benefits, either. Coming down stairs requires about half the energy of going up, which beats the zero energy expended in an elevator or an escalator.

At work

Less than a century ago, one-third of the energy used in American economic pursuits was human muscle power; today, it's less than 1 percent. There are still a few jobs, such as carpentry, that demand a lot of muscle power. If you have such a job, and stick to a low-fat diet, that's probably all the activity you'll need to remain lean and mean. Other jobs, like serving as a mail deliverer, waitress or waiter, nurse, etc., still require a lot of activity, and give you a definite fitness and leanness bonus. But jobs like that are a fast-dwindling minority. So, even for the blue-collar worker, it may be important to find ways to get in some extra activity during the work day. For the office worker, it's a must.

As we've seen, commuting to work can offer a tremendous exercise opportunity, but the possibilities don't stop the minute you walk into the office.

The major way to turn your job into a workout is to make your breaks involve some work—physical work, that is. We don't know what sort of work environment you're in, but one or two work breaks a day are required by law. And in many places you can more or less set your own breaks. If you're lucky, you can walk outside during that time—if you are hungry and want a snack, bring it along. You may be able to walk inside your building. If you want, climb up and down a few flights of stairs (since so few people use the stairs, you can probably do this for months before anyone in your building figures out where you go on your break).

Try taking "minibreaks." After an hour of slaving over a hot computer, just go walk down the hall, up and down a flight of stairs, or whatever. Four minutes of walking four or five times a day adds up to a set point that is three or four pounds lower.

You may work at home, either in a regular job or as a homemaker. Either way, you have almost limitless possibilities for activity. You are in charge of your own time, and you should take advantage of that. So do it. Set a kitchen timer, or your watch, and every hour, without fail, take a break. Go out the door and walk down the block for a few minutes. Or hop on your stationary bicycle.

Covert Bailey, the author of the best-selling *Fit or Fat?* books and host of a television series on fitness, practices what he preaches. When he is working on a book, he will take a break every hour, hop on his exercise bicycle, and pedal for several minutes. Not only does it clear his head for another hour of writing, but he reports that in the winter he saves on his heating bill; the exercise keeps him warm! You don't have to invest in a stationary bike. Try rope jumping, which rivals stair climbing as one of the most intense exercises available. Or hula-hooping. Or keep a few cassettes of music that you like to dance to with your Walkman, and spend ten minutes each hour dancing. Buy some light dumbbells (you don't need anything heavier than two to five pounds) and do some weight exercises each hour.

In fact, even if you now do a workout each day, you may find yourself getting more exercise during your home work breaks than during your workout. If you take, say, seven minutes every hour to exercise, over the course of an eight-hour workday that adds up to almost an hour. You might spend that time all on the stationary bike, or you might mix up a bunch of different activities. Any way you look at it, you've put in an hour of activity. Over the course of a year, that will lower your set point by ten to twenty pounds.

At home with the baby? Use the stroller a few times a day. Toddle with your toddlers. Kids are naturally moving animals, if you give them half a chance. All you have to do is follow them to give yourself an exhausting workout. They also love to be lifted, spun around, thrown in the air, given horseback rides; to play catch, tag, hide-and-go-seek, kick-the-can, and hopscotch. Play along.

Like our commuting example, taking work breaks is a win/win proposition. You get significant amounts of exercise, without taking any time from your day. And this kind of hourly break has been shown in innumerable studies to *increase* productivity. The quality of your work will be higher, your concentration sharper. You may feel guilty the first few times you allow yourself a respite from work during the day to rejuvenate. But you'll soon be convinced that working a few minutes less each hour actually allows you to get more done during the day as your efficiency increases.

And if the break is for exercise rather than just a gossip-and-doughnut opportunity, you get an energy bonus. In one study, for example, people were more alert after taking a brief walk than they were after eating a candy bar. So skip the doughnuts and head out the office door for a four-minute walk around the halls.

Gardening

We often run into our neighbor Lily (not her real name) when we walk around the block. She is usually out in her garden, weeding, trimming, or watering. Lily, it turns out, spends two hours a day working in her garden. She doesn't really do much else in the form of exercise. Yet she is neat and trim, without an extra ounce of fat on her, and looks fifteen years younger than her seventy-plus years. She is always energetic, smiling, full of good humor. Lily is an example of what this single activity can do to keep you fit, energetic, and youthful at any age.

That's because serious gardening is a serious workout. Turning the earth, planting, hauling bags of soil or fertilizer, pruning, weeding are all major efforts. Consider even the humble chore of mowing the lawn. If you get rid of your power mower and use a hand mower (a good one, well oiled, with sharp blades), you will experience a whole new set of sensations. You, not fossil fuels, provide the power to cut those leaves of grass, and you can feel the cutting. There's a satisfaction you don't get with the power mower. It takes very little more time and is certainly a workout. For a bonus, rake the grass rather than using a grass-catcher.

Vegetable gardening gives you the added reward of garden-fresh produce, the tastiest vegetables that you will ever eat. Anyone who has eaten a vine-ripened tomato from his or her own garden has a hard time going back to the mushy lumps masquerading as tomatoes in the supermarket. And freshly picked corn is so sweet it's sinful. Vegetable gardening not only lowers your set point due to the physical activity involved, but provides you with foods that are among the lowest in fat, most nutritious, and most tasty.

Housework

Housework, too, can be seen in a whole new light. Mopping floors, vacuuming rugs, cleaning windows—they're the same in terms of muscle use as light aerobics. So, if you find yourself putting off scrubbing the kitchen floor because it takes too much time, think of it instead as a nudge to lower your set point. The bonus is that your house will be considerably cleaner. You can even consider hanging part of your laundry to dry rather than using the drier. You save on the gas or electricity that the drier uses, and there is nothing like the smell of a sundried towel. Do you have a wood stove for heating, or do you just like a fire in the fireplace? Remember the old adage: wood that you chop yourself warms you twice, once in the chopping and once in the burning. Not to mention that it lowers your set point.

Take advantage of idle time

There are minutes, sometimes hours, in every day when we are simply waiting for something to happen. Use that time to activate your muscles. Rather than standing in front of the elevator, waiting for it to stop at every floor on the way up to yours, walk down the stairs. If you arrive early for an appointment, walk around the block a few times.

One marvelous opportunity, especially if you travel a lot, is in airports. Most are big enough so that you can walk half a mile or more without repeating a step. Just take your carry-on luggage with you. Airport delays can stop being nuisances and start being your chance to get in your activity for the day.

Opportunistic exercise is child's play

Children are naturally active. Any parent can tell you: when a child learns to crawl, watch out! The kid is all over the house, up the stairs, in the bathroom, under the tables. When it learns to walk, then run, a child does both, constantly.

Of course, with a little help from you, your child can become one of the growing number of obese children in America. It's simple, really. When your kid is bored, plunk him down in front of the TV or the video game. The child will become hypnotized, passive. He'll be out of your hair—and getting fat.

If the last paragraph caused a pang of guilt, there is more to consider. Fat children have an excellent chance of becoming fat adults. Research shows that the chances are three out of four that an obese adolescent will be an obese adult. And *you* are the adult from whom your child is going to get the most direct lesson in fitness. Are you leading your child into habits that will lead him or her into fitness, or into fatness? Even more disturbing, are you contributing to a heart attack several decades in the future? Forty percent of American children display a major risk factor for heart disease by the age of eight. Heart disease is rare at any age among active societies that eat a traditional moderate-to-low-fat diet. We have to face the fact that the health habits we instill in our children, even by the age of eight, are the ones that will either cause or prevent the heart attack at age fifty, the breast cancer at age fifty-five, or the osteoporosis at age sixty. Our children can't make the choices that will lead to prevention. We, as parents, must face the responsibility for the right choices.

So you may want to take some time to play with your children. Young children, as we mentioned, love to use adults as "human jungle gyms." Older kids like to play tag, and you can play, too. There's also hopscotch, jumping rope, rollerblading, bike riding, nature hikes, swimming at the neighborhood pool. . . .

As your child matures, he or she may become interested in organized sports such as soccer, basketball, swimming, tennis, volleyball, football, wrestling, baseball, track, cross country. . . . We encourage you to encourage this. Both of us feel tremendous debts to the sports we played in grade school, high school, and college. Not only did they instill a lifelong fitness habit, but many of the clichés about organized sports are true. They really do instill the values of working hard toward a distant goal, subordinating your ego to the goals of the team, taking losing as well as winning in stride. Your child will also end up lean, fit, and healthy, almost as a byproduct.

Your participation doesn't have to be limited to cheering on the sidelines, either. Play soccer with your budding soccer star. Set up a basketball hoop in the driveway. Play catch in the back yard or in the park. Play tennis, or volleyball, or baseball with your children. If you play against them while they are still young, you may even have a chance to win occasionally. Volunteer to coach a team, and lead the team through its warmups and drills.

We can't pretend that playing with your children rather than plunking them down in front of the TV is necessarily the most efficient way to get household chores done. And as parents we certainly are aware of the annoyance that occasionally goes along with choosing to be active with your children. But you'll form a closer relationship with your children in a single hour-long one-on-one basketball game than you will in a month of watching their favorite TV programs with them. You'll learn more about each other on a weekend camping trip than you would in a lifetime of watching Disney videos.

Warning: activity can be addictive and you may require increasing doses

Fitness from everyday activities makes you want to be more active, and makes you more comfortable with the idea of activity. Don't be surprised if, after incorporating activity into every day, you start to feel that's it's not enough. You may start getting off the train or the bus one stop before your usual stop and walking the rest of the way. You may stop driving to the store and instead wheel your groceries home in one of those folding grocery-bag carriers.

Don't worry, all you've done is turn on your genetic program for activity, something that has been in the genes of humans for tens of thousands of years. What do primitive tribes the world over do at night, after the day's chores are through? When there has been little hunting or gathering in a given day (hunter-gatherers typically hunt and gather only two or three days a week), the evening entertainment may sometimes be storytelling (the hunting-gathering equivalent, at least in terms of exercise levels, of watching a video). But instead, it is often dancing! It's hard to sit still when you're used to moving all day. A few hours of dancing at night may be needed to get in at least the minimal amount of activity that your body desires.

The same effect can occur when you start putting aside your "labor-saving" devices. You may start exercising by the strategies that we have suggested in this chapter. But that may soon not be enough. Your body, awakened from its long sleep, may begin to crave even more activity. At this point, you are ready to add structured exercise to your day.

13

Structured Exercise

• • • • •

You may already have experienced some of the pleasures of exercise if you have been diligently taking advantage of opportunistic exercise, as outlined in the last chapter. Perhaps you have found that stair climbing has started to be a challenge, and you take five minutes of your lunch break to climb several flights in your building. Or perhaps when you go to a movie you are parking your car a half-mile away from the theater so you can get in a brisk ten-minute walk before and after the film. Watch out. You are starting to crave larger doses of activity, and you are starting to schedule time in your day to do something that is specifically exercise. You are moving into the second level of an exercise program: *structured exercise.* This is the exercise you set aside time for, probably dress differently for, perhaps shower after—your workout. It's what most people think of when they consider an exercise program.

When, or even if, you reach this point depends a lot on your lifestyle and where you live. If you are homesteading in the wilderness of Alaska, the idea of a brisk thirty-minute stint on the cross-country-ski machine at the end of the day may seem ludicrous. But if you live in an apartment in New York, you may quickly reach a point where, even though you are climbing every stair in sight and eschewing taxis in order to walk, your body starts demanding more exercise than you can fit into your day-to-day activities.

If you decide to add structured exercise to your day, you will probably encounter the fitness establishment, and some entrenched misconceptions about exercise. A common scenario goes something like this:

It's January 7, and Matilda walks into the health club, where, as part of her New Year's resolution to start exercising more, she has just bought a three-month membership. She asks at the front desk if there is someone available to help her with a fitness program.

"Certainly," replies the frighteningly lean and beautiful young woman at the desk. "Bruno will help you."

Bruno turns out to be in his twenties, chiseled from granite, ever smiling. Matilda begins to wonder if there is anyone in this place over the age of twenty-five, or at least with more than twenty-five ounces of fat. Oh well, they're so fit they must be the experts. She'll listen to what they tell her and do just what they say.

"Well, Matilda," says Bruno, "in order to start an exercise program, you must understand target heart rates, minimum exercise duration, number of exercise sessions per week, the difference between aerobic and anaerobic exercise, and proper footwear." He then launches into fifteen minutes of technical talk more suited to a computer class than to a health club. Matilda tries to pay attention, but her mind wanders. This is a lot more complicated than she bargained for.

At last, Bruno suggests that, as her first workout, she should pedal the stationary bicycle for twenty minutes, at a target heart rate of between 120 and 135 beats per minute. There follows another ten minutes of explanation and demonstration on how to find her pulse, count it for a set time, and multiply by the proper factor to get beats per minute. But finally she is on the bike for her twenty-minute ride.

Bruno has assured Matilda that this workout is above her "aerobic threshold" but below her "anaerobic threshold." "As long as you stay in the proper heart-rate range, you should experience a good, almost pleasant workout," he says, as he leaves to help another client.

Matilda starts pedaling and diligently takes her pulse every few minutes. In five minutes she's in her target-heart-rate range. She's had to pedal a bit harder than she really wanted to in order to get her heart beating this fast. In fact, her legs are definitely burning. Is this what they mean by "feel the burn"? After a few more minutes of downright unpleasantness, she checks her pulse again. This time it's not so easy, because the pain in her legs makes it hard to keep track of her heartbeat. After a couple of tries, she gets it—110? She's slipped below the proper range. How can that be, when her legs hurt so much? She starts pedaling harder. She grits her teeth and makes it to twenty minutes. It's an odd combination of pain and boredom, with a dash of elation at the end when the timer bell rings.

Bruno comes over and asks how it went.

"Well, actually it kind of hurt," says Matilda, grimacing.

"Oh yes, it will take a few workouts for your muscles to adjust, but soon you will love it as much as I do," Bruno assures her. "Come back the day after tomorrow and we'll do it again."

But Matilda never goes back. When she thinks about the health club, her legs hurt and her head swims with all the instructions. She can understand how Bruno can pedal the bike for hours, but she's just not built like him. She'll just forget the whole thing.

Meanwhile, Bruno wonders what happened to Matilda, but only briefly. So many of them don't come back.

He can't understand it. He loves exercise. He discovered how pleasant it could be almost by accident. He'd been a fat boy, but in high school he discovered basketball. He wasn't very good his first year, but, then, neither was anyone else. It was fun being part of the team, practicing every day and playing in games, even if they did lose most of the time. And he noticed at the end of the season that he wasn't very fat anymore. He decided to stay in shape for the next basketball season by running his high school's cross-country course every other day after school. It was three miles through the hills, and would have been impossible if he hadn't played basketball for three months before trying it. But now, with his fitness from the sport, running the course in twenty-five minutes or so was an agreeable jog.

Bruno played basketball throughout high school, and his off-season running turned into a lifelong fitness habit. In college, he studied exercise physiology to understand more about what had happened to change that fat little boy into the lean adult. The job at the health club seemed a natural when he graduated. He loves explaining to people all the intricacies of training. He just wishes that more people would understand the benefits they would reap if they would only stick with it. He has seen so many, like Matilda, quit before they even really get started.

The story of Bruno and Matilda illustrates a few of the pitfalls that both exercise instructors and beginning exercisers can face. Bruno doesn't know how painful it can be to start a fitness program too quickly. In fact, he has never started a "fitness program" himself. He forgets that when he began playing basketball he never took his pulse or worried whether he was "aerobic" or "anaerobic." He forgets that he got hooked on exercise because he was doing an activity that he enjoyed. All the information about training came later, after he was already in the exercise habit. If someone had taken the fat little boy Bruno and put him on a stationary bicycle to "get him in shape," chances are he would have ended up as just another exercise dropout, the same as Matilda. But now he truly looks forward to his half-hour on the bike at the end of the day. Exercise has become a lifelong friend that he enjoys meeting in any guise.

Matilda, for her part, is accustomed to myths and media images of exercise, and *expects* the experience to be painful. She expects it to be foreign, even bizarre, with people dressed in skimpy outfits straight out of Victoria's Secret pumping away at weird machines more suited to a science-fiction movie. She gets what she expects; then she quits, because there is nothing enjoyable in the experience.

Our job in this chapter is now to show you a different approach, one more likely to be successful.

Make It a Pleasure, Not a Pain

Your main goal with structured exercise is to *make it a pleasant habit.* Note that we're not saying just to make it a habit. You can make a boring activity like brushing your teeth a habit, because it's short and it doesn't hurt. If brushing teeth were painful and lasted thirty minutes, not many people would do it on a daily basis, no matter what the benefits to their teeth. Any activity on which you're going to spend a significant portion of your time *must* be pleasant, as well as beneficial. There are four guidelines to achieving this goal:

1. Choose the optimum form of exercise for you.
2. Ease into each individual workout as you would ease into a hot tub.

3. Ease into your exercise program slowly.
4. Buy at least one piece of high-quality, durable indoor-exercise equipment.

The first three guidelines are aimed at making each workout a pleasure, something you look forward to and make time for as willingly as you would make time for going to see a good movie. The fourth guideline is to help the pleasure become a habit, to help you maintain it in the face of hectic schedules that don't always allow you to pursue the first choice of exercise for you.

We've focused on eliminating the factors that cause structured exercise to be perceived as boring, painful, or too much trouble, and accentuating the factors that make it engaging, enjoyable, and easy. Once you start seeing structured exercise in this light, it becomes simple to adjust your life to fit it in. In fact, as you'll see, some types of structured exercise don't necessarily require extra time in your day, if you are a bit creative about it.

Guideline 1: Like It, You'll Try It

In our workshops, we ask the participants to name *the* optimal type of workout. We get dozens of answers—running, cross-country skiing, soccer, rowing, walking, weight training, etc., etc. And they are all correct.

The optimal type of workout is the one you like enough to do for years. This consideration overrides all others.

People are sometimes disappointed by this answer. They expect us, the experts, to tell them exactly what exercise machine to buy to burn fat at the optimal rate, and exactly how many minutes per day they should remain hooked up to it to achieve that effect. But we can't tell them that, nor can anyone else. Only *you* can tell yourself which form of exercise is the one that will last, and *it may take several tries before you find out.* You can join the most expensive, exclusive health club in the Western Hemisphere, but if you hate crowds you will never go to it. For you, the best exercise investment may be a good pair of walking shoes for long walks in the park.

Don't be fooled by the latest fashion into thinking that, at last, the perfect form of exercise has been invented. The latest fad, the form of exercise that's presented as the One True Aerobic Solution, may or may not be *your* solution. Jogging, aerobic dance, Nautilus, all have had their day as *the* way to exercise. They are all excellent forms of exercise, but only if you like them enough to do them.

It's a lot like low-fat eating: reject what doesn't fit with your tastes. Don't give up trying because you haven't found something perfect in the first few activities you try.

Sometimes a form of exercise appeals to you not because of the exercise itself but because of what goes along with it.

One workshop participant began swimming at the local YMCA, doing laps in the pool. It was adequate exercise, and he lost a few pounds, but nothing about it endeared it to him. Then he joined a Masters Swim Team, a group of adults who train and compete together in a pleasant, low-pressure setting. The team had a coach who provided interesting and challenging workouts. The team was divided into several groups of five or six swimmers who swam together each day for an hour. Much of the appeal of a workout was the banter between swimmers as they paused between swims, or as they kicked through the water on kickboards. The attraction of swimming in low-pressure meets, where the only competition was with one's own best time, added spice and focus. Swimming was transformed for this man from a chore performed to stay in shape to an activity that he looked forward to, even though it meant getting up early every morning. This man lost an additional ten pounds, because he was no longer skipping his workouts—he looked forward to the morning swims with his team and rarely missed one.

There are hundreds of types of exercise. Find one you like. Don't give up. If you join an aerobics group and you absolutely hate it, try another group, or try another form of exercise. If walking outside embarrasses you, get a *good* indoor-exercise machine and use it. If you're curious what pumping iron is all about, join a gym and find out.

To get started in your fitness quest, think of the activities that you enjoyed as a child or young adult. Did you like to swim all day at the local pool, or ride your bike? Were you active in sports? Did you dance? Ride horses? Rollerskate? Almost anything you did as a kid is probably still open to you. Try it again.

You don't have to get very fancy. Two of the most effective forms of exercise are the low-tech, perennially popular, and exceedingly effective activities called running and walking. Running will, of course, produce more effect in less time than walking. It also has a very high injury potential, requires changing clothes (unless you are very unselfconscious), and requires time to warm up and to shower. Walking requires no clothes change, can be done almost anywhere, at almost any time, and requires no warmup and no shower. You can, by walking alone, achieve essentially all the health benefits that any exercise program has to offer, and decrease your set point dramatically.

Here's a list of fitness activities that will get your heart rate up and your blood pumping, and lower your set point as well. It's intended merely as a starting point for your explorations, something perhaps to jog your memory or arouse your curiosity. If something on this list appeals to you, try it! If there is an activity that is not on this list that appeals to you, try it! We can't overemphasize the idea that the activity that you enjoy is the optimal activity for you. As you begin to become really fit, you may find that many more activities that seemed impossible now become tantalizing. Try them, too.

Walking	Aerobic dance	Stair machine	Soccer
Hiking	Step aerobics	Scuba diving	Ultimate Frisbee
Backpacking	Basketball	Snowshoe	Badminton
Running	Tennis	walking	Ballroom
Rollerskating	Volleyball	Rock climbing	dancing
In-line skating	Water skiing	Bicycling	Martial arts
Ice skating	Jumping	Mountain biking	Horseback riding
Downhill skiing	rope	Weight training	Squash
Cross-country	Snowboarding	Swimming	Racketball
skiing	Rowing	Wrestling	Boxing
Hula-hooping	Orienteering	Kayaking	Canoeing

Guideline 2: Spurn the Burn

We suspect that many fledgling exercise programs are abandoned because people don't warm up at each exercise session. A proper warmup period, which needn't take more than ten minutes, can be the differ-

ence between a workout that is enjoyable and leaves you feeling relaxed, or one that is painful from start to finish and leaves you feeling
tense. Unfortunately, most people think the agonizing workout is more
effective. We are so accustomed to thinking of exercise as something
painful that we adjust our workout pace until, by God, what we're doing does indeed cause pain. And the best way to do that is to plunge in,
full speed ahead.

"Feeling the burn" is the first step to burnout

If you start an activity too quickly, you catch your muscles by surprise.
When a muscle is not being exercised, its blood flow is very limited. If
you suddenly start using that muscle full-blast, its requirements for fuel
can go up a hundredfold. One second it's relaxed, the next second it's
going all-out. Blood flow to the muscle can't adjust so quickly; it takes
minutes, rather than seconds, for blood vessels to open up to allow new
blood in. The result of this mismatch between energy needs and oxygen-
carrying blood is a quick buildup of lactic acid and other anaerobic
waste products that poison the muscle, making it feel very painful. It
takes a long time for those waste products to be flushed out, even when
blood flow to the working muscle finally catches up to demand. As a result, your entire workout can be one big painful experience.

About 90 percent of the people we've seen at gyms fall into this
trap—and about 90 percent give up on their exercise routine because
they think it's too painful. This is too bad, because it's completely
unnecessary.

Exercise should leave you feeling as relaxed and peaceful as if you
had been soaking in a hot tub. But you have to ease into it, just as you
ease into a hot tub. If you just jumped right into a hot tub, the water
would feel scalding hot, you'd jump right out, and you'd wonder what
all the "hot-tub nuts" see in it. If, instead, you put your toe in, then
your foot, your leg, your other leg, then you slowly sit down, it becomes a luxurious experience—and you're in danger of becoming a
hot-tub nut yourself.

So it is with exercise. Start slowly, much more slowly than you really
think you should. Let your body pick up the pace by itself, without
pushing it. This gives the blood vessels in the working muscles a chance

Guideline 4: Equip Your Home

No matter what form of structured exercise you choose, we strongly recommend that, as a backup, you also buy a well-constructed home exerciser, choosing from one of the five basic types that we will discuss below. Our friend Lori, who chose an aerobics class as her form of structured exercise rather than riding a stationary bike, recently bought a step machine as well. Exercising on a piece of exercise equipment may not be your main workout, but there are several reasons to make the investment.

Why buy home exercise equipment?

First, an exercise machine is always available to you. Rain, snow, sleet, or hail won't stop you. You don't have to get in your car, worry about the roads, worry about how you look. You are completely in control of when you use it; you don't have to fit your workout time to a gym schedule or an aerobics-class schedule. You can exercise at two in the morning if you want. You don't even necessarily have to change into special workout clothes to use it (unless you drench yourself in sweat, or don't bathe for several days, the sweat from a light workout is odorless). You don't have to worry about paying dues each month, and a good machine will last you a lifetime. It allows you to break up your workout into smaller parts—say, three ten-minute easy rides on your stationary bicycle rather than one half-hour workout. Or even just one ten-minute ride, rather than skipping exercise altogether because of lack of time.

Second, an exercise machine allows you to exercise in the privacy of your own home. You probably want to lose weight because you find the extra fat you're carrying around to be unattractive. You may be embarrassed by your body. Perhaps that is not the "correct" way to feel, but it is certainly understandable, and you may prefer to exercise, at least at first, in a place where you feel safe and un-self-conscious. Home-exercise equipment allows you to do that and still get a world-class workout.

Third, exercising on a home-exercise machine is the one way to perform structured exercise without necessarily making any extra time in your day. Many types of home-exercise equipment allow you to do

to open up, to allow more blood and oxygen in, so that you don't produce the painful lactic acid. After about ten minutes, you will be up to the same level of work as you would have been if you had plunged right in, but you will never have experienced the acid burning that accompanies the fast start.

If you're feeling pain or even moderate discomfort at the start of your workout, you are starting too fast. Ease up. Give yourself ten to fifteen minutes to get warm, to start to sweat, to start to breathe more deeply. Many top athletes spend half an hour to an hour just warming up for their workout. You can't properly get warmed up in less than ten minutes. If you give yourself that time, you will find that the workout is much smoother, easier, and more pleasant.

Some days you have it, some days you don't

The warmup serves another purpose by telling you how your body is doing on that particular day. You can adjust the pace of your workout accordingly. Some days you will simply "click" right into the motions of your activity almost immediately, with every muscle and tendon feeling oiled and smooth. That's a day when you can go pretty hard and enjoy it. Other days you may feel old and creaky during your warmup, perhaps finding that even a low level of activity is a struggle. That's a day to keep your effort low, not to push yourself, maybe to end your workout early.

How to warm up

The warmup activity should be the same as the workout activity itself, just slower. For example, on the stationary bike, start out with almost no resistance on the pedals. It should be no effort at all to turn them. After a minute or so, turn up the resistance just a notch. It should still be ridiculously easy. Each minute, raise the resistance a tiny amount. At the end of ten minutes, or, better yet, fifteen, you should finally be at the resistance that you will use for the rest of the workout. If you've never tried this approach, you may be amazed at how much easier your workout is. If you can't do the same activity as your workout for a warmup, do something that uses the same muscles.

Incidentally, stretching is *not* a warmup. It is a wonderful, pleasant activity that can help prevent or heal injuries by increasing flexibility, but stretching does *not* send a signal to the muscles to increase blood flow. Warmup through activity before your workout. Stretch for relaxation and injury prevention *after* your workout, or at least after your warmup, when you are already warm.

If you are in an exercise class or on a team, and your instructor does not follow these principles, talk to him or her about it. If he still rushes into the workout at a pace faster than you can handle, you should probably consider finding another instructor. The best instructors merge the warmup with the workout so imperceptibly that you're not sure exactly when you crossed the border.

Guideline 3: If You Want It to Last, Don't Start Out Fast

You should not only ease into each workout slowly, but ease into your entire program slowly. As with warming up, the idea here is to nurture your exercise habit. And, as with warming up, this goes against our cherished notions of what exercise really is. If you're not stiff and sore the day after you begin exercising, you must not have done it right. If the first few workouts aren't torture, leaving you exhausted and wrung out, you must not have worked hard enough. Right?

Wrong. If you push your muscles too hard initially, they will scream bloody murder. After several weeks or months of training, these same muscles will handle heavy workloads easily, with minimum discomfort. But you're in danger of never getting to that point if you start out too fast.

The reason is that an out-of-shape muscle doesn't have a lot of blood vessels to bring blood to the muscle cells, and it isn't very good at using the oxygen in that blood to burn fuel. Thus, when you place a demand on that unconditioned muscle, even after you've warmed up, it will produce lactic acid, which is painful.

This leads to a dilemma for the beginner. You want to get into your new exercise program, yet you find that exercising even at the lowest

levels is painful, because the muscles that are called on to do the exercise are producing lactic acid like crazy. Impatient to make progress, you fight through the pain. And, secretly, you feel that this is correct: you've always associated exercise with pain; it wouldn't really *be* exercise if it weren't painful. The trouble is that no one *likes* pain, and after a half-dozen experiences of burning muscles, you give up, certain that exercise is only for masochists.

What you've missed is the truly miraculous phenomenon of getting in shape. Starting with the very first workout, the muscles involved in the exercise are changing their architecture and their operation. They're building new blood vessels to shunt more blood to themselves during exercise. They're extracting more oxygen from that blood. And they're radically altering their cellular machinery to use that oxygen efficiently, without producing lactic acid. You don't need to go to the point of pain for the muscles to get the message, either. Using them more vigorously than they are normally used will do the trick.

The trouble with exercising hard in the first few workouts and gritting your teeth through the pain is that, just about the time your muscles have changed enough to make a significant difference in the comfort level of your exercise, you quit your workout program. Paradoxically, forcing your muscles to make the fastest changes is also the best way to get yourself to quit.

Instead, start your program slowly. Do not tolerate pain. The sensations of exercise may be new, and sometimes mildly uncomfortable, but overall, *at the end of a workout, you should feel like you could* *another one immediately.* If you don't feel that way, if you feel performing your workout again would be impossible, you have too hard. A bit of soreness in the few days after exercising is mal with unaccustomed activity, but if you can't get out of bed gone *too far.*

You want to avoid pain in your workouts. It isn't necessary, you are an athlete training for high-level competition. It isn't ne to lower your set point, and it isn't necessary for you to experie matic health benefits.

to open up, to allow more blood and oxygen in, so that you don't produce the painful lactic acid. After about ten minutes, you will be up to the same level of work as you would have been if you had plunged right in, but you will never have experienced the acid burning that accompanies the fast start.

If you're feeling pain or even moderate discomfort at the start of your workout, you are starting too fast. Ease up. Give yourself ten to fifteen minutes to get warm, to start to sweat, to start to breathe more deeply. Many top athletes spend half an hour to an hour just warming up for their workout. You can't properly get warmed up in less than ten minutes. If you give yourself that time, you will find that the workout is much smoother, easier, and more pleasant.

Some days you have it, some days you don't

The warmup serves another purpose by telling you how your body is doing on that particular day. You can adjust the pace of your workout accordingly. Some days you will simply "click" right into the motions of your activity almost immediately, with every muscle and tendon feeling oiled and smooth. That's a day when you can go pretty hard and enjoy it. Other days you may feel old and creaky during your warmup, perhaps finding that even a low level of activity is a struggle. That's a day to keep your effort low, not to push yourself, maybe to end your workout early.

How to warm up

The warmup activity should be the same as the workout activity itself, just slower. For example, on the stationary bike, start out with almost no resistance on the pedals. It should be no effort at all to turn them. After a minute or so, turn up the resistance just a notch. It should still be ridiculously easy. Each minute, raise the resistance a tiny amount. At the end of ten minutes, or, better yet, fifteen, you should finally be at the resistance that you will use for the rest of the workout. If you've never tried this approach, you may be amazed at how much easier your workout is. If you can't do the same activity as your workout for a warmup, do something that uses the same muscles.

Incidentally, stretching is *not* a warmup. It is a wonderful, pleasant activity that can help prevent or heal injuries by increasing flexibility, but stretching does *not* send a signal to the muscles to increase blood flow. Warmup through activity before your workout. Stretch for relaxation and injury prevention *after* your workout, or at least after your warmup, when you are already warm.

If you are in an exercise class or on a team, and your instructor does not follow these principles, talk to him or her about it. If he still rushes into the workout at a pace faster than you can handle, you should probably consider finding another instructor. The best instructors merge the warmup with the workout so imperceptibly that you're not sure exactly when you crossed the border.

Guideline 3: If You Want It to Last, Don't Start Out Fast

You should not only ease into each workout slowly, but ease into your entire program slowly. As with warming up, the idea here is to nurture your exercise habit. And, as with warming up, this goes against our cherished notions of what exercise really is. If you're not stiff and sore the day after you begin exercising, you must not have done it right. If the first few workouts aren't torture, leaving you exhausted and wrung out, you must not have worked hard enough. Right?

Wrong. If you push your muscles too hard initially, they will scream bloody murder. After several weeks or months of training, these same muscles will handle heavy workloads easily, with minimum discomfort. But you're in danger of never getting to that point if you start out too fast.

The reason is that an out-of-shape muscle doesn't have a lot of blood vessels to bring blood to the muscle cells, and it isn't very good at using the oxygen in that blood to burn fuel. Thus, when you place a demand on that unconditioned muscle, even after you've warmed up, it will produce lactic acid, which is painful.

This leads to a dilemma for the beginner. You want to get into your new exercise program, yet you find that exercising even at the lowest levels is painful, because the muscles that are called on to do the exercise are producing lactic acid like crazy. Impatient to make progress, you fight through the pain. And, secretly, you feel that this is correct: you've always associated exercise with pain; it wouldn't really *be* exercise if it weren't painful. The trouble is that no one *likes* pain, and after a half-dozen experiences of burning muscles, you give up, certain that exercise is only for masochists.

What you've missed is the truly miraculous phenomenon of getting in shape. Starting with the very first workout, the muscles involved in the exercise are changing their architecture and their operation. They're building new blood vessels to shunt more blood to themselves during exercise. They're extracting more oxygen from that blood. And they're radically altering their cellular machinery to use that oxygen efficiently, without producing lactic acid. You don't need to go to the point of pain for the muscles to get the message, either. Using them more vigorously than they are normally used will do the trick.

The trouble with exercising hard in the first few workouts and gritting your teeth through the pain is that, just about the time your muscles have changed enough to make a significant difference in the comfort level of your exercise, you quit your workout program. Paradoxically, forcing your muscles to make the fastest changes is also the best way to get yourself to quit.

Instead, start your program slowly. Do not tolerate pain. The sensations of exercise may be new, and sometimes mildly uncomfortable, but overall, *at the end of a workout, you should feel like you could do another one immediately.* If you don't feel that way, if you feel that performing your workout again would be impossible, you have gone too hard. A bit of soreness in the few days after exercising is normal with unaccustomed activity, but if you can't get out of bed you've gone *too far.*

You want to avoid pain in your workouts. It isn't necessary, unless you are an athlete training for high-level competition. It isn't necessary to lower your set point, and it isn't necessary for you to experience dramatic health benefits.

Guideline 4: Equip Your Home

No matter what form of structured exercise you choose, we strongly recommend that, as a backup, you also buy a well-constructed home exerciser, choosing from one of the five basic types that we will discuss below. Our friend Lori, who chose an aerobics class as her form of structured exercise rather than riding a stationary bike, recently bought a step machine as well. Exercising on a piece of exercise equipment may not be your main workout, but there are several reasons to make the investment.

Why buy home exercise equipment?

First, an exercise machine is always available to you. Rain, snow, sleet, or hail won't stop you. You don't have to get in your car, worry about the roads, worry about how you look. You are completely in control of when you use it; you don't have to fit your workout time to a gym schedule or an aerobics-class schedule. You can exercise at two in the morning if you want. You don't even necessarily have to change into special workout clothes to use it (unless you drench yourself in sweat, or don't bathe for several days, the sweat from a light workout is odorless). You don't have to worry about paying dues each month, and a good machine will last you a lifetime. It allows you to break up your workout into smaller parts—say, three ten-minute easy rides on your stationary bicycle rather than one half-hour workout. Or even just one ten-minute ride, rather than skipping exercise altogether because of lack of time.

Second, an exercise machine allows you to exercise in the privacy of your own home. You probably want to lose weight because you find the extra fat you're carrying around to be unattractive. You may be embarrassed by your body. Perhaps that is not the "correct" way to feel, but it is certainly understandable, and you may prefer to exercise, at least at first, in a place where you feel safe and un-self-conscious. Home-exercise equipment allows you to do that and still get a world-class workout.

Third, exercising on a home-exercise machine is the one way to perform structured exercise without necessarily making any extra time in your day. Many types of home-exercise equipment allow you to do something else—like watch TV, read, listen to music, or even talk on the phone—while you work out. If you're normally doing these anyway, you can combine the two activities, with no extra time drain.

Fourth, home-exercise machines are one of the most cost-effective ways of exercising. The initial investment for a good machine may run into hundreds of dollars. You can even spend more than a thousand dollars if you insist on every bell and whistle. But if you make the initial investment in a high-quality machine, it will last virtually forever. Over the course of a single year, an exercise machine will usually cost less than joining a health club. Over the course of several years, it will cost less than a serious runner spends on shoes in the same period of time. In fact, you can often find used equipment in perfect condition at a fraction of the cost of new equipment (a result of New Year's resolutions that didn't make it to February).

The five proven types of home exercise equipment

If you step into an exercise-equipment shop, you may be overwhelmed by a veritable jungle of machines. Every square foot seems to be occupied by ever more complex and outlandish-looking devices. How can you decide which is right for you?

Fortunately, you can make sense of this scene by realizing that indoor-exercise machines come in only five basic varieties. (We will not discuss weight-training machines here, which often make up a lot of the stock of an exercise-equipment store—they will be discussed in the next section.) These are the ones that have stood the test of time, that have proved themselves after use by hundreds of thousands of people for cumulative totals of millions of years of exercise. These are:

- stationary bicycles
- step machines (stair climbers)
- treadmills
- cross-country-ski machines
- rowing machines

The immediate impulse of most people is to buy the type of machine that will exercise the most muscles in the least possible amount of time, because that way you will get the "optimum" workout. If you think only in those terms, cross-country-ski machines and rowing machines win, hands down.

But remember, a machine does you no good if you never use it. There are many other factors to consider. Size and portability are important: Will you have room for it in your one-bedroom apartment? Can you move it in front of the TV, or by the phone? Do you have to spend time setting it up? The noise the machine makes during its operation can be a factor in determining whether you can do anything else while you're using it, as can be whether it leaves your hands free or not. For most people, price will be a consideration, as well as durability. You want something that will last decades. The ease of learning to use the machine is also important: Is learning to use it so frustrating that you will give up before you ever get the benefits? Is it hard to adjust, so that you have to interrupt your workout to change the difficulty level? That can be important in allowing you a proper warmup, during which you will want to be able to adjust the difficulty level upward several times as you become warmer and able to exercise harder. And some machines, if not used properly, have potential for injury.

The optimal machine *for you* will be the one that has the best combination, *for you,* of all these features. No one machine is perfect in every way. The cross-country-ski machines and rowing machines, which look so good when you just consider whole-body workout, rank very low in many of these other categories. As one exercise-equipment expert told us, "If you look in the classified ads in the paper, the exercise machine you see for sale the most is the cross-country-ski machine. That tells you something about how many people actually use them."

To make the choice easier, we've created the table below. Each of the five types of machine is ranked from 1 (best) to 5 (worst) in various categories. Please note that these rankings only rate the machines relative to each other; a machine can rank 5 in a category and still be excellent in that category—it's just that the others are better. For example, step machines rate 4 in "ease of adjustment," because on less expensive models you have to stop momentarily to adjust the difficulty of the workout. It's simple and quick, but it's not as simple and quick as the process is for some other exercise machines, on which you can continue to exercise as you adjust the difficulty. Also note that the rankings are for the solid, basic model of each type of machine, not for the high-end health-club versions.

You can see that no single type of machine ranks as the best in all the categories. To help you sort out the pros and cons, we will also discuss each machine individually. In a few cases, where a brand name has become synonymous with quality, we will recommend specific brands. Between the two of us we've spent anywhere from a few dozen to a few thousand hours on each of the types of machines we'll discuss.

	Stationary bicycle	Step machine	Treadmill	Cross-country skier	Rowing machine
Price	1	2	5	3	4
Ease of learning to use	1	2	3	5	4
Ease of adjustment	2	5	3	4	1
Quietness	2	1	3	4	5
Size	1	2	4	3	5
Portability	1	2	5	3	4
Allows other activities	1	2	3	4	5
Durability	1	4	5	3	2
Potential for injury	1	2	3	4	5
Number of muscles worked	5	4	3	1	2

Stationary bicycles

The classic, and in many ways the best, piece of indoor-exercise equipment is the stationary bicycle. In all categories but one (and we'll discuss that issue in the next paragraph), it ranks first or second among the five types of indoor exercisers. Sturdy basic models cost about $200 brand-new, take up as much space as an end table (about two feet by three feet), and are easy to move by tilting the bike onto its wheel, grasping the frame, and rolling it like a wheelbarrow. You need almost no skill to ride one: just put your feet on the pedals and push. Because construction and materials are simple, even a $200 model will last you the rest of your life, and probably your children's, grandchildren's, and great-grandchildren's lives, with a minimum of maintenance. You can ride without holding the handlebars, which means you can read, talk on the phone, talk in sign language, or juggle, if you want to. It's quiet enough to allow TV watching or stereo listening. The injury potential is almost nonexistent; in fact, a stationary bicycle is the standard piece of equipment that athletes use to remain in shape when an injury interferes with their main activity.

The category in which stationary bicycles rank dead last is in the number of muscles exercised. This does not mean they can't give you a great workout. They can: stationary bicycles are what exercise physiologists usually use to bring people to their absolute maximum levels of exertion. But it does mean that most of the power for turning the pedals is supplied by relatively few muscles: the thighs, the buttocks, and, to some extent, the hamstrings (back of the thigh). These are big muscles, and, as we say, are enough to take you right up to the maximum level of exercise you can achieve. But in your first workouts, they don't really have the metabolic machinery set up to do so efficiently. Which means that, even if you go slowly, your legs will probably burn as you ride a bicycle the first few times.

As you start to get in shape, after the first few weeks or couple of months, this problem will start to diminish. Don't be discouraged if at first you can't pedal very hard without pain. Just ease back to a comfortable level. You can adjust a stationary bicycle so that the degree of resistance on the pedals is anywhere from very light—so light that just the weight of your leg will push the pedal down—to extremely heavy—so heavy that you can barely turn the pedals. Find the resistance somewhere between these extremes that requires some effort but does not cause anything more than mild discomfort in your thigh muscles. This is enough of a stimulus to cause the physiological adjustments in the muscles that we described earlier. You will soon find that exercise loads that previously had been too painful to maintain become easy. You are getting in shape.

What to look for: We recommend going with the basics here. A good stationary bicycle has a heavy flywheel (which provides a smooth ride) connected by a chain to a pair of pedals, some way of adjusting the tension on the flywheel, and a padded, adjustable seat. Any other features are frills. Computerized models, pulse monitors, and other accessories can up the price tenfold without providing any additional benefit in terms of your workout, but they do add more parts and electronics that can break. The basic mechanical models are virtually indestructible.

You may see stationary bicycles that have seats with backs and elevated pedals, so that you pedal out in front of your body. These "recumbent bicycles" are said to exercise the buttocks and hamstrings a bit more, and to be easier on the back than upright models. They are also more expensive, take up more space, and obstruct or prevent reading while riding, because your knees come toward your chest, making it difficult to hold a book. We have also found them to be harder on our problem areas (Carol's injured back and Eric's arthritic hips) than upright models. You may find otherwise, but we recommend a long trial period with a recumbent bicycle before you buy one.

The classic brand of this classic home exerciser is Tunturi, which has been around for decades. They produce the least expensive, most basic, and most reliable of the serious stationary bicycles. This is the brand that we own.

Step machines

Also known as "stair-climbing machines" or "steppers." They are the latest exercise-machine fad, but they deserve most of the hype, ranking at or near the top of most categories. Steppers take up only a bit more space than stationary bicycles. They, too, can be tipped and rolled to new locations, though they are a bit harder to maneuver. You can get a good, basic model for under $250. They are almost silent, the quietest of the exercise machines, producing less noise in use than your refrigerator. Even if you have never used one, you'll be an expert by the end of your first lesson, and they are virtually injury-free (unless you have balance problems). They leave your hands free for reading or phone yakking.

Step machines use about the same muscles as stationary bicycles, with a bit more emphasis on the buttocks and hamstrings than stationary bicycles. This means that the same cautions we gave for stationary bikes about being patient in beginning your exercise program also apply to step machines. Steppers are a bit trickier to adjust to low exercise levels than are stationary bicycles, and may require some fiddling before you get to an exercise level that requires some effort but is not painful. Basic models also require that you stop exercising to adjust the difficulty of the workout. The adjustment is very rapid, however, so, even if you have to stop to do it, it's a matter of seconds and won't greatly disrupt your workout. Computerized versions have the tension adjustment on a push-button panel at chest level, so you can continue to exercise as you adjust the tension, which is ideal. They also allow you to program variety into your workout, so that you can climb at various levels at different times, like walking over hilly terrain with sometimes steep, sometimes gentle hills, adding interest to the workout. But computerized models also cost around $1,000 or $2,000.

Step machines generally use hydraulic devices, exactly like the shock absorbers on your car, to provide resistance. Although they should last years, these parts will eventually wear out, so step machines rate lower on durability than other machines, such as stationary bicycles, cross-country-ski machines, and rowing machines which are virtually indestructible. The hydraulic part should be easy to replace if you buy a name brand that is likely to be around for a while (such as Tunturi or Precor). If you buy at an exercise-equipment store, ask about warranty on parts and labor. Ideally, it should be at least two years.

What to look for: You can get models with either dependent or independent steps. With dependent steps, as you push one step down the other goes up, making them easy to learn to use but providing less of a workout. With independent steps, you have to coordinate both legs to get the steps to work properly—more difficult to learn, but ultimately a better workout. Since you can learn to use independent steps in a matter of minutes, and you will be using the machine for years, we recommend independent steps.

Some models have poles that you move with your arms as you step up and down, which means you can work your upper body as well as your lower body (this would, of course, not leave your arms free for reading or phone talking). These turn the exercise into a whole-body workout, making it much more efficient. They seemed awkward to us when we tried them, but may suit you. If you get a version with arm exercisers and decide that you don't like it, or don't want to use them all the time, the machine is still completely usable as a regular stepper.

Computerized models offer the advantage, as we said, that it is easy to adjust the resistance while you are on the steps. They also have more durable means of providing resistance. But, again, they are also five to ten times more expensive, and offer no other significant advantages. On these issues, step machines are inferior to stationary bicycles, which even in noncomputerized versions have easily adjustable resistances and are virtually indestructible.

Treadmills

Once found only in exercise-physiology labs, treadmills have made their way into thousands of home gyms as reliable, durable, reasonably priced models have become available. But they are still relatively expensive, and this, combined with their size, makes them an option only for people with space and money (or the willingness to look for a good used one). Even so, according to an informal survey of exercise-equipment suppliers in our area, treadmills, along with step machines, are the hottest-selling indoor-exercise machines.

Treadmills provide a workout that is every bit as good as running or walking outdoors, a lower-body workout that is slightly more complete than what is available on stationary bicycles and steppers. The hamstrings, in particular, are used in running, although treadmills that allow an incline (so that you can run "uphill") can also work the front muscles of the thighs (the quadriceps) as thoroughly as any step machine. However, as with the bikes and the steppers, you need to start slowly if you are out of shape in order to avoid pain in the muscles being used.

Using a treadmill is not as easy as stepping out your front door for a run. It requires some skill to get started walking or running on the moving belt and then maintain your motion at the constant speed of the belt, whereas in regular running or walking you can slow down or speed up with every step if you wish. This will take a few tries to master, but becomes second nature quickly. Changing the belt speed usually requires no more than punching a few numbers on a control panel located right in front of you as you run. Good models are quiet enough to allow TV watching or music listening, but, even though the treadmill provides no upper-body workout, you must use your hands for balance as you walk or run, so you can't read or otherwise use your hands. Some models come with book stands; these may work for you, or you may find that the fuss of turning pages and rearranging the book in the stand is a distraction.

Treadmills have some drawbacks. The major one, again is price. A low-end model will cost you over $1,000; you will not be able to buy a decent treadmill for under $1,500. This is five times the cost of a good stationary bicycle or stepper, and two to three times the cost of a cross-country ski machine or rowing machine. And that's just for a rock-bottom basic, reliable treadmill. You can spend more than $3,000 on a treadmill that has an electronic incline adjustment, a wide range of belt speeds, and a heart-rate monitor. The second drawback is space. Think of your front door laid flat on the floor. That is the space that you will have to set aside permanently for a treadmill, because once it's there it's difficult to move. This is not an exercise machine that you will be putting in the closet between uses.

Also, walking or running on a treadmill has the same injury potential as doing these activities on a track—that is to say, very low for walking, but rather high for running, because of the impact with the belt at each stride. If you have never engaged in a running program and buy a treadmill expecting to start such a program by using your treadmill, after a few months you may find yourself with the leg problems common to runners and a $2,000 machine that you can't use.

There are two ways to minimize this possibility. First, make sure you get a model with a belt that "gives" somewhat under your weight, so that each foot impact is cushioned. The difference between running on a treadmill with a hard belt and running on one with a cushioned belt is like that between running on concrete sidewalks and running on a leaf-covered forest trail. Second, make sure your treadmill has an incline adjustment. Running uphill puts far less strain on knees, hips, and other joints that suffer from the impact of running, while providing an intense workout. In fact, if the incline is steep enough, *walking* uphill on a treadmill can be a serious challenge even for the most highly conditioned athlete, let alone for us mere mortals. Of course, incline adjustments add to the price of the machine.

A final negative feature is that this is the one exercise machine that requires a motor to operate, since you walk or run on a continuously moving belt. Good models have a tough, solid motor that will last years, but no matter how good it is, it will burn out someday, requiring replacement. Also, because the belt is moving continuously whether you are on the machine or not, there is some danger to pets or children if the belt gets started inadvertently. Most models have a safety interlock so this can't happen.

Because of these drawbacks, especially price, and because it provides only a marginally more complete workout than a stationary bicycle or a stepper (and considerably less complete than a cross-country-ski machine or a rowing machine), the treadmill is not at the top of our list of exercise machines. But if you enjoy walking and running, and have the money and space, this may be the exercise machine for you.

What to look for: Only buy a model in which the belt is moved by an electric motor; don't even consider models in which you move the belt with your own power, since they require awkward and potentially injurious leg motions. The motor should be at least 1.5 horsepower; otherwise it won't have power to keep the belt moving continuously and smoothly.

A treadmill should have a top speed of at least ten miles an hour, which can accommodate most runners. Even if you only plan to walk on it, we recommend this. Who knows? You may be running on it six months from now, and a walking treadmill that goes up to only five miles an hour won't be adequate.

Incline adjustments can be either mechanical, requiring you to turn a knob to move the front of the treadmill up or down, or electronic, doing the job with just the push of a button. Both types can be adjusted while you are using the treadmill. For the ease of electronic push-button adjustment you pay about $400 more. Not only that, you don't get the opportunistic exercise of turning the knob.

Cross-country-ski machines

If you are looking for the one exercise that is considered ideal, that will lower your set point the most quickly for the least amount of time spent exercising, cross-country skiing is the choice. When exercise physiologists measure athletes' fitness—their ability to work at high levels of exertion for long periods of time—cross-country skiers always come out on top.

The reason is simple: cross-country skiing uses just about every muscle in the body, with the possible exception of the ones you use to wiggle your ears. Because all the muscles of the body share the load, no one group gets overstressed and starts to feel painful. This means that you can get a very high quality workout without feeling the burn in any one particular muscle group. If you are used to exercising on a stationary bike, stepper, or treadmill, a workout on a cross-country-ski machine can be a real eye-opener. You find yourself breathing hard, your heart pounding—yet your muscles feel fresh and strong, with no lactic-acid burn. It's easy to work up to long workouts very quickly on these machines. And since all major muscle groups are exercised, all get toned, as well.

But before you run out and buy a cross-country ski machine, look at their ratings in our comparison table for the rest of the categories; they are ranked no higher than third among the five types of machines in any of them.

First and foremost, it takes a little time to master the coordinated motions involved in using the machine—you can't just hop on and go like a pro, as you can on a stationary bicycle. If you already know how to cross-country ski, you'll be able to learn the motions in a single session. If not, count on at least a week to master the coordinated skills involved. Once you learn, it's a smooth, enjoyable activity. Nordic-Track, which has made popular cross-country-ski machines longer than any other company, offers an instructional video with its machine to help novices. But if you're a klutz, or easily frustrated, this machine is going to end up at your next garage sale.

Cross-country-ski machines also put somewhat more of a strain on the back than other machines. This is no problem for healthy backs, and may not even be a concern if you have a back problem now. But if you do, make sure you check out a machine thoroughly before you buy (NordicTrack also allows you to return its machine within thirty days for a full refund if you're not satisfied), and perhaps discuss using such a machine with your doctor or chiropractor.

In terms of size, the complete, set-up machine requires a space about three feet by eight feet. Some fold down into very compact units that take up little more space than an upright vacuum cleaner, and can be wheeled into a closet or a corner for storage. The total time to set up the folding machines is less than a minute. This seems like nothing, but the barrier such setup puts between you and exercise is out of all proportion to the time spent. If the exercise machine isn't out and ready to use at a second's notice, it tends not to get used at all. If possible, find a space where you can keep your machine set up and ready to go.

Cross-country-ski machines are also a bit louder than stationary bicycles and steppers, though still plenty quiet enough for TV watching. And because you're exercising your upper body as well, you can't read or talk on the phone while you're using one, narrowing your options for entertainment while exercising.

Nevertheless, a cross-country-ski machine will give you *the* aerobic workout, second to none. If you can get past the initial learning hump, and if you have room to keep one set up, this machine will reward you with a powerful workout that stresses all parts of the body evenly.

What to look for: There are two types, those that have actual "skis" (short wooden platforms), which you move with your feet as you would real cross-country skis, and those that have only small platforms for the feet. Your arms either pull on cables or on "poles." The resistances for your legs and for your arms are independently adjustable, so that you can provide your upper body and lower body with different levels of work, if you want. The machines with "skis" more closely simulate the actual motion of skiing, but both provide full-body workouts.

As with step machines, your feet can move independently or dependently (as one foot moves, it moves the other side), and, as with step machines, the only machines worth considering have independent movement, so each leg has to do its own work.

Though many models of cross-country-ski machines have computerized accessories, none of these accessories is necessary for smooth operation. Most machines are easy to adjust while you are exercising on the machine.

We have to admit that our prejudice here is toward NordicTrack, which uses the ski-type platforms for your feet and cables for your hands, and which is the type of cross-country-ski machine that we own. Other machines, which include smaller foot platforms, take up less space (because you don't have to allow space for the "ski" to move forward and back in its track) but seemed to us less smooth in their motion and less sturdy in construction. The NordicTrack is also the type that folds into the smallest space, and most models are made from attractive pine or oak materials rather than metal. However, we recommend that you try several brands, if possible, before buying. NordicTrack also allows a free thirty-day trial period.

Rowing machines

When Eric was a college oarsman, the team had periodic tests of stamina and strength. Each oarsman spent six minutes rowing as hard as he could on a "rowing ergometer," a huge machine bolted to the floor of the boathouse, with a sliding seat and an oar handle just like that of a racing shell, the whole contraption connected to a flywheel which was turned by the rower's pull on the handle. The number of times the rower could turn the flywheel in six minutes was a measure of his fitness for rowing. It didn't feel much like actual rowing, and the machines were noisy and unreliable, but there was no other way to gauge a rower's fitness precisely. They were available only in boathouses of serious crews, since they were expensive, bulky, and temperamental.

Then a couple of ex-oarsmen started to think about alternatives to these monsters, something that anyone—from Olympic oarsman to harried housewife—could use at home with a minimum of training. The result was the Concept II Rowing Ergometer, a machine that has virtually revolutionized indoor rowing training. It takes a minimum of space (compared to the old Goliaths), very precisely simulates the smooth sensations of propelling a racing shell through the water, and is relatively inexpensive and easy to use. It has become so popular that Indoor Rowing Competitions are held every year in cities around the world, with thousands of oarsmen and other "Concept II jockeys" competing, quite seriously, on these machines in a variety of categories. We cycling, etc.; it is intense and specific to one muscle group. You perform eight to twelve repetitions of a movement (this is called a "set"), then rest and do it again, and usually a third time (three sets). You do four to ten different movements in a complete workout. It's not the rhythmic, almost hypnotic type of workout that you would get on, say, a step machine. It takes more concentration, especially for beginners; this is one form of exercise where you really do want to "feel the burn." It's a different feeling. The muscle "pump" from weight training is as addictive in its way as the exercise "high" from continuous aerobic activities.

In addition, training with weights is different from other, continuous types of exercise because rest is vital. You must rest between sets. And you must rest between days of weight training. This doesn't mean you can't do other forms of exercise on your weight-training rest days, but you should not weight-train every day. Whereas you can perform low-level continuous exercise every day of the week, you should train with weights no more than three times a week, and you can make impressive gains in strength with as few as two workouts a week.

No other form of exercise packs the same sort of conditioning punch. This extends to set point, too. Two to three workouts a week are the optimum with this form of exercise for lowering set point, often dramatically.

What you need for a home-weight-training workout. We recommend dumbbells, the small, hand-held weights, rather than barbells, the types of weights you see Olympic weight lifters using, which consist of a long bar with weights on each end, lifted with both hands. You can do the same exercises with dumbbells, they are safer to use, and they are smaller and easier to store. All you need is a set of dumbbells, ranging from two pounds to ten or twelve pounds, which can be kept inconspicuously in the corner of a living room, study, or bedroom.

You can get adjustable-weight dumbbells, the weight of which you change by sliding plates on or off, or solid, one-piece, nonadjustable dumbbells. The adjustable ones allow you to use a single set of dumbbells for almost any weight (making them less bulky to store, because you have only one pair). But moving plates on and off takes time. And the collars that hold the plates are not tightly secured, they can slip off, causing injury. We recommend that you get a set of pairs of solid,

have no idea what "Concept I" was, but "Concept II" is pretty strange—people sitting indoors, on solid ground, rowing nowhere. But ask people who have used one of these machines and they'll all tell you how strangely addictive it is.

Rowing is second only to cross-country skiing in providing a whole-body workout. Since the seat on which the rower sits slides forward and backward, the legs provide much of the power, with the back and arms finishing the stroke. The abdominal muscles and the arms receive even more of a workout than on the cross-country-ski machine, the hamstrings a bit less. All major muscle groups are toned.

But, as with the cross-country-ski machines, rowing machines rate quite low in a number of other categories, lessening their overall appeal. They are not as difficult to master as cross-country-ski machines, but unless you have rowed before, it will take you several sessions to pull smoothly. The most common mistake beginners make is to start to pull with the back and arms before the legs are completely straight, causing the oar "handle" (a piece about the size and shape of a baseball bat cut in half) to bump the knees.

It's especially important to know how to use your back. Ideally, you should seek the advice of someone who has rowed, or of an instructor at a health club. These machines have the highest injury potential of any indoor-exercise machine, because of the strain that can be imposed on the lower back, especially with poor technique. If you have any back problems at all, this machine is probably not for you. They are also the bulkiest and most difficult to move of all indoor exercisers, requiring a space of about three feet by eight feet. Newer versions fold up, but you should count on a rather large space dedicated completely to this machine. They require the use of your hands. The price is moderately high at about $900. To top it all off, they are the loudest of the five types of exercise equipment. This, together with the forward-and-backward movement on the sliding seat, makes it difficult to watch TV while using one, although we've done it (you can still listen to tapes on a portable tape player with headphones).

The only category in which rowing machines come out on top is in ease of adjustment of controls. To get a harder workout, you simply pull harder (just as you would if rowing on the water). The resistance, which is provided by air resistance to blades on a flywheel (a little like the cards that kids put in the spokes of their bicycle wheels), automatically increases as the flywheel's speed increases. In this way, rowing machines provide perhaps the smoothest workout of all the indoor exercisers, with an infinite variety of exercise intensities instantly available.

Despite the drawbacks, many people who have never touched an oar in their lives buy these machines and get hooked on the smooth, repetitive motion of the stroke. There is something about this sport that is pleasantly hypnotic like no other—even if you're doing it in your basement, on a machine.

What to look for: The Concept II Rowing Ergometer has no serious competition from any other rowing machine now available. Rowing clubs, college crews, and individual rowers use this machine exclusively. It's evolved over the years to become ever more sophisticated, but even the very first model will provide you with a smooth, reliable workout. More recent models have minicomputers which show you your pace, time elapsed, etc. Like NordicTrack, Concept II also offers a free thirty-day trial period.

The special case of weights

We have a feeling that when we mention "weight training" to people they conjure up visions of straining, sweaty, smelly men slinging barbells over their heads, then contemptuously dropping them to the floor. Not something the downstairs neighbors would appreciate, you may be thinking.

But we're talking about something much more accessible, enjoyable, and easy to do. You can get a weight workout that will improve your muscle tone, straighten up your posture, and make all aspects of your life easier, without lifting anything more threatening than a five- or ten-pound dumbbell.

And remember, such workouts are as effective at lowering set point as any other type of exercise. They have the added benefit of toning and sculpting your body in ways that other forms of exercise simply can't match.

Some other benefits of weight training:

- increases bone density, lowering your risk of osteoporosis
- decreases risk of diabetes

- lessens the pain of the most common form of arthritis
- raises HDL-cholesterol (the "good" cholesterol, which heart disease)

However, we do consider weight training a special case reasons.

First, you *must* learn how to do it under the instruction of knowledgable.

Done properly, exercises with weights are one of the mos ways of preventing injury and maintaining joint mobility, es otherwise healthy older people. For example, in one study eighty-, and ninety-year-olds trained with weights to streng leg muscles, and in a matter of a few months more tha their muscle strength. Because of this added strength, they their daily activity by 35 percent. Most dramatic, four partici had been using walkers were able to get around with only t cane in *less than ten weeks.* And athletes have known for ye best way to protect a joint is to strengthen the muscles surro

But weight training done *improperly* is one of the surest jure muscles and joints. It's difficult to teach yourself p nique. So find good instruction. If you have a friend wh exercises with weights, ask him or her to show you. Some Y most health clubs offer instruction. Many colleges and univ their students physical-education courses in weight trainin be able to locate a trained exercise physiologist at the car rehabilitation unit of a local hospital, or a local senior-cit or they may know of qualified instructors who can give y instruction.

If you absolutely can't find a qualified instructor, start lously light weights and just go through the motions of e for several workouts before trying even moderate weigh instruction book ever written on weight training is *Gett* by Bill Pearl and Gary T. Moran, Ph.D. (Bolinas, Calif.: S cations, 1986). If you follow the advice in this book, you far wrong.

The second reason weight training is special is that th unlike the continuous, steady, exercise that you get walk nonadjustable dumbbells, from two pounds to about twelve pounds (men may want to go up to fifteen or twenty pounds). You may end up with five or six pairs of dumbbells, but the space to store them is still minimal, as is cost, and they make your workout more efficient, since you are not constantly changing weights, and safer, since nothing can slip off.

There is a dumbbell exercise for every single muscle group in the body. Some are quite ingenious. You can increase the variety of exercises available to you by buying a weight bench (a padded bench about the size and height of a picnic-table bench) and by setting up a pull-up bar in a doorway. If you decide to get a weight bench, find a solid, tough model, one that won't tip, with fabric that won't rip under years of use. We know one couple who have bought an excellent used bench for less than $20 from a fitness club that was going out of business. However, neither a bench nor a pull-up bar is necessary to achieve a whole-body workout. Again, consult someone well versed in the use of weights for options.

How to buy home-exercise equipment

The ideal way to select the type of home-exercise machine that is right for you is to use them all, under the guidance of someone who is familiar with them on a day-in, day-out basis. And the best way to do that is in a health club that has all five types of machines we've discussed. Even if you don't want to join long-term, you can often find short-term "deals," especially around the New Year. A couple of months is really all you need to explore the potential of various machines. For a modest fee, some clubs will even let you use their facilities several times without joining, which probably would be enough for you to try out the more unfamiliar pieces, like cross-country-ski machines.

Whether you choose to try out machines at a health club or not, when it comes to actually buying a machine, try out various brands at an exercise-equipment store, not a sporting-goods store. Sporting-goods stores often have only one or two exercise machines, seemingly selected at random, and personnel generally are not knowledgable about them. Exercise-equipment stores usually stock a variety of brands in a range of qualities, from very basic models to top-of-the-line. The sales personnel know the machines well and can help you try each one, so make sure you dress in loose clothing (preferably the clothes you work out in), and be prepared to huff and puff and sweat a bit. If you buy a machine at an exercise-equipment store, the management are usually helpful about fixing any problems, either doing it themselves or helping you find someone who can.

Two types of equipment that are hard to find in stores are Nordic-Track cross-country skiers and Concept II Rowing Ergometers. Both can be ordered direct from the factory, and, as we said, both allow you a thirty-day trial period, which should be enough time to determine if you like the machine. Phone numbers: 800 245-5676 for Concept II, 800 328-5888 for NordicTrack.

You may also want to consider buying used exercise machines, expecially if you have had a chance to try out different types either in a health club or at an exercise-equipment store. This is an especially good option for stationary bicycles, cross-country-ski machines, and rowing machines. These types of indoor-exercise equipment are mechanical and very basic, which means that, if you find a used machine that feels smooth and has no obvious malfunctions, it will probably last about as long as a new one, yet you can get it at a fraction of the price. Look for machines at flea markets, in thrift shops, at garage sales, and in the classified ads of your local paper or classified flea market. We know several people who have bought good exercise machines for under $20 this way.

Buying used treadmills or steppers is a bit more chancy, since both contain parts (the hydraulics in the stepper and the electric motor in the treadmill) that are difficult for the average person to assess: they can feel great today and fail tomorrow. Still, if you get a name brand, if it does malfunction you can probably get the necessary repair done easily and cheaply, and have a high-quality piece of equipment at a fraction of its cost new. You can also try shopping at a local exercise-equipment store first, to find out what brands it stocks and which feel best to you (and which brands the shop services), then go out in search of those models. You might even want to place an ad in the paper. In a large urban area, where there are probably thousands of barely used indoor-exercise machines sitting in garages and attics, this strategy can save you hundreds or even thousands of dollars for a high-quality machine.

A low-tech, low-cost home-workout alternative

What we've said so far about indoor-exercise equipment may seem a bit overwhelming. We want to emphasize again that you don't *have* to own a single piece of exercise equipment to get plenty of exercise, enough to keep you healthy and lean, if you simply take every advantage of opportunistic exercise.

And even if you do want to start doing some exercises in the privacy of your own home, you don't have to rush out and buy an expensive piece of equipment. In fact, you can get a complete aerobic and strength workout with nothing more than a board, a few cans from your cupboard, and perhaps a couple of plastic gallon milk jugs.

If you place a sturdy board, about three feet by one foot, across two solid supports about six inches high, you have created the world's cheapest step machine. It is every bit as effective as the $5,000 model in you local health club. You use it by stepping up on the board with one foot, bringing your other foot up so that you momentarily stand on the board, then stepping down with the same foot you first stepped up with and bringing the second foot down, so you momentarily stand on the floor. Continue this motion, alternating the foot you lead off with. It will take you a few minutes to learn the sequence. Once you learn it, it's easier to step up and down rhythmically if you put on some music with a beat that matches your pace. Continue for as long as you like, two minutes or two hours, it's up to you. Do one long workout or several short ones during the day.

This is the same basic motion that is used on step machines and in step-aerobics classes (and you can buy fancy platforms, adjustable to several heights, specifically designed for step aerobics—but then we're getting out of the low-tech range). It is relatively injury-free as long as you keep the board low (don't try stepping up on a chair, which puts too much strain on the knee), you are sure the supports are solid, and you step down under control; that is, don't slam down, lower yourself down. You are completely free to adjust the pace to make the workout as easy or difficult as you want.

If you would also like to do a workout for strengthening and toning, you can use cans from your cupboard as "dumbbells." For heavier weights, use plastic gallon milk bottles with various amounts of water in them. There are also all the exercises you can do using your own body weight—for example, push-ups and sit-ups. These are just as effective as exercises on Nautilus machines, and you carry them with you wherever you go.

In fact, one idea for the traveling fitness buff is to carry a jump rope and a couple of ten-foot lengths of surgical tubing. The jump rope provides your aerobic workout. The tubing can be used to provide resistance in doing a wide variety of strengthening and toning exercises, for your "weight workout."

You get the idea. Machines are nice. They certainly make it easier to exercise at home. But they are by no means essential, and a low-tech, low-cost, high-efficiency workout is available to you almost anyplace, with a little imagination.

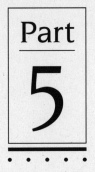

Part

5

Taking Action

14

Measuring Progress

· · · · ·

Anne, Mary, and John came to one of our workshops together driving fifty miles to attend. Mary and John were a wife and husband, both in their mid-thirties, and parents of two-year-old twins, who both found themselves twenty pounds heavier than they had been a decade earlier. Anne, Mary's mother, was a retired schoolteacher, a widow who had been putting on a pound or two every year since her early thirties. Now, at age sixty-six, she was fifty pounds overweight. Her doctor had told her that she needed to lose weight.

They had all been on diet after diet, without success, and were ready for a new approach. And after the workshop, they all chose different combinations of low-fat eating and exercise to achieve their weight-loss goals.

Anne felt that, with fifty pounds to lose, she'd better go all-out. She decided to switch immediately to eating 10 percent fat. And she had been feeling guilty for some time about not giving her two dogs enough exercise—they were looking a little overweight themselves. She decided she could exercise her dogs and herself at the same time by extending their two daily walks to thirty minutes each, from their present length of ten minutes.

Mary and John decided that, with the twins taking up so much time and energy, the transition to eating 10 percent fat might be too much, at least at first. But after they heard us describe Phase 1, eating 20 percent fat, they knew they could make that change right away. Mary saw

from her answers to the diagnostic quizzes that one major area she could change was her habit of eating dairy products made from whole milk. Worried about calcium because of her pregnancy and nursing, she drank two extra glasses of milk a day; she was surprised and pleased to find out that nonfat milk would provide the same amount of calcium. John had gotten into the habit of snacking on several handfuls of walnuts each evening, because he'd heard on the news that walnuts were good for your heart. He decided it might be better for his heart if he lost some weight, and the walnuts were the obvious item to start with. Both Mary and John identified several other areas in their eating habits that they could easily change.

John didn't want to start doing any exercise. He'd had some unpleasant experiences in high-school gym class, and just didn't want to consider it. Mary, on the other hand, had been on her high-school swim team, but had gradually slipped out of the exercise habit, especially since the twins were born. During the exercise part of the workshop, she remembered that the health club in their neighborhood offered child care; one of her friends who also had young children used it and said it was very professional and allowed her to take some time during the day to do something good for *herself*. Mary knew immediately that she was going to do it—an hour a day at the health club, where she planned to swim and maybe take an aerobics class. They were having a special rate reduction right now, and she could join for just $30 a month. And if they could afford $400 for a new printer for John's computer, she figured they could afford the same amount for a high-quality indoor exerciser to use on days when she just couldn't get to her regular workout at the club. She'd decide which type to get after she'd tried them at the health club.

By the end of the workshop, Anne, Mary, and John were enthusiastically planning their fat-loss campaigns. And they all had the same question:

"If we throw away our scales, like you told us to do, how will we be able to keep track of our progress?"

Throw Away the Scale—Really

One way *not* to measure your progress is by daily, or even weekly, weighings. A comment that we get a lot from people who start eating low-fat or exercising: "I've been on your program for two whole weeks now and I haven't lost a single pound!" If you are saying this, you may have missed our discussion of why you should throw away your scale. Go back and read it now (see page 35).

Your scale will not tell you how much fat is on your body. Ever. That is not what it measures—it measures weight. You may actually *gain* weight as you lose fat. This is true for a number of reasons that we went over before: putting on muscle if you are exercising, or replenishing your glycogen stores. You may even gain a little *fat* initially, if you have kept your set point artificially low through constantly restraining your eating. If you see these weight gains initially, it is almost impossible to keep going; we all seem to be locked into blindly following changes in weight as the ultimate indicators of how fat we are.

Your scale is not only useless, it is pernicious. It will encourage impatience and lead you into all sorts of traps. You will start playing games to make sure you can see a weight loss. If you are still going by weight as your measure of progress, your chances of success are decreased, dramatically.

Body-Fat Measurements

If you really *must* have a number by which to measure your progress, get the percentage of your body weight that is fat measured. If you are a woman and over 30 percent of your body weight is fat, you can't hide it from yourself or anyone else. For men, if you're over 25 percent fat you'll start to bulge. The "ideal" percentage of body fat is about 20 percent for females, 15 percent for males. Athletes can be as low as 10 percent body fat for females, and 5 percent (!) for males.

What you want to do in order to measure progress is to be able to measure your percent body fat now, then measure later and compare. If your percentage is going down, you are losing fat, which is what you want.

So a better instrument than a scale to have in the bathroom would be one that measures body fat as easily and accurately as a scale measures weight. Just step onto it and the readout says "Twenty-nine percent body fat, down 1 percent from a month ago."

Alas, such an instrument is not yet available. Several methods *are* currently available to measure body fat, but none of the measurements is quick and only a couple are considered very accurate. We'll discuss the three most common methods. The first two, underwater weighing and electrical-impedance measurements, require that you visit a laboratory that performs these measurements—call your local university, college, or community-college physical-education department or your local hospital's cardiac-rehabilitation unit and tell them that you are interested in having your body composition measured. Most have facilities for doing so at a modest fee; if not, they may be able to direct you to such a facility in your area. Some health clubs are set up to do these tests. The third method, using calipers, you can do yourself with the help of another person, but you must first buy a set of calipers.

If you have your body fat measured at a clinic, they will tell you your weight, your percent body fat, the number of pounds of fat on you, and the number of pounds of lean tissue (bone, muscle, internal organs, etc.—everything but fat).

Underwater weighing

The most accurate way to measure body fat, the one that is considered the gold standard by researchers, is underwater, or full-immersion, weighing. It is based on the fact that fat floats, so fat people weigh less underwater than lean people do; from a comparison of a person's weight underwater with his or her weight on solid ground, you can calculate the percentage of body fat that he or she is carrying around. It is cumbersome, time-consuming, and somewhat frightening to some people: although it is not at all dangerous or painful, you do have to be completely underwater for several seconds. This one definitely requires equipment not available in the home.

Electrical impedance

In this method, a small, harmless electrical current is passed through the body. Fat and lean tissue offer different barriers, or impedances, to the current. Based on this, the amount of fat and lean tissue can be calculated.

This method is almost as accurate as the underwater-weighing method, and the measurement is much easier. But the equipment is expensive and likely to be found only in a research laboratory.

Calipers

A cheaper and easier way to get an idea of percentage body fat is to use calipers, which look and function somewhat like giant clothespins, with which you can pinch (gently) various areas of the body and measure the thickness of the fold of skin and fat that is pinched. The bigger the fold, the more fat. You take several measurements and, by comparing the values with those in tables supplied with the instrument, you can get a rough idea of the percentage of body fat for the whole body.

The nice thing about calipers is that a good pair costs about as much as a good scale (look in the back of runners' magazines or fitness magazines for companies that sell them), so this is one method that you can use at home.

The disadvantage is that measurements are extremely variable, depending on who is using the calipers. So, if you decide to get a pair, make sure the same person takes the measurements each time, and don't trust any measurements until that person has had a lot of experience. (You can't do the measurements on yourself. Some locations, like the middle of your back, are simply impossible to reach.) Have your measuring person take measurements every day for two weeks. When the percentage of body fat agrees each day to within .5 percent every day, the person is taking reliable measurements. You should be able to see body-fat loss *as long as the same person takes the measurements*. If you go to a clinic where they use calipers to measure body fat, the same person *must* take the measurements each time, preferably using the same pair of calipers each time. Otherwise you simply can't trust the results.

For any measurement

Remember that there is a little bit of slop in any measurement. You could have your body fat measured one day and be told you are at 22 percent, then come back the next day and be measured by the same person, same method, same instrument, and be told you are at 24 percent. So, if you want to use these measurements to keep track of fat loss, wait at least six months between measurements. Otherwise you might get discouraged, because the fat you have lost might not show up, given the inevitable inaccuracy of the measurements.

Commonsense Measurements

Sometimes low-tech is better than high-tech. In the case of body fat, this is true. The following questions will give you a better assessment of your body fat than the most modern total-immersion tank. They are easy and completely free, and will tell you what you really want to know—how do I look and how do I feel?

How do your clothes fit?

It's so obvious that people don't believe it—the best instrument you have for keeping track of body fat is your clothes. For men, the best is the belt; as fat leaves the body, the belt has to be moved in a notch, then another notch, just to hold your pants up. That's progress, and it's visible every day. For women, it's the fit of a pair of pants; the same pair may be too tight to get into one month, and too loose to wear six months later.

Perhaps you can't really call this method completely free, because you will have to buy smaller clothes. But most people will be willing to pay that price.

How do you look in the mirror?

Relatively few people who want to lose weight need do so for health reasons. If you wonder whether you are carrying so much fat that it is unhealthy, see the next section. You probably aren't. Most of us want to lose fat for reasons of vanity. You may suppose we would scoff at that, and say you should eat low-fat and exercise for all the wonderful health benefits, but in our experience the *real* reasons most people (including us!) stay on a low-fat-eating-and-exercise life-style are two immediate, short-term benefits. One is the energy, vitality, and optimism that it imparts. And the other is the improved appearance.

So look in your mirror and be vain. Your mirror doesn't lie. Ugly folds hanging down, a belly that sticks out twelve inches—these are not considered attractive in our culture (they are considered attractive in some, including European cultures of the not-too-distant past, but we don't live there or then). These will disappear, given time, if you follow a low-fat-and-exercise life-style.

One warning. A mirror is like a scale. There is one in the bathroom, just waiting for you to look at yourself after each shower, which means every day for most people. It's easy to get impatient for changes. You must be realistic. Change will happen, but it's going to take six months to a year to be really, unequivocally visible. Give it time!

How do you feel?

The most subjective measurement may be the best of all. Are you bouncing out of bed in the morning? Do you find yourself with greater energy and enthusiasm, the feeling that you have enough in reserve to weather any crisis? Are you finding yourself happier, no matter what you look like? If so, you are making the most important progress of all.

A Health Measurement

One very simple measurement will give you a rough idea of whether the amount of fat that you carry around is dangerous, at least to your heart (remember, heart disease is the number-one killer in the United States). Measure your waist when your stomach is relaxed (your waist is considered the thinnest circumference between your hips and your chest). Measure the widest part of your hips. Divide the waist measurement by the hip measurement. If the ratio is *greater* than 0.80 for women, or 0.95 for men, your fatness is putting you at high risk for heart disease. If it is less, you are at low risk. There are many other factors that contribute to heart disease, but this will tell you if *obesity* is likely to be a factor for you.

As for the number-two killer, cancer, the most important factor is not the fat on your body, but the fat in your diet.

You can skip any measurement and go directly to eating low-fat and exercising, if you wish. This will provide you with the optimal health and energy that *you* can have, regardless of body measurements or what our society considers "attractive."

Be Patient

Remember, even if you start eating 10 percent fat and exercising moderately for half an hour a day, you will probably lose no more than one to four pounds of fat a *month*. Some people respond with more fat loss, some with less. But almost no one will see much progress in the first month. Just expect that. A lot of people will see little or no progress in the first three months. So just expect that, too. It will be at about *six months* that almost everyone will see definite progress. Mark the date six months from now on your calendar, and when you get discouraged, look at how far away it still is. And don't forget, fat loss doesn't stop after six months. It will continue until you reach your natural new set point, which can take a year or more.

Anne, Mary, and John After the Workshop . . .

On the way home, Anne, Mary, and John discussed their plans. Reluctantly, they agreed to put their scales in their garages and not look at them for six months. They couldn't bear actually to get rid of them.

As soon as she got home, Anne measured her waist. Forty inches. Then she measured her hips. Forty-five inches. She got out her calculator. Her waist/hip ratio was .89, much higher than the .80 considered to be the upper limit of healthy. And she remembered her doctor telling her that her cholesterol was above 220. Her husband had died of a heart attack without warning just a couple of years earlier. One

minute he was watching TV in his easy chair; the next minute the paramedics were trying in vain to resuscitate him.

Well, she'd had *her* warning. And she was going to do something about it. She went to her cupboard and started pulling out packaged items, reading the labels. At first it took her a while to determine whether they were high- or low-fat. But she followed the label-reading two-step (page 144), and soon she could tell in a matter of seconds what was acceptable and what wasn't. She had some surprises. That microwave popcorn was loaded with fat! And the tortilla chips that she was sure must be more healthful than potato chips turned out to be sky-high, too. She started preparing a food bag to give away to the local food bank. Oh, and she'd need to make a new menu, and a new shopping list . . . and take the dogs for their first half-hour walk. . . .

Meanwhile, John and Mary were at the grocery store. They'd asked the babysitter to watch the twins for another hour so that this first low-fat trip through the store could be uninterrupted. John passed the nuts section with a regretful sigh. Let's see, maybe instead of walnuts before dinner he could try half a bagel with nonfat cream cheese and jam. It seemed like such a sin to eat that instead of the "healthy" nuts. Could he really slim down by eating things that tasted good? Well, what did he have to lose, except his paunch? He looked down at his belt. It was on the next-to-last notch, and even that one was a bit tight. John knew exactly how he was going to keep track of his fat loss.

Mary stood in front of the dairy case. Okay, everything was going to be nonfat now. The store stocked nonfat milk from two different dairies, so she got half a gallon from each to see if there was any difference in taste. She used to buy half-gallons of ice cream—"for the babysitter," she'd told herself—but Mary seemed to be the one who always finished them. This time it was a couple of different brands of nonfat frozen yogurt, and a quart of lemon sorbet.

When John and Mary got to the produce section of the store, they happily bought the same fruits and vegetables they always did. But this time they bought double the usual quantity. The twins both loved apples, so they bought several different varieties. And they all enjoyed their nightly salads, so Mary decided to make double portions and store the extra for the next day's lunches. Oh, and they should try some nonfat salad dressings. . . .

The next day, Mary took the twins with her to the health club. She just hoped Jason and Justin wouldn't start screaming when she left them at the child-care facility. But as soon as they saw the toys and the other children, they ran over to them. They didn't even notice when she slipped out the door. In fact, half an hour later, when she returned fresh from her swim, they didn't want to leave! Keeping them happy during her workout certainly wasn't going to be a problem. At the front desk, Mary pulled out her checkbook and paid for a year's membership. It was cheaper that way, and it symbolized her commitment to getting back into the exercise habit.

And Mary had found out that the health club also had a section that was used by amateur and professional athletes for the rehabilitation of sports injuries. One of the services they offered was underwater weighing to determine body fat. She signed up to be measured the next day. She wanted to know exactly how much fat she was losing in the next six months. . . .

. . . and Six Months Later

It hadn't been easy for Anne at first. Some of the low-fat recipes she tried in her first few weeks had been disastrous. One particularly memorable meal had featured baked beans and sweet-potato bread. The beans had taken hours to prepare and wound up crunchy yet tasteless. And the bread . . . Well, brick was more like it. On the bright side, sawing through that loaf with a knife had provided plenty of exercise. So had chewing it.

But she'd discovered dozens of 10-percent-fat recipes that were tasty and quick, and modifying many of her old standbys had been a snap. Her favorite was spaghetti, the sauce for which she now made with turkey instead of ground beef. And she had never realized before how much she enjoyed fruit. After just a couple of weeks, she was eating 10 percent fat most days, and by one month her new eating habits were well established.

A funny thing happened to her walks with her two dogs. She found that, after eating low-fat for just a couple of weeks, she was bursting with new energy. She knew she couldn't have lost much weight, but she felt so

much *lighter*. She'd thought it would be a chore to add time to her walks with her dogs. Instead, she found herself going farther and farther each day. The walks extended to twenty minutes, then half an hour, then forty-five minutes. After three months, she and her dogs were walking for an hour in the morning and an hour in the evening! Yet the exercise seemed to give her *more* energy, not less. Also at three months, she was really noticing a difference in how her clothes fit. In fact, many of her dresses were getting so loose that they just didn't look right anymore. She decided to reward herself for her new habits by going clothes-shopping.

At six months, Anne didn't know how much weight she'd lost, but she knew exactly how many inches. Her waist measurement was now thirty-two, down eight inches from six months ago. Her hips were forty-one inches, down four. The ratio was now .78. She just barely made it under the .80 limit considered "safe," but, although she wasn't losing fat as fast as she had at first, she could tell by the way her new, smaller clothes were starting to loosen up that she still hadn't reached the limit of her fat loss. She might have to make another shopping expedition when she finally settled into her lower set point. Already she was fitting into dresses smaller than any she'd worn since she was forty-five. Best of all, she had had her cholesterol measured at a local clinic. It was down to 178, from the 220 that her doctor had measured less than a year earlier.

The only thing that worried her was that winter was now approaching. She wouldn't be able to take the dogs out for those long, wonderful walks anymore, but she didn't want to give up the exercise. Maybe she would do something she had never imagined before, and buy an indoor-exercise machine, like John and Mary. They'd bought a step machine, but, frankly, it looked a little outlandish to Anne. On the other hand, she could set up a stationary bicycle in front of the TV and use it while she watched her soap operas. (She felt guilty about watching them. Maybe if she was getting some exercise at the same time she'd feel better about it.) Yes, she was going to go out tomorrow to price stationary bicycles. . . .

• • •

Both Mary and John found that following the eating guidelines of Phase 1, which brought them to eating 20 percent fat, was simple. Almost too simple. After a week or so, they couldn't really tell the difference between the way they'd eaten before and the way they ate now. And the twins never noticed at all, not even when they started getting nonfat milk instead of whole milk with their meals. (Remember, if they had *not* yet been two years old, they would still have needed whole milk.) How could something this easy make any difference?

Mary had her body fat measured by underwater weighing at the start of her new eating and exercise habits. Because of her swimming experience, it didn't bother her at all that she had to breathe out completely underwater, then stay motionless for a few seconds. But it did bother her to discover that she carried 35 percent fat—55 of her 155 pounds were fat! She knew that she had been putting on weight, and she could tell just looking in the mirror that she was losing the battle of the bulge, but . . . 55 pounds?

The technician who did the measurements explained that a lot of the fat was hidden; much of it was stored around internal organs, to provide padding, and a lot of the rest was actually inside her muscles, just like the marbling in a cut of meat. She said that optimum for women was around 20 percent fat, which, at her present body weight, would still leave her with 31 pounds of fat, but if she got down that low she would be looking very slim. Mary wasn't sure she believed her—how could you look slim with the equivalent of two fifteen-pound turkeys' worth of fat on you? But she had to admit that, whatever she would end up with, she was too fat *now*. She was more determined than ever to put aside an hour a day just for herself, and use that time to work out.

She alternated swim days with days on which she took an hour-long aerobics class along with two of her friends. She didn't know whether it was the exercise or the way she was eating, but after a couple of months clothes were starting to loosen. After four months, there was no doubt about it—she was starting to enjoy looking in the mirror, rather than dreading it. And after six months, she had her body fat measured again.

She was startled to learn that she'd only dropped from 155 pounds to 145. Only 10 pounds after six whole months? How could that be, especially since she'd also dropped three dress sizes? It just didn't seem possible. Then the technician calculated her percent body fat and total number of *fat* pounds. Mary had dropped from 35 percent fat to 25 percent. She now carried 37 pounds of fat, compared with 55 pounds the first time she was measured. She'd lost 18 pounds of fat—and *gained* 9 pounds of muscle because of the increase in her exercise levels. She remembered that the fat loss was the equivalent of eighteen one-pound cartons of butter. When she thought about that much fat, the change in her dress sizes made a little more sense. She didn't know where the muscle was going, but, if anything, it was making her shapelier. For the first time in years, she enjoyed getting into her swim suit.

Sure, she was still a little plump. But the change to eating 20 percent fat had been so easy, maybe it was time for her and John to try eating 10 percent fat. She never would have considered it six months ago. But they'd had dinner at her mother's house and eaten meals that were below 10 percent fat. These had actually been very tasty, after a few early fiascos. Seeing the results of the changes she'd made so far made her confident that she could do more. She'd call her mother tonight and ask for some recipes. . . .

• • •

John's engineering firm was on the tenth floor. He remembered how those Johns Hopkins doctors said climbing each step added four seconds to your life. Just for fun, he got out his calculator. Let's see, there were twenty steps between the floors in his building. And he was on the tenth floor. So if he climbed those ten flights he would add a little over thirteen minutes to his life. And it wouldn't take any more time, really, than waiting for the elevator. It was like getting something for nothing. When you looked at it that way, it wasn't really exercise, which he hated—it was just a little bonus each day. So he started climbing stairs, first one flight, then two, then three, until after a month he was climbing up all ten flights each morning, and down all ten at night. And every once in a while he'd get up from his desk, walk to the stairwell, and climb up and down a "bonus" flight. Another minute and a half tacked on to his life.

When Mary insisted they get a home-exercise machine, he liked the step machine at the exercise-equipment store so much he convinced her that this was the one they should get. It was partly because it reminded him of his daily stair climbing, which he now kind of enjoyed.

But mainly because it had a readout displaying minutes elapsed, number of stairs climbed, number of feet climbed, number of calories burned—this was the machine for him! Not that he'd ever use it, of course. He hated exercise.

After three months, John noticed that he had to tighten his belt a notch to keep his pants up. Hey, something really was happening! Could those painless changes in his eating habits really be making a difference? Maybe, with the stair climbing . . . After six months, he tried tightening his belt another notch. No, that was uncomfortable. It looked as if he'd plateaued on his weight loss. It made a difference, though—a few people asked if he'd lost weight. Still, he had another three or four notches to go before he'd really be happy. Mary was talking about dropping down to eating 10 percent fat, and that didn't sound so far-fetched to him anymore.

And he'd gotten on the step machine at home a few times. Mary used it a lot; she said it was a great way to fit in a few minutes of exercise when the twins were napping. And what a change there had been in Mary! She looked almost as slim as when they'd married.

But John wasn't going to do any workouts on the machine. Exercise was not for him. Still, he did want to lose a little more weight. Stair climbing at work was a breeze now. And it really cleared his head. He thought it might be fun to "climb Mount Everest" on the step machine at home. How long would it take? Let's see, Mount Everest was twenty-nine-thousand feet tall. And each "step" you took on the machine was twelve inches (he knew because he'd measured it). And he'd found, according to the digital readout on the machine, that he "climbed" at precisely ninety steps per minute. He'd need his calculator to see how many minutes he'd have to put in before he reached the summit. Of course, he'd "climb Mount Everest" strictly for his own amusement, not for exercise. He had sworn off regular exercise in high school. . . .

• • •

John, Mary, and Anne are composites of dozens of workshop participants, based on comments, letters, and conversations we've had over the years about their progress on the program, as well as on the dozens of scientific studies now available. They represent the range of commitment and response we've seen, from people like Anne, who start right in at a high level of exercise and the lowest level of fat and achieve remarkable reductions in body fat in a relatively short time, to those like John, who try a modest level of change and are willing to accept smaller (but noticeable) losses of fat. Many people find, as John did in our example, that, once the small changes start, they want more. With the different levels of low-fat eating and exercise offered on our program, they know just how to achieve it.

And now so do you. You have the information you need to start living lean in a fat world. Choose the level of low-fat eating and/or exercise you'd like to begin with, take the appropriate diagnostic quizzes, and start! Join the thousands who have used these approaches to live healthier, more energetic—and leaner—lives.

Appendixes

Recipes

· · · · ·

Here are a couple dozen of our tried-and-true everyday favorites, as well as several fancier recipes for entertaining. They are as easy to prepare as their high-fat counterparts, and they all have been taste-tested by ourselves, plus our families, friends, and guests. Any that elicited grim smiles or jokes about rabbit food have been eliminated.

We haven't included an exhaustive number of recipes. It's more like a starter kit. As you begin using the principles for low-fat cooking described in Phase 1 and Phase 2, you will find, as discussed in chapter 8, that almost any recipe, including most of your old favorites, can be modified to be deliciously low-fat. Also, in the bibliography we describe a number of books that may be useful sources of low-fat recipes.

In keeping with our philosophy that low-fat eating should be simple, without a lot of counting of fat grams and squinting at nutritional tables, we analyzed these recipes only for their fat percentage. Eating is not a scientific experiment, and ordinary people do not construct meals by looking at the nutritional analysis for each component; they eat what tastes good. We're not offering a dietetic menu plan but, rather, simple, low-fat dishes that can serve as the centerpieces of nutritionally balanced meals, as well as some side dishes and sauces that can boost the taste without boosting the fat content of your meal. To complete the nutritional picture, just make sure that you are putting together whole meals that help you to eat at least five servings of fruits and vegetables daily. For example, a dinner entree such as spaghetti with turkey sauce can be accompanied by French bread, a tossed green salad, and a vegetable.

The recipes that you will see in this section were created or adapted using only the principles of cooking we have discussed in the recipe section, and are designed to feed five or six people. We had never actually analyzed these recipes until we wrote this book. So it was with some curiosity that we began to analyze the recipes for fat content. To our delight, we have found that the vast majority of the recipes are extremely low in fat (8 percent or less) and the few recipes we considered to be very "rich" were a respectable 15–16 percent fat. It really does work!

One major nutritional concern for many people, especially women, is calcium; their main worry is osteoporosis (thinning of the bones). There is some debate among nutritionists as to the exact daily requirement and the best sources, but mainstream scientists recommend 1,000 milligrams daily for premenopausal women, and 1,500 milligrams daily for postmenopausal women not taking estrogen. Dairy products are still considered the best source, and for that reason we recommend as part of Phase 1 that you simply switch to nonfat dairy products rather than giving them up. Because of this, you will be getting as much calcium on our program as you were on a high-fat diet. If you are concerned that this may not be enough, you may want to take a calcium supplement (calcium carbonate). You should also be aware that weight-bearing exercise, such as walking or jogging, as well as weight training, may be even more effective in building and maintaining strong bones than dietary measures.

A final note: some of the recipes call for Parmesan cheese, mozzarella cheese, Chinese sesame oil, and even chocolate chips. Gasp! Isn't that transgressing on the very foundations of Phase 1 (no oils, only nonfat dairy)? Well, yes and no. Though in the purest sense we should be avoiding such foods, there are exceptions in cooking. As we discussed in Phase 2, you can use some high-fat foods if you treat them like spices—in other words, if you use *very* small amounts in recipes whose other ingredients are all extremely low fat. In the following recipes you'll use small enough amounts of these high-fat foods so that the overall fat content of the food prepared will still be low. So enjoy. Also, if you like to cook, review the section on altering recipes in chapter 8. And feel free to send us any great recipes you discover or create. Have fun!

Relatively quick and easy recipes
Basil Tomato Sauce
Lentil Soup
Mexican Beans
Split Pea Soup
Chili (Vegetarian or with Meat)
Low-Fat Alfredo Sauce
Hearty Vegetable Stew (or with Chicken or Turkey)
Orange Fennel Chicken
Curried Turkey and Rice Salad
Tuna Fish Sandwich Spread
Spaghetti with Turkey Sauce
Linguine with Clam Sauce
Garlicky Cream Cheese Fondue
Pancakes or Waffles
French Toast
Nonfat Vinaigrette
Quick and Easy Salsa
Homemade Low-Fat Cream Cheese
Hot and Sour Vegetable Sauté
Bavarian-Style Vegetable Sauté
Tuscan Bean Soup

Fancier cooking
Chicken or Turkey with Couscous and Vegetables
Stuffed Baked Potatoes
Vegetarian Lasagna, or Ground Turkey Lasagna
Spicy Curried Turkey Breast with Vegetables
Black and White Bean, Tex-Mex Couscous Salad
Bavarian Black Forest Chocolate Cake
Prune Puree (Oil Substitute in Baking)

Basil Tomato Sauce

Time to prepare: 15 minutes
Cooking time: 20 minutes

½ c. water (if you like the taste of red wine, substitute ¾ c. wine)
1 onion, chopped
4 or 5 medium-sized cloves garlic, minced (or ½–¾ tsp. garlic
   powder)
2 15-oz. cans diced tomatoes in juice (or around 3 lbs. fresh
   diced tomatoes)
1 15-oz. can tomato sauce
2–3 tsps. dried basil (6–8 fresh leaves finely chopped)
½ tsp. crushed red pepper (more if you like it spicy)
1 15-oz. can artichoke hearts (in water), cut into chunks
¾ c. chopped green pepper, celery, or other vegetables (optional)

1. In a large saucepan, sauté onion and garlic in water or wine until
   onions are transparent.
2. Stir in tomatoes, tomato sauce, and spices. Bring to a boil, then
   reduce heat so sauce will simmer. Place lid partially off, so steam
   can vent, and allow sauce to simmer for at least 15 minutes.
3. Add artichoke hearts, and any additional vegetables. Allow to simmer for at least another 5 minutes. Serve over low-fat pasta or
   rice (1 lb. dry pasta or 2 c. cooked rice).

% Calories from Fat: 4% (sauce only)
                             8% (sauce with pasta)

Lentil Soup

Time to prepare: 15 minutes
Cooking time: 45 minutes

2½ c. (1 lb.) lentils
8 c. defatted chicken broth* or water, or a combination of both
1 medium onion, diced
3–4 medium carrots, diced
2 15-oz. cans diced tomatoes
1 10-oz. package frozen corn (about 1 ½ c.)
½–1 tsp. garlic powder
½–1 tsp. dried oregano (optional)
½ c. barley (optional)
1–2 medium potatoes, diced

1. Add all ingredients except potatoes to a large saucepan. Bring to a boil, then reduce heat and simmer with lid partially on, for about 30 minutes.
2. Add potatoes, then simmer for about 15 minutes.

% Calories from Fat: 3%

---

*To defat broth with a spoon, skim any fat floating on the surface of the broth, or simply buy a brand of broth that is fat-free.

Mexican Beans

(Adapted from Nathan Pritikin's *The Pritikin Promise*).

Note: Although we encourage the use of canned beans to simplify recipes and hasten preparation, these beans are a worthwhile exception. They are so rich in taste and so simple to prepare. Though the cooking time is lengthy, there is very little work besides occasionally stirring the pot. They also freeze extremely well and make marvelous leftovers.

Time to prepare: 10 minutes
Cooking time: 2–3 hours

2 c. red, pink, or black beans, or a mix of the three
6–8 c. water
1 7-oz. can green-chili salsa
1 15-oz. can tomato sauce
1 tsp. onion powder
1 tsp. chili powder
1 tsp. ground cumin
1 tsp. garlic powder
2 tsps. ground coriander
½–1 tsp. salt

1. Rinse beans and place in a large saucepan. Cover beans with water and bring to a boil.
2. Once beans are boiling, reduce heat to a simmer, cover pot, and allow to simmer for 1–2 hours.
3. Check beans from time to time to be sure water is still covering them. If you need to, you can add more water. Beans should be cooked until very soft.
4. Now add remaining ingredients and stir to mix thoroughly. Simmer beans for an additional 20 minutes to an hour. Add more water if beans become dry.
5. Serve beans on corn tortillas as tacos or tostadas or with rice.

% Calories from Fat: 3%

Split Pea Soup

(Adapted from Mary McDougall's
The McDougall Health Supporting Cookbook)

Time to prepare: 15 minutes
Cooking time: 45 minutes

1¼ c. (½ lb.) **split peas**
4 c. **defatted chicken broth**
4 c. **water**
2 large **carrots, diced**
1 medium **onion, diced**
2–3 cloves **garlic, minced, or** ¼ tsp. **garlic powder**
½ tsp. **dried oregano**
2 **bay leaves**
½–1 tsp. **salt**
1 T. **bacon bits or bacon-flavored bits (optional)**
Potatoes (optional)

1. Toss all ingredients in a pot, bring to a boil, then reduce heat and allow to simmer with the lid partially off. Simmer for 30–45 minutes.
2. If you wish to add potatoes, do so 10–15 minutes into the cooking time.

% Calories from Fat:　　4% **(without bacon bits)**
　　　　　　　　　　　　　　7% **(with bacon bits)**

Chili (Vegetarian or with Turkey)

Time to prepare: 20 minutes
Cooking time: 15–40 minutes

½ c. water or red wine
1 lb. ground turkey breast (optional)
1 onion, chopped
3–4 cloves garlic, crushed, or ½ tsp. garlic powder
2 carrots, shredded
1 stalk celery, chopped
½ green pepper, diced
1 15-oz. can diced tomatoes in juice (add a second can of
     tomatoes in juice if you like more tomatoes)
1 15-oz. can tomato sauce
2 15-oz. cans cooked beans (kidney, pinto, or black)
½ c. frozen corn
1 8-oz. can sliced water chestnuts (optional)
1–2 T. chili powder
½ tsp. cumin powder
½ tsp. onion powder (optional)

1. Sauté ground turkey in water or wine, breaking it into bite-sized pieces. Add onion, garlic, carrot, celery, and green pepper and continue sautéing for about 5 minutes.
2. Stir in all other ingredients, partially cover, and allow to simmer for at least 15 minutes. The longer it simmers, the tastier it gets. Serve with crusty French bread or steamed corn tortillas and a green salad.

% Calories from Fat: 4% (without turkey)
                             6% (with turkey)

Low-Fat Alfredo Sauce

(Adapted from Molly Katzen's *Still Life with Menu Cookbook*;
Berkeley, Calif.: Ten Speed Press, 1988)

Time to prepare: 10 minutes
Cooking time: 10 minutes (or time it takes to cook the noodles)

1 16-oz. container nonfat sour cream
8 oz. nonfat cottage cheese (small-curd, or puree large-curd)
½–1 tsp. salt
¼–½ tsp. black pepper
2 cloves garlic, minced, or ¼ tsp. garlic powder (optional)
2–4 T. nonfat or regular Parmesan cheese
2 T. minced fresh parsley (optional)

1 lb. dry pasta noodles

1. Mix all ingredients for the sauce, whipping it till mixed thoroughly.
2. Cook and drain pasta. Toss hot pasta with Alfredo sauce. Alfredo sauce is also very tasty on cooked vegetables, such as cauliflower, broccoli, or baked potatoes.

% **Calories from Fat:**   6% (sauce only, using nonfat
                                 Parmesan cheese)
                             5% (sauce with pasta, using nonfat
                                 Parmesan cheese)
                            13% (sauce only, using regular
                                 Parmesan cheese)
                             7% (sauce with pasta, using regular
                                 Parmesan cheese)

(Most white pasta is extremely low in fat, around 3%, thus it can dilute the overall fat content nicely.)

Hearty Vegetable Stew
(or with Chicken or Turkey)

Time to prepare: 15 minutes
Cooking time: 30–40 minutes

3 15-oz. cans defatted chicken broth
1 c. water
2 chicken breasts, diced, or 1 lb. turkey-breast strips (optional)
3–4 carrots, chopped
1 onion, chopped
2–3 cloves garlic, crushed, or ¼ tsp. garlic powder
2 potatoes, in 1-in. dice
1 c. frozen corn
1 c. green beans, chopped in ¼-inch pieces
1 T. cornstarch
2 T. water

1. In a large saucepan, bring chicken broth and water to a boil, add chicken, and simmer for 5 minutes.
2. Stir in carrots, onion, and garlic and simmer for 10 minutes.
3. Stir in remaining vegetables and simmer for another 20–30 minutes.
4. Mix together cornstarch and water, then add it to the stew, stirring constantly. Allow to cook for another 5 minutes, till sauce thickens.

% Calories from Fat: 5% (vegetables only)
                             7% (with turkey breast)
                             11% (with chicken breast)

Orange Fennel Chicken

(Adapted from *Jane Brody's Good Food Book*)

Time to prepare: 15 minutes
Cooking time: 30 minutes

Sauce (enough for 8–10 breasts)

1 12-oz. can orange-juice concentrate
1 c. water
4 cloves garlic, minced, or ½ tsp. garlic powder
3 tsps. fennel seeds
¾ tsp. ground ginger
1 tsp. salt
¼ tsp. ground pepper
2 T. cornstarch mixed with 2 T. water

8–10 chicken breasts (skinless, boneless chicken breast halves)

1. Mix all sauce ingredients except cornstarch mixture in a sauce-pan. Bring mixture to a boil, then reduce heat and simmer for 5 minutes.
2. Add cornstarch mixture and simmer for 1 minute more. Remove sauce from heat.
3. Preheat oven to 325 degrees.
4. Place skinless chicken breasts in a baking dish and spoon sauce over them. Cover dish with aluminum foil and bake for 30 minutes. Halfway through the baking time, spoon sauce over chicken, then cover again for the rest of the baking time.
5. Serve chicken with sauce spooned over it. It goes beautifully with rice.
6. The great thing about this dish is that the *extra sauce freezes quite well,* and this recipe makes a lot of sauce, enough for at least 10 breasts.

% Calories from Fat: **1% (sauce only)**
                            16% (sauce with chicken)

Curried Turkey and Rice Salad

(Adapted from George Mateljan's *Cooking Without Fat*,
Health Valley Foods Company, 1992

Time to prepare: 10 minutes (once rice is cooked)
Cooking time: 20–55 minutes (for rice)

3 c. cooked brown or white rice
3–4 c. (1–1½ lbs.) diced cooked turkey breast
2 c. seedless green grapes
3 T. white-wine vinegar
1 c. nonfat mayonnaise
3 tsps. curry powder
½ tsp. salt
¼ tsp. pepper

1. Prepare rice as instructed on the package.
2. In a large bowl, combine rice, turkey, and grapes. Add vinegar and mix.
3. Combine mayonnaise, curry powder, salt, and pepper. Add to turkey mixture and mix thoroughly.

% Calories from Fat: 6%

Tuna Fish Sandwich Spread

Time to prepare: 5 minutes

1 6-oz. can chunk white tuna packed in water only (or suitable
**   low-fat canned tuna)**
1 heaping T. nonfat mayonnaise
1 T. spicy brown mustard
1 tsp. dried minced onions or 2 tsps. fresh diced onion

Mix all ingredients, and use in sandwiches or on nonfat crackers.

% Calories from Fat: **a range of 8–16%**

(The % fat will depend on the fat content of tuna used, which varies greatly from brand to brand because of the way they are cleaned and packaged, and because some types of tuna are fattier than others.)

Spaghetti with Turkey Sauce

(Courtesy of Beth Witt)

Time to prepare: 20 minutes
Cooking time: 50 minutes

Turkey Sauce

1 large onion, chopped
2–3 cloves garlic, minced, or 1 tsp. garlic powder
1 can defatted chicken broth (15-oz.)
1 lb. ground skinless turkey breast
salt and pepper to taste
1–1½ tsps. dried oregano
1 26–32-oz. jar low-fat pasta sauce (spaghetti sauce, marinara, etc.)
1 4-oz. can mushrooms, stem and pieces, drained

1 lb. spaghetti or other pasta

1. Sauté onion and garlic in a large nonstick skillet in about ⅓ can chicken broth for about 10 minutes over medium heat. Add ground turkey broken up into small pieces, add about ⅓ of the remaining chicken broth, and brown for about 10 minutes, adding more broth if pan becomes dry.
2. Remove from heat. Salt and pepper lightly. Mix in oregano. Add pasta sauce and mushrooms, mixing thoroughly. Simmer on low heat, covered, for 20 to 30 minutes.

3. While meat mixture is cooking, prepare spaghetti according to package directions. Serve sauce and pasta topped with a small amount of Parmesan cheese or a large amount of fat-free Parmesan.

% Calories from Fat: 8% (sauce only)
5.5% (sauce with pasta)

Linguine with Clam Sauce

(Courtesy of Sharon Correia)

Time to prepare: 20 minutes
Cooking time: 30 minutes

1 10-oz. bottle clam juice
2 6.5-oz. cans clams (in their juices)
1 onion, finely chopped
⅓ c. fresh parsley, chopped
3 cloves garlic, minced, or 1–1½ tsps. garlic powder
½ tsp. salt
¼ tsp. pepper
1–1½ cups fresh basil, chopped (loosely packed), or
1–1½ T. dried basil

1 lb. linguine noodles

1 T. cornstarch, dissolved in 2 T. water

1. To a large saucepan, add clam juice, clams, onion, parsley, garlic, salt, and pepper. Bring to a boil, and lower the heat until the mixture simmers. Simmer for about 25 minutes with the lid off, stirring occasionally. Add basil, and allow to simmer 5 minutes more.
2. While the sauce simmers, cook the pasta.

3. Mix the cornstarch and water. Slowly add it to the clam mixture while constantly stirring. Within a few minutes, the sauce should thicken slightly. Remove from heat.
4. Place the pasta in a large bowl, pour the sauce over the pasta, and mix thoroughly. Serve with nonfat Parmesan cheese, or small amounts of regular Parmesan.

% Calories from Fat: **9.5% (sauce only)**
                             5% (sauce with pasta)

Garlicky Cream Cheese Fondue

(Courtesy of Shelly McKeirnan)

Time to prepare: 3 minutes
Cooking time: 3–5 minutes

1 8-oz. container nonfat cream cheese
¼ c. nonfat or regular Parmesan cheese
1 tsp. garlic powder
1 tsp. onion powder
salt and pepper to taste
¼–½ c. nonfat milk

1. In a heavy saucepan, whip all ingredients to a thick, creamy consistency. Heat over a low flame to warm completely. You may need to add more milk. You may also heat this in a covered microwavable dish for 2 minutes or so, on the high setting.
2. Serve with bread sticks or cut vegetables. It is also delicious over cooked vegetables, such as broccoli, cauliflower, or baked potatoes.

% Calories from Fat: **3.6% (with nonfat Parmesan cheese)**
                             14% (with regular Parmesan cheese)

Pancakes or Waffles

(Adapted from *Jane Brody's Good Food Book*)

Time to prepare: 10 minutes
Cooking time: 15 minutes

Dry Ingredients

1 c. whole-wheat flour
¼ c. corn meal
2 tsps. sugar
1 tsp. baking powder
½ tsp. baking soda
¼ tsp. salt

Wet Ingredients

1¼ c. buttermilk or nonfat milk
4 egg whites
¼ c. applesauce or prune puree (see page 348
    on how to make prune puree)
½ tsp. vanilla
¼ tsp. cinnamon

For Pancakes
1. Mix dry ingredients in one bowl. Add all wet ingredients, then mix all ingredients together.
2. Heat nonstick pan over medium heat. Use nonstick spray or nothing. Pour sufficient amount of batter onto pan to make the size of pancake you want. Pancake is ready to flip when top begins to bubble and bottom is golden brown. Flip to cook other side.
3. Serve with maple syrup, fruit spread, or fresh fruit.

For Waffles
Use a nonstick waffle iron. Heat iron to the appropriate temperature indicated on your iron. Use a small amount of nonstick spray, if you

wish. Pour sufficient amount of batter to cover approximately ⅔ of the iron surface. Close the iron immediately to cook. Steam will be emitted from the area where the iron comes together. When the waffle has stopped steaming, it is finished. Remove waffle and enjoy.

% Calories from Fat: 5%

French Toast

Time to prepare: 15 minutes
Cooking time: 10 minutes

6 egg whites
¼ c. nonfat milk
1 tsp. vanilla
1 tsp. cinnamon
5–6 slices bread
nonstick spray or oil (optional)

1. Heat nonstick pan over medium heat. If you wish to use nonstick spray or oil, wipe the pan with a paper towel after adding the oil, to pick up any extra.
2. Whisk all ingredients except bread in a shallow dish. Dip both sides of each slice of bread, one slice at a time, in the egg-white mixture. Cook in pan till golden brown, flip, and cook till golden on other side.
3. Serve with maple syrup, fruit spread, or fresh fruit.

% Calories from Fat: 8%

Nonfat Vinaigrette

Time to prepare: 5 minutes

1 T. pectin
¾ c. boiling water
½ tsp. Italian spice, dried oregano, or paprika, depending on
 your tastes
1 tsp. garlic powder
1 tsp. onion powder
½ tsp. salt
½ c. vinegar (red-wine or balsamic is great)

Dissolve pectin in hot water. Place all ingredients in a cruet, or other container with a tight-fitting lid. Shake vigorously. *Ta dah!*

% Calories from Fat: 0%

Quick and Easy Salsa

Time to prepare: 10 minutes

juice of ½ lemon or lime
2 cloves garlic, whole, or ¼–½ tsp. garlic powder
1–2 serrano chilis or jalapeño peppers, or ⅛ tsp. cayenne pepper
½ small red onion, cut in 4 pieces
2 T. loose fresh cilantro
½ tsp. cumin and ½ tsp. ground coriander
½–1 tsp. salt
4 large ripe tomatoes, each cut in 4 pieces

In a blender, combine lemon or lime juice, garlic, chilis, and onion. Blend till it becomes a slurry. Add spices and tomatoes. Puree. You will finish with a very blended salsa. If you prefer the chunky style, chop the ingredients by hand.

% Calories from Fat: 5%

Homemade
Low-Fat Cream Cheese

Time to prepare: 10 minutes
Standing time: 1–4 days

32 oz. (2 lbs.) nonfat plain yogurt

1. Place a moistened paper filter or cheesecloth into Melitta-type coffee funnel or strainer.
2. Set the funnel over a deep bowl, place the yogurt into the funnel, cover airtight, chill, and drain until the yogurt is the consistency of whipped cream cheese, about 1–4 days.
3. Before adding the yogurt to the strainer, you can add any flavoring you wish. A nice combination is: 2 T. fresh chopped basil, 1 clove crushed garlic, ½ tsp. salt, and ¼ tsp. pepper.

% Calories from Fat: 2%

Hot and Sour Vegetable Sauté

Time to prepare: 20–30 minutes
Cooking time: 5 minutes

Sauce

½ c. defatted chicken broth
1–2 T. soy sauce
¼–½ tsp. ground ginger
½–1 tsp. garlic powder, or 2 cloves fresh garlic, minced
1 tsp. honey
¼ c. rice-wine vinegar
⅛ tsp. cayenne pepper or ground white pepper
½ tsp. dark Chinese sesame oil
1–1½ T. cornstarch

¼ c. defatted chicken broth or water
¼ c. sliced bamboo shoots
¼ c. sliced water chestnuts
8 c. assorted fresh vegetables suitable for sauté, such as: napa
  cabbage, bok choy, celery, broccoli, Chinese pea pods,
  zucchini, mushrooms, very thinly sliced carrot, thinly
  sliced cauliflower, diced tomatoes

1. Wash and chop vegetables into bite-size pieces. Set aside.
2. Combine all the sauce ingredients and set aside.
3. In a large nonstick skillet, sauté vegetables in ¼ c. chicken broth
   or water on high heat for 2–3 minutes, stirring constantly.
4. Add the sauce, stirring constantly until sauce thickens and vegetables are coated. If sauce thickens too much, add a little extra
   chicken broth. Remove from heat, cover, and let stand a few minutes before serving.
5. Serve over rice or pasta.

% Calories from Fat: 10% (vegetables with sauce)
                             4% (vegetables with sauce and rice)

Bavarian-Style Vegetable Sauté

Time to prepare: 20 minutes
Cooking time: 25–30 minutes

1½ c. defatted chicken broth
1 tsp. garlic powder, or 3 cloves fresh garlic, minced
⅛ tsp. cayenne pepper or white ground pepper
½–1 tsp. caraway seeds
1 medium onion, diced
3–4 carrots, chopped
2 potatoes, chopped
2–3 c. chopped white cabbage

1. Wash and chop vegetables into bite-size pieces. Set aside.
2. In a large nonstick skillet, add and mix the chicken broth, spices, onion, and carrots. If you need to, add more chicken broth. Simmer with the lid on for 10 minutes, or until the carrots are almost tender. Add the remaining ingredients, cover, and simmer until the potatoes and carrots are tender, about 15 minutes. The chicken broth should develop into a thin sauce.
3. If you wish to thicken the sauce: mix 1 T. cornstarch with 2 T. cold water, and add a little of this mixture to the sauce, and stir over heat until the desired thickness is achieved.
4. This can be served alone with a large loaf of crusty brown or rye bread, or over rice.

% Calories from Fat: 3%

Tuscan Bean Soup

(Adapted from Molly Katzen's *Still Life with Menu Cookbook*)

Time to prepare: 15 minutes
Cooking time: 35–40 minutes

4 cans white beans (or 1½ c. dried beans, cooked)
2–3 cloves garlic, minced, or 1 tsp. garlic powder
2 stalks celery, chopped
3 large carrots, sliced
1 medium onion, diced
3 14.5-oz. cans defatted chicken broth (4–5 cups)
1 tsp. salt
3 tsps. dried basil
2 c. green beans cut in ½-inch pieces
2 tsps. butter or margarine (optional; the butter adds a lot of
    flavor, and yet the entire recipe is still under 15% fat, since
    the butter is used like a spice)

1. In a large saucepan, combine all ingredients except green beans and
   butter. Simmer mixture for about 30 minutes without covering.
2. Add remaining ingredients and simmer for 5 minutes. Serve with
   sourdough bread and topped with low-fat Parmesan cheese.

% Calories from Fat: 11% (with butter)
                        4% (without butter)

Chicken or Turkey with Couscous and Vegetables

(Adapted from *Jane Brody's Good Food Book*)

Time to prepare: 35 minutes
Cooking time: 25–30 minutes

1 onion, chopped
2 large cloves garlic, minced, or ¼ tsp. garlic powder
4–5 boneless skinless chicken breast halves or 1 lb. turkey breast, cut in strips
salt and pepper to taste
½–1 c. water or defatted chicken broth
1 15-oz. can diced tomatoes
3 large carrots, cut in 1-in. chunks
2 large stalks celery, cut in 1-in. chunks
1 turnip, peeled and cut in ½-inch cubes
½ tsp. cinnamon
½ tsp. cumin
¼–½ tsp. turmeric
dash of cayenne pepper
2 tsps. honey
2 medium zucchini, cut in half and sliced in 1-in. chunks
3–4 small yellow squash, cut in 1-in. chunks
½ red bell pepper, cut in 1-in. chunks
8–10 snow peas, cut in half or in thirds
½ c. raisins, chopped, or currants
1 15-oz. can cooked garbanzo beans
¼ c. fresh parsley, finely minced
¾ c. quick-cooking couscous

1. In a large deep skillet, sauté the onions and garlic over medium heat with about 2 T. water or broth till the onions are transparent.
2. Rinse chicken or turkey breast and remove any fat. Cut in 1-in.-thick strips.

3. When the onions are cooked, add the chicken and ¼ c. water or broth to the skillet, cover, and simmer the chicken for 3–4 minutes. Turn the chicken over, cover, and simmer for 3–4 more minutes. Salt and pepper chicken to taste.
4. Add tomatoes and their liquid, carrots, celery, turnip, all spices, and honey. Stir ingredients gently, but try to leave the chicken pieces at the bottom of the pan. Bring the liquid to a boil, reduce heat, and simmer for 25–30 minutes. Check occasionally and add a little water or broth if liquid is mostly gone.
5. Add the remaining ingredients except couscous and simmer for another 10–15 minutes.
6. Add 1⅓ c. boiling water to ¾ c. quick-cooking couscous, cover the container with plastic wrap or a lid, and allow it to steam for five minutes. Fluff with a fork.
7. Place warm couscous in the bottom of a serving dish (or place portions on each person's plate) and top the couscous with the chicken-vegetable mixture.

% Calories from Fat: **13% (with chicken)**
                              8% (with turkey)

Stuffed Baked Potatoes

(Adapted from *Jane Brody's Good Food Book*)

Time to prepare: 25 minutes
Cooking time: 25–30 minutes

4 large baked potatoes
½ c. nonfat milk, warmed
1 c. nonfat cottage cheese
1 clove garlic, minced, or ⅛ tsp. garlic powder
salt and pepper to taste
2 c. chopped broccoli, steamed for 5 minutes
½ onion, minced, steamed for 5 minutes
4 T. grated Parmesan cheese, regular or nonfat

1. Cut the potatoes in half while warm. With a teaspoon, scoop out the flesh (white part) without tearing the skins. Place the flesh in a mixing bowl and arrange the skins in a baking dish.
2. Mash the potato flesh with the warm milk. Mix in the cottage cheese, garlic, salt and pepper, broccoli, onion, and half the Parmesan cheese.
3. Mound the potato-flesh mixture in the potato-skin halves, piling it high. Sprinkle the stuffed potatoes with the remaining Parmesan cheese.
4. Place potatoes back in baking dish, and bake them in a preheated 350-degree oven for 20–25 minutes.

% Calories from Fat: **7% (with regular Parmesan cheese)**
                              2% (with nonfat Parmesan cheese)

Vegetarian Lasagna, or Ground Turkey Lasagna

(Adapted from *Jane Brody's Good Food Book*)

Time to prepare: 20–25 minutes
Cooking time: 50 minutes

Vegetarian Sauce

2 tsps. minced garlic
1 small onion, finely chopped
1 carrot, shredded
¾ c. green beans, chopped into ¼-in. pieces
2 15-oz. cans tomato sauce
2 15-oz. cans tomato puree
1½ tsps. dried oregano
1½ tsps. dried basil
½–1 tsp. salt

Ground Turkey Sauce

1 lb. ground turkey breast
2 tsps. minced garlic
1 small onion, finely chopped
2 tsps. dried oregano
2 tsps. dried basil
1 tsp. dried rosemary
2 tsps. chili powder
½–1 tsp. salt
2 15-oz. cans tomato sauce
2 15-oz. cans tomato puree

Other Ingredients

¾ lb. uncooked lasagna noodles
2 c. nonfat cottage cheese
2–3 oz. part-skim mozzarella
2 T. grated Parmesan cheese, or 4 T. grated nonfat
    Parmesan cheese

To Prepare Vegetarian Sauce
Prepare sauce by sautéing vegetables over medium heat in ¼ c. water.
Add chopped beans and cook the mixture, stirring it, for several more
minutes. Add tomato sauce and puree and spices. Bring sauce to a boil
and simmer for 5–10 minutes.

To Prepare Ground Turkey Sauce
Sauté the ground turkey over medium heat in ¼ c. water, breaking
turkey into small pieces, sprinkling meat with the spices and diced
onion and garlic as it cooks. Add tomato sauce and puree. Bring sauce
to a boil and simmer for 5–10 minutes.

To Assemble Lasagna
   1. Spread a thin layer of the sauce of your choice on the bottom of a
      9 × 13–in. baking pan. Arrange a layer of uncooked noodles to
      cover the sauce in such a way that they touch but do not overlap.

2. Cover the noodle layer with half the cottage cheese, half the mozzarella, and one-third of the remaining sauce.
3. Repeat with a layer of noodles, cottage cheese, mozzarella, and sauce.
4. Finish off with layers of the remaining noodles and sauce.
5. Sprinkle the Parmesan cheese on top

To Cook Lasagna
Cover pan tightly with foil. Bake in a preheated 350-degree oven for about 50 minutes, or until pasta is cooked. If there is too much liquid remaining in the pan, remove the foil and bake the lasagna for another 10 minutes. Let lasagna rest for 5 minutes before cutting and serving.

% Calories from Fat: 9% (with turkey)
                             8% (vegetarian)

Spicy Curried Turkey Breast with Vegetables

(Adapted from George Mateljan's *Cooking Without Fat*)

Time to prepare: 35 minutes
Cooking time: 35–40 minutes

1 lb. turkey breast, cut in strips
¼–½ c. water or defatted chicken broth
1 14.5-oz. can defatted chicken broth
1 14.5-oz. can diced tomatoes
1 tsp. ground turmeric
1 medium onion, chopped
4 large carrots, cut in ½-in. pieces
3 large potatoes, cut in ½-in. chunks
2 medium turnips, cut in ½-in. chunks
3 stalks celery, cut in ½-in. pieces
½ large green pepper, diced
2 small zucchini, cut in ½-in. pieces
1 c. frozen peas

Curry Sauce

**1 15-oz. can low-fat vegetable soup (any brand will do
    as long as it's low-fat)**
1–2 T. curry powder (to taste)
2 tsps. honey
1 tsp. garlic powder
1 tsp. onion powder
salt and pepper to taste

1. In a very large nonstick saucepan or skillet, sauté the turkey strips in water or chicken broth over medium heat until the outside of the strips are cooked.
2. Add to the skillet the chicken broth, diced tomatoes, turmeric, onion, and carrots. Bring contents to a boil, and reduce heat to a simmer. Cover pan and simmer for 10 minutes.
3. Add the potatoes, turnips, and celery, making sure the vegetables are mostly submerged in liquid. Bring to a boil and reduce heat to a simmer. Cover pan and simmer for 20–25 minutes, or until potatoes and turnips are well cooked. Stir in the green pepper and zucchini. Cover and allow to simmer an additional 5 minutes.
4. To assemble the sauce, place all sauce ingredients in a blender and puree. Add the sauce to the other ingredients and stir thoroughly. Add frozen peas and allow mixture to simmer another 5 minutes.
5. Serve over rice. This recipe can be prepared without the turkey and still makes a delicious and filling main course.

% Calories from Fat: **5%**

Black and White Bean, Tex-Mex Couscous Salad

Time to prepare: 35–40 minutes
Cooking time: 5 minutes (couscous)

Dressing

⅔ c. hot water
3 T. pectin
juice of 1 lemon or 1 lime (about 2 T.)
⅔ c. rice wine or white vinegar
1 tsp. dark Chinese sesame oil (optional)
1 T. ground coriander
1 T. garlic powder
1 T. onion powder
¼ tsp. cayenne pepper
½–1 tsp. salt

1 c. uncooked couscous
2 c. boiling water
4 fresh medium roma tomatoes, diced, or 2 15-oz. cans
    diced tomatoes, drained
¾ c. corn kernels, canned or frozen
1 small zucchini, diced
1 small onion, diced
½ c. green bell pepper, diced
½ c. celery, diced
1 14.5-oz. can black beans, drained
1 14.5-oz. can white beans, drained
½–¾ c. fresh cilantro, chopped

1. Dissolve the pectin in hot water, being careful to mix vigorously to eliminate any lumps. In a jar or other container, mix all ingredients for the dressing. Set aside.
2. Place couscous in a bowl large enough to accommodate at least

3 c. Pour boiling water over couscous, stir, and then quickly cover the container with plastic wrap or a lid. Allow the couscous to steam this way for at least 5 minutes. Remove the plastic wrap or lid, and fluff the couscous with a fork.

3. Mix all ingredients except dressing in a large bowl. Pour dressing over salad ingredients. Mix and chill. Serve slightly chilled.

% Calories from Fat: 6% (with sesame oil)
3% (without sesame oil)

Bavarian Black Forest Chocolate Cake

(Adapted from *Environmental Nutrition*, September 1994)

Time to prepare: 25 minutes
Cooking time: 55–65 minutes

Dry Ingredients

2 c. cake or all-purpose white flour
1 c. unsweetened cocoa powder
1½ c. brown sugar
1 tsp. baking powder
2 tsps. baking soda
½ tsp. salt

Wet Ingredients

1 cup prune puree (recipe follows)
¾ c. nonfat milk
4 tsps. vanilla
5 egg whites
2 T. instant coffee, dissolved in 1 c. hot water

Additional Ingredients

¾ c. mini chocolate chips
2 c. frozen, pitted, unsweetened dark sweet cherries, coarsely
    chopped and drained
powdered sugar for dusting (optional)
additional cherries and mint sprigs for garnishing (optional)

1. Preheat oven to 350 degrees. Coat a 3–4-quart bundt pan with nonstick spray, then wipe the inside with a paper towel, making sure all surfaces are lightly coated with the spray. Dust a small amount of flour in the pan, just enough to stick to the oil. Discard any extra flour.
2. In a large bowl, mix together thoroughly all dry ingredients.
3. In another bowl, whisk together all wet ingredients except coffee. Slowly add hot coffee to wet ingredients, mixing constantly, until completely blended. (Make sure the coffee is not too hot, or you may cook the egg prematurely.)
4. Stir wet ingredients into dry ingredients; mix just until blended.
5. Add chocolate chips and cherries; mix just until blended.
6. Pour batter into bundt pan. Bake about 55 minutes, or until toothpick inserted into cake comes out clean.
7. Set pan on rack and cool cake for 15 minutes; then invert onto rack, remove pan and cool completely.
8. Dust with powdered sugar. Fill cake center with additional cherries and garnish with mint.

% Calories from Fat: 15%

(Remember that although chocolate chips are a very high fat food, we can use them here as a spice and still produce a cake that overall is 15% fat.)

Prune Puree (Oil Substitute in Baking)

Time to prepare: 10 minutes

2⅔ c. (1 lb.) pitted prunes
¾ c. water

1. Combine prunes and water in food processor or blender; process 2–3 minutes, or until pureed.
2. Puree may be covered and refrigerated for up to 2 months. Makes 2 c.

% Calories from Fat: **0.9%**

Bibliography

· · · · ·

Books denoted with an asterisk (*) include recipes.

Set-Point Theory

The Dieter's Dilemma, by William Bennett, M.D., and Joel Gurin (New York: Basic Books, 1982). A fascinating, humorous, and highly readable description of set-point theory and its scientific basis, as well as the sociology and psychology of fatness and body image. This book will absolutely convince you of the futility of conventional dieting and the reality of set point. Includes an entire chapter on exercise as a method of "resetting" the set point to a lower amount of fat. The book was written before any research on the effect of dietary-fat content on set point had been conducted, so it contains little information on the influence of diet composition on set point. Nonetheless, an extremely valuable and entertaining book.

How to Lower Your Fat Thermostat, by Dennis Remington, M.D., Garth Fisher, Ph.D., and Edward Parent, Ph.D. (Provo, Ut.: Vitality House International, 1983). Another discussion of set point, which includes many studies done on animals that support the idea. These authors recognize the importance of a low-fat diet, but don't think people can go below 20 or 25 percent fat. They also emphasize behavior control a bit more than we do. However, this book provides another perspective on this important idea.

Low-Fat Eating for Fat Loss

Eat More, Weigh Less, by Dean Ornish, M.D. (New York: Harper Collins, 1993). Dean Ornish is well known as the man who has conducted the most convincing research to date indicating that heart disease can be reversed by life-style changes, including low-fat diet. In this outstanding book he explores the connection between fat content of the diet and weight loss, offering a wealth of scientific evidence supporting the idea that a low-fat diet leads to a low-fat body. He also emphasizes the psychological aspects of eating and the idea of establishing a sense of community and using various stress-reduction techniques as means to pay more attention to diet and eating. He places little emphasis on exercise. The recipes were created by some of the finest gourmet chefs in the world; they take more effort than most but also promise the richest low-fat culinary experience.

The Fit or Fat Target Diet, by Covert Bailey (Boston: Houghton Mifflin, 1984). Covert Bailey has probably done more than anyone else in America to promote exercise as a method of attaining a leaner, healthier body (i.e., lowering set point). Here he tackles the fat in our diets, with a wealth of practical, sensible, and funny advice on how and why to lower the fat content of your diet. Oddly enough, he misses the boat on the effect of low-fat diet in reducing body fat—he flatly states, ". . . you still have to decrease calorie intake for effective fat loss." Say it ain't so, Covert! Oh well, this book was written before much solid information was available on the effects of low-fat diet on body fat, so we suppose he can be forgiven. Except for that one glitch, this is one of the best books around on the how-to and why-to of low-fat eating.

The Pritikin Permanent Weight Loss Manual, by Nathan Pritikin (New York: Grosset and Dunlap, 1981). Nathan Pritikin was the first to challenge accepted dietary ideas, and his initial efforts were aimed at people who wanted to be healthier. But he saw that people on his program of low-fat eating and exercise also lost weight, sometimes astonishing amounts of weight. So he wrote this book. However, even Pritikin was fooled into thinking that low-calorie diets would be successful, and this book contains a few such diets, as well as the standard Pritikin diet. Stick with the standard diet and forget the low-calorie nonsense. The second half of the book is "nuts and bolts," and contains some good recipes.

*The McDougall Program for Maximum Weight Loss, by John Mc-Dougall, M.D. (New York: Dutton, 1994). Contains an excellent discussion of how cutting calories activates hunger mechanisms. McDougall advocates a low-fat diet similar to that of Ornish and Pritikin, except he recommends no animal products whatsoever. There is a (short) chapter on exercise.

Exercise for Fat Loss

The New Fit or Fat, by Covert Bailey (Boston: Houghton Mifflin, 1991). This revised edition of Covert Bailey's classic, *Fit or Fat?*, is probably *the* best book on exercise, fat, and muscle. It is certainly the funniest and easiest to read. Bailey leads you painlessly through the basic ideas of biochemistry, metabolism, and exercise physiology, and gets you fired up enough to start an exercise program this minute. He emphasizes that pounds don't count, only pounds of fat, and that the best way to take fat off the body is exercise, *not* dieting. He then clearly explains what types of exercise will do this best, how to start, how to keep track, how to know if you're doing too much, etc. He has a (somewhat muddled) chapter on set-point theory, and almost no mention of the effect of fat in the diet on body fat. But, for the exercise part of resetting your set point, this book is great! Highly, highly recommended.

*Fitness Without Exercise, by Bryant A. Stamford, Ph.D., and Porter Shimer (New York: Warner Books, 1990). Okay. You read Covert Bailey's *The New Fit or Fat* (see above). You are completely committed to exercise. You work out three times a day. You take your pulse seventeen times during each exercise session. Your training diary is thicker than the Manhattan phone book (which, by the way, you can rip in two). Then, one day, you realize that you *hate* exercise. Should you give up completely on the idea of moving your body farther than from the bed to the car? No! Read *Fitness Without Exercise*. Its authors are two self-confessed exercise junkies, one of them a respected exercise physiologist, the other a well-known health writer, who burned out on structured exercise routines, yet still manage to keep fit *and* slim. They explain the real benefits of exercise, some of the myths that have grown up around exercise, and how to achieve the activity levels that are right for *you*. They also explain the benefits of a low-fat diet and offer dozens of tips on how to be active without being obsessive. The ideas in this

book may surprise you, but they are supported by a number of studies. An alternative to structured exercise routines.

Health Benefits of Low-Fat Diet and Exercise
Food for Life, by Neal Barnard, M.D. (New York: Harmony Books, 1993). Good background, with a wealth of scientific evidence on the benefits of a low-fat diet. Some coverage of exercise and stress reduction, but by far the major emphasis is on diet. Dr. Barnard devotes separate chapters to the effects of diet on aging, heart disease, cancer, and weight control, then discusses the "four new food groups," first proposed in 1991 by the Physicians' Committee for Responsible Medicine. These are grains, beans, fruits, and vegetables. Good suggestions on switching over to a low-fat diet, including a twenty-one-day menu plan, as well as dozens and dozens of additional menus. All around, this is probably the best book currently available on the benefits of low-fat diet and how to change over.

The 10% Solution for a Healthy Life, by Raymond Kurzweil (New York: Crown, 1993). The 10% refers to the fat content of the diet that Kurzweil recommends to ". . . eliminate virtually all risk of heart disease and cancer." The book is about the various "diseases of civilization" (heart disease, cancer, diabetes, arthritis) that are caused or exacerbated by our modern, high-fat, high-protein diet. The author is a scientist who became interested in the subject because of his own risk factors for cardiovascular disease. The book is thoroughly researched and documented, and very accessible to the layman. Kurzweil writes in a question-answer format that is easy to follow and fun to read. He is very precise in his guidelines for achieving 10 percent fat in the diet—maybe too precise for some, but if you have perfectionist tendencies you might be interested in knowing the fat content of your diet down to the tenth of a percent. There is a chapter on weight control in which caloric intake levels are recommended. Ignore it. Again, *don't count calories.*

The Pritikin Promise, by Nathan Pritikin (New York: Simon and Schuster, 1983). Nathan Pritikin wrote several books about his program. This one is the best. The book covers all aspects of Pritikin's program, from the scientific basis to tips on low-fat cooking to step-by-step instructions for starting to exercise. There are many stories from people who have gone on this type of program and experienced enormous changes, including weight loss, lowering of blood pressure, and control of diabetes. The core of the book is a twenty-eight-day program designed to introduce you to the benefits of low-fat eating and exercise. We especially recommend the chapters "Run and Die on the American Diet" and "Runners' Death" for anyone who thinks that an active life-style will protect them from nutritional excesses.

The McDougall Plan, by John A. McDougall, M.D., and Mary A. McDougall (Piscataway, N.J.: New Century, 1983). McDougall covers the same ground as Pritikin but focuses more on specific diseases. His documentation is, if anything, even more complete than Pritikin's. The diet he recommends is completely free of animal products (thus no milk, chicken, or eggs), taking things one step further than Pritikin.

Stress, Diet, and Your Heart, by Dean Ornish, M.D., (New York: Holt, Rinehart and Winston, 1982). Dean Ornish was the first to conduct research showing that heart disease may be reversed through diet and life-style changes. This book is the first that he wrote about his results (he has written another since, *Dr. Dean Ornish's Program for Reversing Heart Disease*). He emphasizes dietary changes and stress reduction to treat cardiovascular disease. At the time this book came out, the ideas were highly controversial, and many cardiologists reviled Dr. Ornish. Now the largest insurer in the U.S. is paying for heart patients to go on Dr. Ornish's program, because it costs about one-tenth as much as conventional medical care and is likely, if followed rigorously, to be more effective.

The Paleolithic Prescription, by S. Boyd Eaton, M.D., Marjorie Shostak, and Melvin Konner, M.D., Ph.D. (New York: Harper and Row, 1988). An evolutionary perspective on low-fat eating and exercise. One interesting idea that the authors stress is that our ancestors were much more robustly muscled than we are, because of the incredible demands on their strength that their daily living imposed. For that reason, these authors emphasize weight training in their exercise recommendations much more than most authorities did at the time their book was written. They are now being proved right: study after study indicates the health benefits of weight training, even for very elderly people.

Restaurant Eating

The Official Pritikin Guide to Restaurant Eating, by Nathan Pritikin and Irene Pritikin (New York: Berkley Books, 1984). If you eat out a lot, you may find this book useful. It is a complete course on ordering low-fat under just about any imaginable circumstance. It includes a chapter called "A Practical Course in Menu Literacy," with sample menus from a variety of types of restaurants, and complete commentary on what's "good" and "bad" in each one.

Recipes

*Jane Brody's Good Food Book, by Jane Brody (New York: W. W. Norton, 1985). Wonderful, thorough, complete book on nutrition, food preparation, weight control, plus hundreds of *good* recipes that range from quick and easy to truly gourmet. Anyone who cooks a lot, or even a little, will want to get this book. Just be careful—Ms. Brody recommends a diet around 20–30 percent fat, which is high for optimum health and body-fat loss. You will have to modify the recipes to cut out most or all of the added fat, but most of them taste just as good after modification. A gold mine.

*Eating Well in a Busy World, by Francine Allen (Berkeley, Calif.: Ten Speed Press, 1986). The outstanding feature of this book is that it presents complete meals, not just single recipes, along with the exact preparation time for each meal. Some are low-fat as is; most of the others are easily modified.

*Target Recipes, by Covert Bailey and Lea Bishop (Boston: Houghton Mifflin, 1985). Recipes to accompany Bailey's *Fit or Fat Target Diet*. Many of the recipes in the book are excessively high in fat, but can be modified to low-fat.

*The McDougall Health Supporting Cookbook, by Mary McDougall (Piscataway, N.J.: New Century, 1985). For those who wish to eat very low fat and completely vegetarian meals, there are over one hundred recipes in this book.

Miscellaneous

The Complete and Up-to-Date Fat Book, by Karen J. Bellerson (Garden City Park, N.Y.: Avery Publishing Group, 1991). Okay, you burned your calorie charts, but you still want to get obsessed with something.

Great! Get obsessed with the *fat* content of foods. This book contains over fifteen thousand foods, by brand name, and their percentage of fat content. Here you will learn fascinating tidbits such as: Hershey's Baking Chocolate is 76 percent fat, whereas Hershey's Syrup is only 11 percent fat. By the time you read this, there may even be a nonfat chocolate syrup on the market, as manufacturers respond to consumer demand.

Notes

• • • • •

Introduction

Page

xi Even doctors and scientists: The National Task Force on the Prevention and Treatment of Obesity, "Weight Cycling," *Journal of American Medical Association* 272: 1196–1202, 1994.

Chapter 1: Our Dinner with Lori

18 "40 percent of American women and 25 percent of American men": D. F. Williamson, M. K. Serdula, R. F. Anda, A. Levy, and T. Byers, "Weight Loss Attempts in Adults: Goals, Duration, and Rate of Weight Loss," *American Journal of Public Health* 82: 1251–57, 1992.

20 In a classic 1964 study: E. A. H. Sims, R. F. Goldman, C. M. Gluck, E. S. Horton, P. C. Kelleher, and D. W. Rowe, "Experimental Obesity in Man," *Transactions of the Association of American Physicians* 81: 153–70, 1968.

21 By three years after their "reverse diet": P. Pasquet and M. Apfelbaum, "Recovery of Initial Body Weight and Composition After Long-term Massive Overfeeding in Men," *American Journal of Clinical Nutrition* 60: 861–63, 1994.

21 Lest you think that this applies only to men: R. L. Leibel, M. Rosenbaum, and J. Hirsch, "Changes in Energy Expenditure Resulting from Altered Body Weight," *New England Journal of Medicine* 232: 622–28, 1995.

22 Your metabolic rate goes up: ibid.

22 "But ancient cave paintings show": S. B. Eaton, M. Shostak, and M. Konner, *The Paleolithic Prescription* (New York: Harper and Row, 1988).

24 Fat people have been found to eat: E. Danforth, Jr., "Diet and Obesity," *American Journal of Clinical Nutrition* 41: 1132–45, 1985; I. Romieu, W. C. Willett, M. J. Stampfer, G. A. Colditz, L. Sampson, B. Rosner, C. H. Hennekens, and F. E.

Speizer, "Energy Intake and Other Determinants of Relative Weight," *American Journal of Clinical Nutrition* 47: 406–12, 1988; D. M. Dreon, B. Frey-Hewitt, N. Ellsworth, P. T. Williams, R. B. Terry, and P. D. Wood, "Dietary Fat: Carbohydrate Ratio and Obesity in Middle-aged Men," *American Journal of Clinical Nutrition* 47: 995–1000, 1988; W. C. Miller, A. K. Linderman, J. Wallace, and M. Niederpruem, "Diet Composition, Energy Intake, and Exercise in Relation to Body Fat in Men and Women," *American Journal of Clinical Nutrition* 52: 426–30, 1990; B. L. Heitmann, L. Lissner, T. I. A. Sorensen, and C. Bengtsson, "Dietary Fat Intake and Weight Gain in Women Genetically Predisposed for Obesity," *American Journal of Clinical Nutrition* 61: 1213–17, 1995.

24 For example, in one study: L. Lissner, D. A. Levitsky, B. J. Strupp, H. J. Kalkwark, and D. A. Roe, "Dietary Fat and the Regulation of Energy Intake in Human Subjects," *American Journal of Clinical Nutrition* 46: 886–92, 1987.

28 In his first study, done in the 1970s: D. Ornish, *Stress, Diet, and Your Heart* (New York: Holt, Reinhart, and Winston, 1982), pp. 337–58.

29 "So it's unlikely that your doctor knows": M. Winick, "Nutrition Education in Medical Schools," *American Journal of Clinical Nutrition* 58: 825–27, 1993.

31 "While foods like pasta": *New York Times*, Oct. 19, 1994.

31 "I went from a size 8": Spokane *Spokesman-Review*, Oct. 30, 1994.

Chapter 2: Heresies

40 At the end of World War II: A. Keys et al., *The Biology of Human Starvation*, 2 vols. (Minneapolis: University of Minnesota Press, 1950).

Chapter 3: Side Effects

47 listed by the National Institutes of Health: NIH Technology Assessment Conference Panel, "Methods for Voluntary Weight Loss and Control," *Annals of Internal Medicine* 119: 764–70, 1993.

49 These people died: T. A. Wadden, A. J. Stunkard, and K. D. Brownell, "Very Low Calorie Diets: Their Efficacy, Safety, and Future," *Annals of Internal Medicine* 99: 675–84, 1983.

49 Ironically, this is the time: M. A. Crawford, "The Role of Essential Fatty Acids in Neural Development: Implications for Perinatal Nutrition," *American Journal of Clinical Nutrition* (suppl.): 703S–710S, 1993.

49 In fact, some experts think: M. Wynn and A. Wynn, *The Prevention of Handicap of Early Pregnancy Origin* (London: Foundation for Education and Research in Child Bearing, 1981).

52 If you eat a high-fat meal: P. T. Kuo, A. F. Whereat, and O. Horwitz, "The Effect of Lipemia upon Coronary Circulation and Peripheral Arterial Circulation in Patients with Essential Hyperlipidemia," *American Journal of Medicine* 26: 68–75, 1959; M. Friedman, R. H. Rosenman, and S. Byers, "Serum Lipids and Conjunctival Circulation After Fat Ingestion in Men Exhibiting Type-A Behavior Pattern," *Circulation* 29: 874–86, 1964; M. Delamaire and F. Durand, "Erythrocyte

Aggregation and Vascular Pathology," *Journal des Maladies Vasculaires* 15: 344–45, 1990 (in French).

52 Many common antidepressants work: P. D. Kramer, *Listening to Prozac* (New York: Viking Penguin, 1993).

52 By a complicated biochemical chain: Serotonin is built from an amino acid called tryptophan that is a normal component of protein. How would a low-fat diet affect an amino acid, which comes from protein? The effect has to do neither with fat nor (directly) with protein. It's caused by carbohydrate.

If you decrease the amount of fat in your diet, you have to replace it with something (because, remember, you're not cutting calories, only fat). You replace the missing fat in your diet with carbohydrate. So a low-fat diet is also a high-carbohydrate diet. These carbohydrates are ultimately broken down to glucose, which is carried in your bloodstream. Because on a low-fat diet you are eating more carbohydrates, there is more glucose circulating for a longer time. Glucose signals the pancreas to release insulin. Insulin tells the cells to take up the glucose, to get it out of the bloodstream and into the cells, where it will do some good. Insulin also tells the cells to take up amino acids from the blood. This makes sense, because any meal made from natural foods (which is what our body evolved to run on) will have *both* carbohydrates and protein in it. But insulin does not tell the cells to take up all amino acids equally—some, such as tryptophan, tend to remain in the bloodstream. Tryptophan can be taken up by the brain, and it is. Because other amino-acid levels have been lowered (they have been taken up by other cells), the brain gets a relatively large dose of tryptophan. In the brain, tryptophan is converted to serotonin, where it exerts its mood-elevating effects.

The effects of antidepressants that operate by increasing brain levels of serotonin can even be *reversed* by dietary manipulation. When people who have been taking these drugs, and who have recovered from their depression as a result, are given a laboratory-prepared diet designed to *deplete* tryptophan (the building block of serotonin) in their blood, they become depressed again within hours (because their brain levels of serotonin are dropping). When they are put back on a normal diet, their depression disappears. The people in these experiments were clinically depressed, possibly because of malfunctions of their serotonin pathways. But even when ordinary volunteers are fed an artificial amino-acid mixture containing all the amino acids *except* tryptophan, they experience a deterioration in mood that has been described by one researcher as "remarkable." You can swing your mood either way, depending on the foods you eat.

And we've only discussed tryptophan—at least four other amino acids may influence brain chemistry. Even the situation with tryptophan isn't so simple—the effect of the high-carbohydrate meal in raising the levels of tryptophan in the blood is abolished if you eat too much protein at the same time.

For a further discussion of these concepts, see: P. L. Delgado, D. S. Charney, L. H. Price, G. K. Aghajanian, H. Landis, and G. R. Heninger, "Serotonin Function and the Mechanism of Antidepressant Action," *Archives of General Psychiatry* 47: 411–18, 1990; J. D. Fernstrom, "Dietary Amino Acids and Brain Function," *Journal of the American Dietetic Association* 94: 71–77, 1994; J. D. Fernstrom,

"Effects of the Diet and Other Metabolic Phenomena on Brain Tryptophan Uptake and Serotonin Synthesis," *Advances in Experimental Medicine* 294: 369–76, 1991; J. D. Fernstrom, R. J. Wurtman, W. B. Hammarstrom, W. M. Rand, H. N. Munro, and C. S. Davidson, "Diurnal Variations in Plasma Concentrations of Tryptophan, Tyrosine, and Other Neutral Amino Acids: Effect of Dietary Protein Intake," *American Journal of Clinical Nutrition* 32: 1912–22, 1979; I. Blum, L. Nessiel, E. Graff, A. Harsat, U. Gabbay, J. Sulkes, O. Raz, and Y. Vered, "Food Preferences, Body Weight, and Platelet-poor Plasma Serotonin and Catecholamines," *American Journal of Clinical Nutrition* 57: 486–89, 1993.

52   Exercise stimulates the release of endorphins: L. Schwarz and W. Kindermann, "Changes in Beta-endorphin Levels in Response to Aerobic and Anaerobic Exercise," *Sports Medicine* 13: 25–36, 1992.

53   When people exercise after taking such a blocking agent: M. Daniel, A. D. Martin, and J. Carter, "Opiate Receptor Blockade by Naltrexone and Mood State After Acute Physical Activity," *British Journal of Sports Medicine* 26: 111–15, 1992.

53   two of the most effective ways of decreasing: R. Stamler, J. Stamler, F. C. Gosch, J. Civinelli, J. Fishman, P. McKeever, A. McDonald, and A. R. Dyer, "Primary Prevention of Hypertension by Nutritional-hygienic means: Final Report of a Randomized, Controlled Trial," *Journal of the American Medical Association* 262: 1801–7, 1989; M. H. Alderman, "Non-pharmacological Treatment of Hypertension," *Lancet*, July 30, 344 (8918): 307–11, 1994; G. H. Blake and D. K. Beebe, "Management of Hypertension: Useful Nonpharmacologic measures," *Postgraduate Medicine* 90: 151–54, 1991; P. O. Kwiterovich, Jr., "Detection and Treatment of Elevated Blood Lipids and Other Risk Factors for Coronary Artery Disease in Youth," *Annals of the New York Academy of Science* 748: 313–30, 1995.

53   helping some diabetics: B. Braun, M. B. Zimmermann, and N. Kretchmer, "Effects of Exercise Intensity on Insulin Sensitivity in Women with Non-insulin-dependent Diabetes Mellitus," *Journal of Applied Physiology* 78: 300–306, 1995; M. Kjaer, C. B. Hollenbeck, B. Frey-Hewitt, H. Galbo, W. Haskell, and G. M. Reaven, "Glucoregulation and Hormonal Responses to Maximal Exercise in Non-insulin-dependent Diabetes," *Journal of Applied Physiology* 68: 2067–74, 1990; J. T. Devlin, M. Hirschman, E. D. Horton, and E. S. Horton, "Enhanced Peripheral and Splanchnic Insulin Sensitivity in NIDDM Men After Single Bout of Exercise," *Diabetes* 36: 434–39, 1987.

54   dramatic effect from low-fat eating on Type II diabetes: R. J. Barnard, L. Lattimore, R. G. Holly, S. Cherny, and N. Pritikin, "Response of Non-insulin-dependent Diabetic Patients to an Intensive Program of Diet and Exercise," *Diabetes Care* 5: 370–74, 1982; R. J. Barnard, M. R. Massey, S. Cherny, L. T. O'Brien, and N. Pritikin, "Long-term Use of a High-complex-carbohydrate, High-fiber, Low-fat diet, and Exercise in the Treatment of NIDDM Patients," *Diabetes Care* 6: 268–73, 1983.

57   Exercise will also help: P. D. Wood, M. L. Stefanick, P. T. Williams, and W. L. Haskell, "The Effects on Plasma Lipoproteins of a Prudent Weight-reducing Diet, With or Without Exercise, in Overweight Men and Women," *New England Journal of Medicine* 325: 461–66, 1991.

60 As the Japanese adopt more Western food habits: W. Insull, Jr., A. Silvers, L. Hicks, and J. L. Probstfield, "Plasma Lipid Effects of Three Common Vegetable Oils in Reduced-fat Diets of Free-living Adults," *American Journal of Clinical Nutrition* 60: 195–202, 1994.

60 The Japanese rate of death from breast cancer: D. P. Rose, "Dietary Fat, Fiber, and Cancer," in *Nutrition in the '90s*, vol. 2., ed. F. N. Kotsonis and M. A. Mackey (New York: Marcel Dekker, 1994), pp. 1–14.

60 Almost a hundred experiments have been done with mice and rats: C. W. Welsch, "Interrelationship Between Dietary Lipids and Calories and Experimental Mammary Gland Tumorigenesis," *Cancer* 74: 1055–62, 1994.

61 Certain forms of the female hormone estrogen: B. E. Henderson, R. K. Ross, and M. C. Pike, "Toward the Primary Prevention of Cancer," *Science* 254: 1131–38, 1991.

61 Women who eat a lot of fat in their diets: H. Merzenich, H. Boeing, and J. Wahrendorf, "Dietary Fat and Sports Activity as Determinants for Age at Menarche," *American Journal of Epidemiology* 138: 217–24, 1993.

61 Eating a high-fat diet increases estrogen levels: D. M. Ingram, F. C. Bennett, D. Willcox, and N. de Klerk, "Effect of Low-fat Diet on Female Sex-hormone Levels," *Journal of the National Cancer Institute* 79: 1225–29, 1987.

61 also leads to obesity: P. C. MacDonald, C. D. Edman, D. L. Hemsell, J. C. Porter, and P. K. Siiteri, "Effect of Obesity on Conversion of Plasma Androstenedione to Estrone in Postmenopausal Women With and Without Endometrial Cancer," *Obstetrics and Gynecology* 130: 448–55, 1978.

62 Not only are fruits and vegetables low in fat: D. D. Kitts, "Bioactive Substances in Food: Identification and Potential Uses," *Canadian Journal of Physiological Pharmacology* 72: 423–34, 1994.

62 But if they were also given sulforaphane: Y. Zhang, T. W. Kensler, C. G. Cho, G. H. Posner, and P. Talalay, "Anticarcinogenic Activities of Sulforaphane and Structurally Related Synthetic Norbornyl Isothiocyanates," *Proceedings of the National Academy of Sciences* 91: 3147–50, 1994.

63 There were such headlines in 1992: *Los Angeles Times*, Oct. 21, 1992.

63 The research study that generated the confusion: W. C. Willet, D. J. Hunter, M. J. Stampfer, G. Colditz, J. E. Manson, D. Spiegelman, B. Rosner, C. H. Hennekens, and F. E. Speizer, "Dietary Fat and Fiber in Relation to Risk of Breast Cancer: An 8-year Follow-up," *Journal of the American Medical Association* 268: 2037–44, 1992.

64 Exercise not only will help: L. Bernstein, B. E. Henderson, R. Hanisch, J. Sullivan-Halley, and R. K. Ross, "Physical Exercise and Reduced Risk of Breast Cancer in Young Women," *Journal of the National Cancer Institute* 86: 1403–8, 1994.

Chapter 5: What to Expect

77 Researchers who examined: D. L. Ballor, and R. E. Keesey, "A Meta-analysis of the Factors Affecting Exercise-induced Changes in Body Mass, Fat Mass, and Fat-free Mass in Males and Females," *International Journal of Obesity* 15: 717–26, 1991.

79   We found about twenty studies: R. D. Mattes, "Fat Preference and Adherence to a Reduced-fat Diet," *American Journal of Clinical Nutrition* 57: 373–81, 1993; M. Shah, P. McGovern, S. French, and J. Baxter, "Comparison of a Low-fat, Ad Libitum Complex-carbohydrate Diet with a Low-energy Diet in Moderately Obese Women," *American Journal of Clinical Nutrition* 59: 980–84, 1994; L. Lissner, D. A. Levitsky, B. J. Strupp, H. J. Kalkwarf, and D. A. Roe, "Dietary Fat and the Regulation of Energy Intake in Human Subjects," *American Journal of Clinical Nutrition* 46: 886–92, 1987; R. L. Hammer, C. A. Barrier, E. S. Roundy, J. M. Bradford, and A. G. Fisher, "Calorie-restricted Low-fat Diet and Exercise in Obese Women," *American Journal of Clinical Nutrition* 49: 77–85, 1989 (this study included a group that ate as much as they wanted of a low-fat selection of foods); A. Kendall, D. A. Levitsky, B. J. Strupp, and L. Lissner, "Weight Loss on a Low-fat Diet: Consequence of the Imprecision of the Control of Food Intake in Humans," *American Journal of Clinical Nutrition* 53: 1124–29, 1991; T. T. Shintani, C. K. Hughes, S. Beckham, and H. K. O'Connor, "Obesity and Cardiovascular Risk Intervention Through the Ad Libitum Feeding of Traditional Hawaiian Diet," *American Journal of Clinical Nutrition* 63(6 suppl.): 1647S–1651S, 1991; L. Sheppard, A. R. Kristal, and L. H. Kushi, "Weight Loss in Women Participating in a Randomized Trial of Low-fat Diets," *American Journal of Clinical Nutrition* 54: 821–28, 1991; T. E. Prewitt, D. Schmeisser, P. E. Bowen, P. Aye, T. A. Dolecek, P. Langenberg, T. Cole, and L. Brace, "Changes in Body Weight, Body Composition, and Energy Intake in Women Fed High- and Low-fat Diets," *American Journal of Clinical Nutrition* 54: 304–10, 1991; I. M. Buzzard, E. H. Asp, R. T. Chlebowski, A. P. Boyar, R. W. Jeffery, D. W. Nixon, G. L. Blackburn, P. R. Jochimsen, E. F. Scanlon, W. Insul, Jr., R. M. Elashoff, R. Butrum, and E. L. Wynder, "Diet Intervention Methods to Reduce Fat Intake: Nutrient and Food Group Composition of Self-selected Low-fat Diets," *Journal of the American Dietetic Association* 90: 42–50, 1990; D. Ornish, *Stress, Diet, and Your Heart* (New York: Holt, Rinehart and Winston, 1982), pp. 337–58; D. Ornish, *Eat More, Weigh Less* (New York: HarperCollins, 1993); D. A. Levitsky, "Imprecise Control of Food Intake on Low-fat Diets," *Nutrition in the '90s: Current Controversies and Analysis*, vol. 2, ed. F. N. Kotsonis and M. A. Mackey (New York: Marcel Dekker, 1994), pp. 45–60; D. Bagga, J. M. Ashley, S. Geffrey, Hei-Jing Wang, J. Barnard, R. Elashoff, and D. Heber, "Modulation of Serum and Breast Ductal Fluid Lipids by a Very-low-fat, High-fiber Diet in Premenopausal Women," *Journal of the National Cancer Institute* 86: 1419–21, 1994; A. H. Lichtenstein, L. M. Ausman, W. Carrasco, J. L. Jenner, J. M. Ordovas, and E. J. Schaefer, "Short-term Consumption of a Low-fat Diet Beneficially Affects Plasma Lipid Concentration Only When Accompanied by Weight Loss, Hypercholesteremia, Low-fat diet, and Plasma Lipids," *Arteriosclerosis and Thrombosis* 14: 1751–60, 1994; D. G. Schlundt, J. O. Hill, J. Pope-Cordle, D. Arnold, K. L. Virts, and M. Katahn, "Randomized Evaluation of a Low Fat Ad Libitum Carbohydrate Diet for Weight Reduction," *International Journal of Obesity* 17: 623–29, 1993; E. White, M. Hurlich, R. S. Thompson, M. N. Woods, M. M. Henderson, N. Urban, and A. Kristal, "Dietary Changes Among Husbands of

Participants in a Low-fat Dietary Intervention," *American Journal of Preventive Medicine* 7: 319–25, 1991; W. Insull, Jr., M. M. Henderson, R. L. Prentice, D. J. Thompson, C. Clifford, S. Goldman, S. Gorbach, M. Moskowitz, R. Thompson, and M. Woods, "Results of a Randomized Feasibility Study of a Low-fat Diet," *Archives of Internal Medicine* 150: 421–27, 1990; N. F. Boyd, M. L. Cousins, S. E. Bayliss, E. B. Fish, E. Fishnell, W. R. Bruce, "Diet and Breast Disease: Evidence for the Feasibility of a Clinical Trial Involving a Major Reduction in Dietary Fat, in *Cancer, Nutrition, and Eating Behavior,* ed. T. G. Burish, S. M. Levy, and B. E. Meyerowitz (Hillsdale, N.J.: Lawrence Earlbaum Association, 1985), pp. 165–86.

80 One of the longest (six months): Shah et al., "Comparison of a Low-fat, Ad Libitum Complex-carbohydrate Diet."

81 We already told you about his earliest study: Ornish, *Stress, Diet, and Your Heart*, pp. 337–58.

81 Researchers at UCLA: Bagga et al., "Modulation of Serum and Breast Ductal Fluid Lipids."

82 At Tufts University: Lichtenstein et al., "Short-term Consumption of a Low-fat Diet."

83 The most incredible example: Shintani et al., "Obesity and Cardiovascular Risk Intervention."

84 In a few studies: Buzzard et al., "Diet Intervention Methods"; Sheppard et al., "Weight Loss in Women"; White et al., "Dietary Changes Among Husbands."

84 Fortunately, two brave researchers: Ballor and Keesey, "Meta-analysis of the factors."

85 That's no small matter: G. W. Gleim, "Exercise Is Not an Effective Weight Loss Modality in Women," *Journal of the American College of Nutrition* 12: 363–67, 1993.

86 Moderately overweight women were asked: A. Tremblay, J.-P. Despres, J. Maheux, M. C. Pouliot, A. Nadeau, S. Moorjani, P. J. Lupien, and C. Bouchard, "Normalization of the Metabolic Profile in Obese Women by Exercise and a Low Fat Diet," *Medicine and Science in Sports and Exercise* 23: 1326–31, 1991.

86 the case of Mike Stroud and Sir Ranulph Fiennes: M. Stroud, *Shadows on the Wasteland: Crossing Antarctica with Ranulph Fiennes* (Woodstock, N.Y.: Overlook Press, 1993), pp. 27, 41, and 99.

88 One good, controlled scientific study: Hammer et al., "Calorie-restricted Low-fat Diet" (despite the title, one group in this experiment did not restrict calories; that is the group from which we take the data for this section).

89 It's true for exercise: Ballor and Keesey, "Meta-analysis of the factors."

90 one long-term exercise study: Tremblay et al., "Normalization of the Metabolic Profile in Obese Women."

91 such as in Papua New Guinea: P. Sinnett and M. Whyte, "Lifestyle, Health and Disease: A Comparison Between Papua New Guinea and Australia," *Medical Journal of Australia* 1: 1–5, 1978.

91 in places such as rural China: J. Chen, T. C. Campbell, J. Li, and R. Peto, *Diet, Lifestyle, and Mortality in China: A Study of the Characteristics of 65 Chinese Counties* (Oxford: Oxford University Press, 1990).

Chapter 6: Principles of Low-Fat Eating

100 The average American works: J. Schor, *The Overworked American: The Unexpected Decline of Leisure* (New York: Basic Books, 1993).

100 thirty minutes a day in the kitchen: L. S. Burns, *Busy Bodies: Why Our Time-obsessed Society Keeps Us Running in Place* (New York: W. W. Norton, 1993).

101 The typical fish dish: Jacques Pépin, *Everyday Cooking with Jacques Pépin* (New York: Harper and Row, 1982).

Chapter 7: Phase 1 of Low-Fat Eating—20 Percent Calories from Fat

115 We've included a recipe for Bavarian Black Forest Chocolate Cake: recipe and information about prune puree are from *Environmental Nutrition*, Sept. 1994.

122 espresso drinks from a number of different espresso bars: *Tufts University Diet and Nutrition Letter* 12 (5), July 1994.

123 *The average nineteen-to-fifty-year-old woman: Nutrition Action Healthletter*, April 1994.

125 In a study reported in 1990: J. Rodin, "Comparative Effects of Fructose, Aspartame, Glucose, and Water Preloads on Calorie and Macronutrient Intake," *American Journal of Clinical Nutrition* 51: 428–35, 1990.

126 Those who eat five or more servings: G. Block, B. Patterson, and A. Subar, "Fruit, Vegetables, and Cancer Prevention: A Review of the Epidemiological Evidence," *Nutrition and Cancer* 18: 1–29, 1992.

Chapter 10: Twenty Questions

196 Prisoners have been fed diets: M. Winitz, D. A. Seedman, and J. Graff, "Studies in Metabolic Nutrition Employing Chemically Defined Diets, I, Extended Feeding of Normal Human Adult Males," *American Journal of Clinical Nutrition* 23: 525–45, 1970.

196 developing children were fed the same diet: C. M. McKean, "Growth of Phenylketonuric Children on Chemically Defined Diets," *Lancet*, Jan. 17, 1 (638): 148–49, 1970.

196 Some experts think: J. A. McDougall, *The McDougall Program for Maximum Weight Loss* (New York: Dutton, 1994), pp. 44–45.

197 recommended by some authors: A. L. Gittleman and J. M. Desgrey, *Beyond Pritikin* (New York: Bantam Books, 1988).

198 Dr. Frank Sacks at Harvard: quoted in J. Carper, *Food—Your Miracle Medicine* (New York: Harper Perennial, 1993), pp. 66–67.

199 Tarahumara Indians: W. E. Connor, M. T. Cerqueira, R. W. Connor, R. B. Wallace, M. R. Malinow, and H. R. Casdorph, "The Plasma Lipids, Lipoproteins, and Diet of the Tarahumara Indians of Mexico," *American Journal of Clinical Nutrition* 31: 1131–42, 1978.

199 But Dean Ornish has shown: D. Ornish, S. E. Brown, L. W. Scherwitz, J. H. Billings, W. T. Armstrong, T. A. Ports, S. M. McLanahan, R. L. Kirkeeide, R. J.

Brand, and K. L. Gould, "Can Lifestyle Changes Reverse Coronary Heart Disease? The Lifestyle Heart Trial," *Lancet*, July 21, 336 (8708): 129–33, 1990.

199 In the Framingham study: N. Barnard, *Food for Life* (New York: Harmony Books, 1993). p. 34.

200 The Recommended Dietary Allowance: National Research Council, *Recommended Dietary Allowances*, 10th ed. (Washington, D.C.: National Academy of Sciences, 1989).

201 The idea that all the essential amino acids: F. M. Lappé, *Diet for a Small Planet* (New York: Ballantine Books, 1971).

201 It can lead to such conditions as osteoporosis: J.-F. Hu, X.-H. Zhao, B. Parpia, and T. C. Campbell, "Dietary Intakes and Urinary Excretion of Calcium and Acids: A Cross-sectional Study of Women in China," *American Journal of Clinical Nutrition* 58: 398–406, 1993; J. Lutz and H. M. Linkswiler, "Calcium Metabolism in Postmenopausal and Osteoporotic Women Consuming Two Levels of Dietary Protein," *American Journal of Clinical Nutrition* 34: 2178–86, 1981; B. J. Abelow, T. R. Holford, K. L. Isogna, "Cross-cultural Association Between Dietary Animal Protein and Hip Fracture: A Hypothesis," *Calcified Tissue International* 50: 14–18, 1992.

201 One effective treatment for existing kidney disease: A. J. Williams, S. E. Bennett, G. I. Russell, and J. Walls, "Alteration of the Course of Chronic Renal Failure by Dietary Protein Restriction," *Proceedings of the European Dialysis and Transplant Association—European Renal Association* 21: 604–7, 1985.

201 Experiments conducted at Cornell University: L. Youngman and T. C. Campbell, "Inhibition of Aflatoxin B1-induced Gamma-glutamyltranspeptidase Positive (GGT+) Hepatic Preneoplastic Foci and Tumors by Low Protein Diets: Evidence That Altered GGT+ Foci Indicate Neoplastic Potential," *Carcinogenesis* 13: 1607–13, 1992.

201 Other studies show the same results: Committee on Diet, Nutrition, and Cancer, *Diet, Nutrition, and Cancer* (Washington D.C.: National Academy Press, 1982); S. K. Clinton, C. R. Truex, and W. J. Visek, "Dietary Protein, Aryl Hydrocarbon Hydroxylase, and Chemical Carcinogenesis in Rats," *Journal of Nutrition* 109: 55–62, 1979; F. R. White and M. Belkin, "Source of tumor proteins, I, Effect of Low-nitrogen diet on the Establishment and Growth of a Transplanted Tumor," *Journal of the National Cancer Institute* 5: 261–63, 1945; A. L. Babson, "Some Host-tumor Relationships with Respect to Nitrogen," *Cancer Research* 14: 89–93, 1954.

201 Rural Chinese eat only 6–7 percent: J. Chen, T. C. Campbell, J. Li, and R. Peto, *Diet, Life-Style, and Mortality in China: A Study of the Characteristics of 65 Chinese Counties* (Oxford: Oxford University Press, 1990).

201 Here in America, we eat 14–18 percent: *Nationwide Food Consumption Survey 1977–1978, Food Intakes: Individuals in 48 States, Year 1977–1978*, report no. 1-I (Hyattsville, Md.: U.S. Department of Agriculture, 1983); *Nationwide Food Consumption Survey, Continuing Survey of Food Intakes by Individuals, Men 19–50 Years, 1 Day*, report no. 85–3 (Hyattsville, Md.: U.S. Department of Agriculture, 1986); *Nationwide Food Consumption Survey, Continuing Survey of Food Intakes*

by Individuals, Women 19–50 Years and Their Children 1–5 Years, 4 Days, report no. 85-4 (Hyattsville, Md.: U.S. Department of Agriculture, 1985).

203 Four out of ten people are reluctant: Survey by Princeton Survey Research Associates, cited in *Tufts University Diet and Nutrition Letter* 12 (2), April 1994.

203 But researchers have found: "Healthier and Wealthier, the Wise Eater," *Tufts University Diet and Nutrition Letter* 12 (2), April 1994.

204 For example, it's been suggested that Olestra: T. Adler, "Designer Fats," *Science News* 145: 296–97, 1994.

204 An experiment at the University of Pennsylvania: R. D. Mattes, "Fat Preference and Adherence to a Reduced-fat Diet," *American Journal of Clinical Nutrition* 57: 373–81, 1993.

205 There is some evidence that moderate alcohol use: P. M. Suter, Y. Schutz, and E. Jequier, "The Effect of Ethanol on Fat Storage in Healthy Subjects," *New England Journal of Medicine* 326: 983–87, 1992.

205 Women who drink even *one drink a day:* W. C. Willett, M. J. Stampfer, G. A. Colditz, B. A. Rosner, C. H. Hennekens, and F. E. Speizer, "Moderate Alcohol Consumption and the Risk of Breast Cancer," *New England Journal of Medicine* 316: 1174–80, 1987.

206 In 1994, scientists discovered: Y. Zhang, R. Proenca, M. Maffei, M. Barone, L. Leopold, and J. M. Friedman, "Positional Cloning of the Mouse Obese Gene and Its Human Homologue," *Nature* 372: 425–32, 1994.

214 "New Star in the Diet World": San Francisco *Chronicle*, Jan. 3, 1994.

214 He found only one careful study: D. Hasten, E. P. Rome, B. D. Franks, and M. Hegsted, "Effects of Chromium Picolinate on Beginning Weight Training Students," *International Journal of Sport Nutrition* 2: 343–50, 1992.

215 "New Cream Shrinks Women's Thighs": San Francisco *Chronicle*, Oct. 21, 1993.

215 Another of the researchers bragged: San Francisco *Examiner*, Oct. 31, 1993.

215 A major reason that women give for smoking: San Francisco *Chronicle*, July 11, 1994.

216 Not to mention the damage to fetuses: ibid.

218 Indeed, in areas of the world: D. L. Hachey, "Benefits and Risks of Modifying Maternal Fat Intake in Pregnancy and Lactation," *American Journal of Clinical Nutrition* 59 (suppl.): 454S–64S, 1994; H. L. Delgado, R. Martorell, R. E. Klein, "Nutrition, Lactation, and Birth Interval Components in Rural Guatemala," *American Journal of Clinical Nutrition* 35: 1468–76, 1982; M. Lawrence, J. Singh, F. Lawrence, and R. G. Whitehead, "The Energy Cost of Common Daily Activities in African Women: Increased Expenditure in Pregnancy," *American Journal of Clinical Nutrition* 42: 753–63, 1985; K. Tontisirin, U. Booranasubkajorn, A. Hongsumarn, and D. Thewtong, "Formulation and Evaluation of Supplementary Foods for Thai Pregnant Women," *American Journal of Clinical Nutrition* 43: 931–39, 1986; W. M. van Steenbergen, J. A. Kusin, S. Kardjati, and C. de With, "Energy Supplementation in the Last Trimester of Pregnancy in East Java, Indonesia: Effect on Breast-milk Output," *American Journal of Clinical Nutrition* 50: 274–79, 1989.

219 Most women take in about half that amount: E. Moyer, *Vitamins and Minerals* (Allentown, Pa.: People's Medical Society, 1993), pp. 106–7.

220 no detrimental effects of low-fat diets during lactation: National ·Cholesterol Education Program, "Report of the Expert Panel on Population Strategies for Blood Cholesterol Reduction," *Circulation* 83: 2154–2232, 1991.

220 about one-third of your baby's energy needs: Food and Agriculture Organization/World Health Organization, *Report of an Expert Consultation: The Role of Dietary Fats and Oils in Human Nutrition* (Rome: FAO, n.d.).

220 researchers at the University of California at Davis: K. G. Dewey, M. J. Heinig, and L. A. Nommsen, "Maternal Weight-loss Patterns During Prolonged Lactation," *American Journal of Clinical Nutrition* 58: 162–66, 1993.

221 The fat in breast milk seems to be specially "formulated": S. M. Innis, "Essential Fatty Acid Requirements in Human Nutrition," *Canadian Journal of Physiology and Pharmacology* 71: 699–706, 1993.

221 infants may not be able to use these two essential fatty acids: M. A. Crawford, "The Role of Essential Fatty Acids in Neural Development: Implications for Perinatal Nutrition," *American Journal of Clinical Nutrition* 57 (suppl.): 703S–10S, 1993.

221 But at least one study shows: A. Lucas, R. Morley, T. J. Cole, G. Lister, and C. Geeson-Payne, "Breast Milk and Subsequent Inteligence Quotient in Children Born Preterm," *Lancet*, Feb. 1, 339 (8788): 261–64, 1992.

222 no significant difference in the milk of regular exercisers: C. A. Lovelady, B. Lonnerdal, K. G. Dewey, "Lactation Performance of Exercising Women," *American Journal of Clinical Nutrition* 52: 103–9, 1990; K. G. Dewey, C. A. Lovelady, L. A. Nommsen-Rivers, M. A. McCrory, and B. Lonnerdal, "A Randomized Study of the Effects of Aerobic Exercise by Lactating Women on Breast-milk Volume and Composition," *New England Journal of Medicine* 330: 449–53, 1994.

222 "Almost no data exist": L. Finberg, "Modified Fat Diets: Do They Apply to Infancy?" *Journal of Pediatrics* 117 (suppl.): S132–S133, 1990.

224 People may actually burn fewer calories while watching TV: R. C., Klesges, M. L. Shelton, L. M. Klesges, "Effects of Television on Metabolic Rate: Potential Implications for Childhood Obesity," *Pediatrics* 91: 281–86, 1993.

224 It's no accident: F. Falkner, "Obesity and Cardiovascular Disease Risk Factors in Prepubescent and Pubescent Black and White Females," *Critical Reviews of Food Science and Nutrition* 33: 397–402, 1993; L. A. Tucker and M. Bagwell, "Television Viewing and Obesity in Adult Females," *American Journal of Public Health* 81: 908–11, 1991.

Chapter 11: Don't Make a Myth-Guided Attempt at Exercise

237 people who lift weights are compared with people who walk, jog, or cycle: D. L. Ballor and R. E. Keesey, "A Meta-analysis of the Factors Affecting Exercise-induced Changes in Body Mass, Fat Mass, and Fat-free Mass in Males and Females," *International Journal of Obesity* 15: 717–26, 1991.

240 one study compared women walking at different paces: J. J. Duncan, N. F. Gordon, and C. B. Scott, "Women Walking for Health and Fitness: How Much Is Enough?" *Journal of the American Medical Association* 266: 3295–99, 1991.

243 People who regularly engage in walking: R. S. Paffenbarger, Jr., A. L. Wing, and R. T. Hyde, "Physical Activity as an Index of Heart Attack Risk in College Alumni," *American Journal of Epidemiology* 108: 161–75, 1978.

243 Ticket takers in England's double-decker buses: J. N. Morris, J. A. Heady, P. A. B. Raffle, C. G. Roberts, and J. W. Parks, "Coronary Heart Disease and Physical Activity of Work," *Lancet*, Nov. 21, 2 (6795): 1053–57, 1953.

243 Longshoremen suffer less heart disease: R. S. Paffenbarger, Jr., M. E. Laughlin, A. S. Gima, and R. A. Black, "Work Activity of Longshoremen as Related to Death from Coronary Heart Disease and Stroke," *New England Journal of Medicine* 282: 1109–14, 1970.

243 A study of 13,334 men and women: S. N. Blair, H. W. Kohl, R. S. Paffenbarger, Jr., D. G. Clark, K. H. Cooper, and L. W. Gibbons, "Physical Fitness and All-cause Mortality: A Prospective Study of Healthy Men and Women," *Journal of the American Medical Association* 262: 2395–2401, 1989.

244 Bassler claimed, in the late 1970s: see, for example, T. J. Bassler, "More on Immunity to Atherosclerosis in Marathon Runners," *New England Journal of Medicine* 299: 201, 1978; T. J. Bassler, "Prevention of Coronary Heart-disease," *Lancet*, June 1, 1 (866): 1106–7, 1977.

245 "Running provides at least": Jim Fixx quoted in B. A. Stamford and P. Shimer, *Fitness Without Exercise* (New York: Warner Books, 1990), p. 126.

245 But several studies show: G. F. Watts, B. Lewis, J. N. H. Brunt, E. S. Lewis, D. J. Coltart, L. D. R. Smith, J. I. Mann, and A. V. Swan, "Effects on Coronary Artery Disease of Lipid-lowering Diet, or Diet Plus Cholestyramine, in the St. Thomas' Atherosclerosis Regression Study (STARS)," *Lancet*, Mar. 7, 339 (8793): 563–69, 1992; D. Ornish, S. E. Brown, L. W. Scherwitz, J. H. Billings, W. T. Armstrong, T. A. Ports, S. M. McLanahan, R. L. Kirkeeide, R. J. Brand, and K. L. Gould, "Can Lifestyle Changes Reverse Coronary Heart Disease? The Lifestyle Heart Trial," *Lancet*, July 21, 336 (8708): 129–33, 1990; D. H. Blankenhorn, R. L. Johnson, W. J. Mack, H. A. El Zein, and L. I. Vailas, "The Influence of Diet on the Appearance of New Lesions in Human Coronary Arteries," *Journal of the American Medical Association* 263: 1646–52, 1990.

246 "... in a man 69 years old": J. D. Hubbard, S. Inkeles, and R. J. Barnard, "Nathan Pritikin's Heart," *New England Journal of Medicine* 313: 52, 1985.

Chapter 12: Opportunistic Exercise

247 in the few remaining primitive societies in the world: S. B. Eaton, M. Shostak, and M. Konner, *The Paleolithic Prescription* (New York: Harper and Row, 1988), pp. 168–95.

247 studies of existing traditional societies: ibid., p. 160; P. Sinnett and M. Whyte, "Health and Disease: A Comparison Between Papua New Guinea and Australia," *Medical Journal of Australia* 1: 1–5, 1978.

247 The Masai: N. Pritikin, *The Pritikin Promise* (New York: Simon and Schuster, 1983), p. 88.

248 *eighteen-to-thirty-year-olds:* University of California, Berkeley, *Wellness Letter,* July 1994.
248 Those numbers are actually increasing: C. Bailey, *The New Fit or Fat* (Boston: Houghton Mifflin, 1991), p. 6.
258 Two doctors from Johns Hopkins Medical School calculated: B. G. Petty and D. M. Herrington, "Physical Activity and Longevity of College Alumni" (letter), *New England Journal of Medicine* 315: 399–400, 1986.
259 Less than a century ago: B. A. Stamford and P. Shimer, *Fitness Without Exercise* (New York: Warner Books, 1990), p. 89.
260 people were more alert after taking a brief walk: ibid., p. 85.
262 Research shows that the chances are three out of four: ibid., p. 100.
263 Forty percent of American children: ibid.

Chapter 13: Structured Exercise

291 For example, in one study: M. A. Fiatarone, E. F. O'Neill, N. D. Ryan, K. M. Clements, G. R. Solares, M. E. Nelson, S. B. Roberts, J. J. Kehayias, L. A. Lipsitz, and W. J. Evans, "Exercise Training and Nutritional Supplementation for Physical Frailty in Very Elderly People," *New England Journal of Medicine* 330: 1769–75, 1994.

Chapter 14: Measuring Progress

301 If you really *must* have a number: comparisons of various methods based on H. C. Lukaski, "Methods for the Assessment of Human Body Composition: Traditional and New," *American Journal of Clinical Nutrition* 46: 537–56, 1987.
305 One very simple measurement: *Consumer Reports,* June 1993, p. 348.

Index

• • • • •